BIOSTATISTICS:
How It Works

Steve Selvin

University of California, Berkeley

PEARSON EDUCATION, INC.
Upper Saddle River, New Jersey 07458

Library of Congress Cataloging-in-Publication Data
   Selvin, S.
   Biostatistics: How it works/Steve Selvin
     p. cm.
   Includes bibliographical references and index.
   ISBN 0-13-046616-6
   1. Medical statistics. 2. Biometry. 3. Statistics.
     4. Medicine–Research–Statistical methods. I. Title.

   RA409.S326   2004
   610.7′27–dc21   2003048620

Editor in Chief: *Sally Yagan*
Acquisitions Editor: *George Lobell*
Production Editor: *Lynn Savino Wendel*
Vice President/Director of Production and Manufacturing: *David W. Riccardi*
Senior Managing Editor: *Linda Mihatov Behrens*
Assistant Managing Editor: *Bayani Mendoza DeLeon*
Executive Managing Editor: *Kathleen Schiaparelli*
Assistant Manufacturing Manager/Buyer: *Michael Bell*
Manufacturing Manager: *Trudy Pisciotti*
Marketing Manager: *Halee Dinsey*
Marketing Assistant: *Rachel Beckman*
Art Director: *Jayne Conte*
Editorial Assistant: *Jennifer Brady*
Cover Designer: *Bruce Kenselaar*
Cover Photo Credits: *Squeak Carnwath, Art Practice, Berkeley, California*

 © 2004 by Pearson Education, Inc.
Pearson Education, Inc.
Upper Saddle River, New Jersey 07458

Printed in the United States of America
10 9 8 7 6 5 4 3 2

ISBN 0-13-046616-6

Pearson Education Ltd., *London*
Pearson Education Australia Pty, Limited, *Sydney*
Pearson Education Singapore, Pte. Ltd.
Pearson Education North Asia Ltd., *Hong Kong*
Pearson Education Canada, Ltd., *Toronto*
Pearson Educacion de Mexico, S.A. de C.V.
Pearson Education—Japan, *Tokyo*
Pearson Education Malaysia, Pte. Ltd.

for Nancy and Liz

Statistical thinking will one day be as necessary for efficient citizenship as the ability to read and write.

H. G. Wells

If at first you don't succeed, you're about average.

Anonymous

Contents

Preface

The study of statistics begins with potential confusion—the word "statistics" has two different meanings. Statistics is the name of the process used to summarize collected observations to describe essential properties of a sampled population, frequently leading to a better understanding of a specific topic or issue. The analytic tools used to create this description are also called statistics. This text is about both kinds of statistics but primarily it is about one specific statistical tool, the sample mean value. The principles underlying this fundamental and relatively simple way to explore data are at the center of this text.

The study of statistics is not always well received by students enrolled in an introductory and sometimes required course. Part of the explanation may be the kind of textbook used in introductory classes. Many modern introductory books are extensive (in the neighborhood of 800–1000 pages) and contain a large number of data sets (usually a computer disk is included). They are numerous problems/exercises for each of many sections (one popular text contains more than 1200 problems). These texts generally minimize the role of even simple mathematics to make the presented material accessible to a wide audience. Whether these texts are written for students in public health, business, biology, economics, or social science, they contain a large variety of topics aimed at creating an extensive toolbox of statistical techniques. In addition, these techniques are usually supported with one or more statistical computer packages (for example, Stata, SAS, Excel, Statistica, or Minitab).

This text has a different objective. The goal here is to provide a sophisticated introduction of how statistics works at a beginning level. As in all statistics texts, a number of useful and important statistical techniques are discussed but this text sharply focuses on the sample mean as a way of understanding the statistical process in general. The book is short (less than 400 pages), contains only a limited number of problems, uses elementary mathematics, and makes no mention of computer applications.

A few problems at the end of each chapter (many adapted from research journal articles) are not a series of "practice" problems. These small hands-on data sets are intended to encourage the reader to work carefully through the details of the statistical process as part of the text's how-it-works philosophy. Most of the data used throughout the text also come from actual research projects and consist of only a few representative observations (usually less than 30) so that the reader can readily duplicate the results using a handheld scientific calculator, a spreadsheet program such as Excel, or any statistical system. The reader should work all the problem sets included. While small in number, these problems are quite focused on key ideas.

The reason statistical analysis tools are useful is concisely and unambiguously expressed in the language of symbols. In addition, elementary mathematics frequently demonstrates clearly the logic of a specific approach. Simple algebraic explanations (enclosed in boxes) are one of the several ways the statistical concepts are presented. (This mathematical material is not necessary for a first reading and can be skipped without disrupting the logic or flow of the text.) Parallel numeric examples also concretely demonstrate the important features of each concept. Graphic displays, included wherever possible, provide visual interpretations. Elementary mathematics, worked examples, and graphic illustrations brought together with detailed discussions potentially provide a keen insight into the statistical process.

After introducing the sample mean and a few other descriptive statistics, the text turns to a bit of elementary probability theory. The introduction to probability is then extended to characterize samples selected from populations. The text next explores the accuracy and precision of the mean value calculated from samples (hypothesis testing and confidence intervals). Then, digressing slightly from the discussion of the properties of the mean value, the chi-square analytic technique is presented. A mastery of elementary chi-square techniques adds perspective to statistical testing and, in general, illustrates the process of evaluating the impact of random variation on specific kinds of data. The remainder of the text deals with summarizing and analyzing bivariate data (regression and correlation analysis).

The material in this text was developed for a large (over 300 students) one-semester course taken by a mixture of graduate and undergraduate students, primarily from the School of Public Health and the biological sciences at the University of California, Berkeley. These students are not required to have a previous statistics course or a mathematical background beyond usual high school algebra. The text is designed to appeal to two kinds of students: those who plan to continue on to more data analysis-oriented courses and others who will not be directly analyzing data but wish to understand a process that frequently makes modern and complex issues more comprehensible. An introductory text that traces the thread of statistical logic for the narrow but important case of a sample mean provides both kinds of students with a foundation for understanding how and why the statistical process works.

There are many students and colleagues who have contributed to the material and spirit of this text, particularly Ms. Carol Langhauser and Dr. Chin Long Chiang who created some of the examples and problems, and Dr. Mark Hudes who carefully read the text and made helpful suggestions. I also want to thank the reviewers whose suggestions improved the manuscript: Peter Mac Donald, McMasters University; William Briggs, Weill Cornell Medical College; and P. K. Pathak, Michigan State University.

Steve Selvin
selvin@stat.berkeley.edu

PART ONE

PROBABILITY: PROPERTIES OF SAMPLES

CHAPTER 1

Descriptive Statistics

In the beginning

Measurement is a cornerstone of statistical analysis and a key to much of human knowledge. When someone says, "Billy is smarter than Sally" things immediately get complicated—on what scale?, does it matter?, in what context?, in relation to what? and, of most importance, by what measure?

The fundamental element of a statistical analysis is called a *variable*. A statistical variable, defined in its simplest terms, is the thing measured, counted, or identified; the thing of interest. It can be the birth weight of a newborn infant, the count of coronary heart disease cases, the number of whales caught each year, the time a clock fails or practically any definable quantity. The process of organizing and summarizing measurements collected to study the properties of a variable is called *descriptive statistics*. In their book *Beginning Statistics with Data Analysis*[1] the authors state, "Although we often hear that data speak for themselves, their voices can be soft and sly." Descriptive statistics makes these voices loud and bold by using a few summary measurements to identify and characterize the properties of collected data.

Four kinds of variables

Variables are classified conveniently as categorical or quantitative. Categorical variables are further classified as nominal or ordinal and quantitative variables are further classified as discrete or continuous. To a large extent, the kind of variable dictates the kind of analysis.

Nominal variable.   A categorical variable is *nominal* when it results from naming or labeling. Nominal variables have no natural order. Some examples of nominal variables are:

the sex of a newborn child: male or female,

the ethnicity of an individual: white, African-American, or Asian-American,

the species of a tree: redwood, cedar, pine, or oak, and

the jersey numbers of players on a basketball team: numeric values used as labels.

Ordinal variable. A categorical variable is *ordinal* when it results from ordering observations into a series of categories when no appropriate numerical scale is available. Some examples of ordinal variables are:

intensity of pain: none, mild, moderate, or severe,

muscle tone: limp, some flex, or active motion,

smoking status: never, former, or current, and

injury: none, mild, moderate, severe, or death.

Ordinal values are frequently ordered (ranked) based on nonnumeric criteria. For example, vintage wines can be ranked from low to high by the quality of their taste. The classification of olives, perhaps, pushes an ordinal scale to its limits with the classification: small, medium, large, extra large, jumbo, colossal, and supercolossal.

Discrete variable. A quantitative variable is *discrete* when it results from counting. More technically, a discrete variable takes on zero or a positive integer value. Some examples of discrete variables are:

the number of male children in a family with three children (0, 1, 2, or 3),

the number of spots on the up-face of a die (1, 2, 3, 4, 5, or 6),

the number of salmon caught per boat (0, 1, 2, 3, $\cdots$), and

the number of red blood cells in a cubic milliliter of blood (0, 1, 2, 3, $\cdots$).

Continuous variable. A quantitative variable is *continuous* when it results from measuring. The accuracy of a continuous variable depends on the refinement of the measurement process. In other words, a continuous variable theoretically takes on an infinite number of possible values and its reported value is limited only by physical measurement accuracy. Some examples of continuous variables are:

the time a clock stops,

the birth weight of a newborn infant,

the amount of carbon monoxide in a person's lungs, and

the level of cholesterol in a cubic milliliter of blood.

Not all variables fit cleanly and unambiguously into one of these four categories. For example, an individual's age is a continuous measurement that is almost always reported in number of complete years lived (a discrete value), frequently classified into ordered age categories such as less than 1 year, 1–5 years, 6–10 years, 11–15 years, $\cdots$ and often spoken of as young, teenage, middle-age, and old.

DESCRIPTIVE STATISTICAL SUMMARIES

Symbolic representation

Table 1.1 contains 80 body weights from a sample of children measured as closely as possible to their fifth birthday and serves to illustrate a few fundamental descriptive statistical summaries. These data are a small part of a large (2000$^+$ participants) longitudinal study of child growth and development.[2]

A necessary part of the statistical process is the representation of the collected data with symbols. For example, the letter x could stand for the variable weight and $x_1 = 33.1$ lbs, $x_2 = 33.5$ lbs, $\cdots$ etc. $\cdots$, $x_{80} = 52.7$ lbs would then represent the 80 specific body weight measurements. The abstract symbols $x_1, x_2, \cdots, x_{80}$ denote the sampled data. The letter stands for weight and the subscript indicates different sampled individuals. Any letter can represent an observation or a property of the observations. For example, every collection of data contains a specific number of observations, the *sample size*. The sample size is traditionally represented by the abstract symbol n rather than a specific number that would vary from situation to situation. For the body weight data, the value represented by n is 80. Once a symbol is defined, it is possible to describe its properties in general terms. If the sample size is doubled, it is represented as $2n$ or a 60% reduction in number of observations as $0.6n$. Without abstract symbols, a general description of a statistical process becomes awkward and in most cases impossible. The material in this text is not concerned with the mathematics of statistical theory but

TABLE 1.1: Body weights (pounds) of 80 five-year-old white male children (ordered from lowest to highest values for convenience).

33.1	33.5	34.7	35.2	35.5	35.7
36.1	36.5	37.0	37.0	37.2	37.5
38.2	38.5	38.7	38.7	38.8	38.9
39.2	39.2	39.2	39.5	39.5	39.7
39.7	39.7	40.0	40.0	40.2	40.7
40.7	41.0	41.0	41.0	41.2	41.2
41.2	41.7	42.1	42.1	42.2	42.2
42.5	42.7	43.0	43.0	43.2	43.5
43.5	43.5	43.5	44.0	44.0	44.2
44.5	44.8	44.9	45.1	45.2	45.3
45.3	45.5	46.0	46.0	46.5	46.7
47.0	47.0	47.0	47.2	47.6	47.8
48.1	48.2	49.0	50.0	50.2	50.5
51.6	52.7				

rather the use of symbols as a language to describe how and why statistical methods work.

Summary measures of location

Descriptive methods are part art and part science intended to summarize many numeric values, such as the 80 body weight measurements, with a few representative numbers that reveal succinctly the properties of the sampled data. These summaries are not the "whole-story" but reflect essential aspects of the collected data. One such summary is a *measure of location*. A measure of location indicates the center of the distribution of the collected observations. It designates a "typical" value. Three common measures of location or central tendency are: the mean, median, and mode (in order of importance).

Sample mean

The *sample mean*, sometimes less formally called the average, is usually represented by the symbol $\bar{x}$ and is the sum of a series of numbers (denoted by x) divided by the number of values in the sum (denoted by n). In symbols, the process of calculating a sample mean value is described by

$$\bar{x} = \frac{x_1 + x_2 + \cdots + x_n}{n} = \frac{1}{n}\left[\sum_{i=1}^{n} x_i\right].$$

The notation $\sum_{i=1}^{n} x_i$ is a shorthand version of the more extensive expression $x_1 + x_2 + \cdots + x_n$ where $i = 1$ represents the starting point and n represents the ending point of the sum. The summation symbol $(\sum)$ is an efficient and abstract representation of the addition process. Appendix B.1 contains a more complete explanation of the summation notation.

From the example body weight data (Table 1.1),

$$\bar{x} = \frac{33.1 + 33.5 + \cdots + 52.7}{80} = \frac{1}{80}\left[\sum_{i=1}^{80} x_i\right] = \frac{1}{80}[3385.3] = 42.316 \text{ lbs}$$

is the mean weight of five-year-old males calculated from the 80 sampled individuals. Again, the symbol x_i denotes each body weight but it could be any letter. The symbols defining the mean value $\bar{x}$ show how it is calculated but indicate little about its properties or why it is important.

The sample mean value is the "balancing point" of a set of observations where each value serves as its own weight. In physics, this balancing point is called the *center of gravity*. Thus, the value that causes the sum of all deviations to be exactly zero is the mean of the sampled values. In symbols, if

$\sum_{i=1}^{n}(x_i - a) = 0$, then $a = \bar{x}$. For example, the numbers

1, 3, 7, 8, and 11

have a mean of $\bar{x} = 6$ because

$$(1-6) + (3-6) + (7-6) + (8-6) + (11-6) = -5 - 3 + 1 + 2 + 5 = 0.$$

Only the value 6 has this property. Graphically, where each dot represents equal weight,

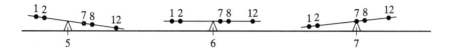

For the 80 body weights, the mean is $\bar{x} = 42.316$ because $\sum_{i=1}^{80}(x_i - 42.316) = 0$.

Polls show consistently that about three-quarters of adults interviewed report that they are above-average drivers, have above-average good looks, believe they will live longer than average, and look younger than average. Remember that only in Lake Wobegon, "all the women are strong and all the men good-looking and the children are all above average." Elsewhere, the sum of deviations from the mean value equals zero, which requires that some of the averaged values be above the mean and some below.

The children of Israel took 40 years to cross the Sinai desert to reach the promised land, about 200 miles. The mean speed was less than a snail's pace or about 3 feet/hour. Of course, this summary value is meaningless since it combines values that are not consistent or uniform measurements of progress. Presumably, on most days no progress was made and other days were spent wandering in the wrong direction. A mean value is an effective summary and amenable to statistical analysis only when it summarizes separate and consistent observations of the same phenomenon. A sample mean value then characterizes all the collected observations with a single "typical" value. The question as to what is meant by "typical" is fundamental to statistical analysis and is pursued extensively in the following chapters.

Median

The *median* (denoted by the symbol $M_{0.5}$) of n observations is the value that divides the ordered sample into two equal pieces. Equal in the sense that the same number of observations (50%) are above and below the median value. Unlike the sample mean, the magnitude of each observation is relatively unimportant. If the number of observations n is odd, then the position of the median value is

$$M_{0.5} = \left(\frac{n+1}{2}\right)^{\text{th}} \text{ ordered observation.}$$

The value $(n + 1)/2$ is not the median value but the location of the median value. The median of the seven ordered numbers 5, 8, 9, 12, 15, 18, and 77 is the $(7 + 1)/2$th or the 4th value, namely $M_{0.5} = 12$. There are three values below and three values above the median value 12. To repeat, the numbers must be ordered. If the number of ordered observations n is even, then

$$M_{0.5} = \text{the average of the two middle values, the } (n/2)^{\text{th}} \text{ and}$$
$$\text{the } (n/2 + 1)^{\text{th}} \text{ observations.}$$

For example, the median of the six numbers 5, 8, 9, 12, 15, and 18 is $M_{0.5} = (9 + 12)/2 = 10.5$, which is the average of the 3rd and 4th observations. Again, there are three values below and three values above the median value 10.5. The median weight of the five-year-old boys is $M_{0.5} = (42.1 + 42.2)/2 = 42.150$ lbs, which is the average of the 40th and 41st observations in the ordered sample (Table 1.1). Half (40) of the 80 body weights are below and half (40) are above the median value 42.150.

The median value is the balancing point of a set of data where each observation has equal weight regardless of its numeric value. Each observation counts equally whether it is 6 or 600. The median, therefore, divides the total number of observations into two equal pieces based strictly on counting the sampled values. The median, like the sample mean, is a single "typical" value again characterizing the entire data set. Occasionally, one hears or reads statements such as, "half the apartments surveyed are below the median rent-code standards." This is not "news."

For a symmetric sample of observations, the mean and median coincide (Figure 1.1, on the left). When a distribution is not symmetric, these two measures of central location differ (Figure 1.1, on the right). Such a distribution

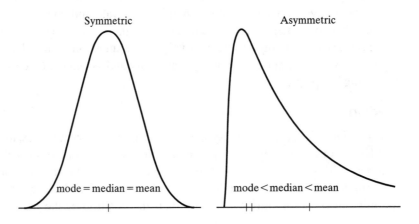

FIGURE 1.1: A symmetric and nonsymmetric representation of a set of observations.

is called *skewed*. Figure 1.1 (right side) shows a distribution "skewed to the right" or "positively" skewed. The phrase "skewed to the right" indicates that the most extreme values are to the right, shifting the mean value to the right of the median value (as illustrated). The comparison of mean and median values, therefore, is one indication of the degree of asymmetry in the collected data.

The following two sets of numbers have the same median but different mean values:

$$4, 4, 8, 14, 15 \quad \bar{x} = 9 \quad M_{0.5} = 8$$

$$4, 4, 8, 14, 150 \quad \bar{x} = 36 \quad M_{0.5} = 8.$$

The median is not sensitive to extreme values where the mean value is influenced by both large and small values. One measure of central location is usually preferred to the other, depending on its use. Personal income data are summarized frequently by a median, so that the summary value is not highly affected by a few superrich or by the extremely poor making it more representative of the entire group. In other situations, a summary that is influenced by the magnitude of each observed value is desired. The mean is then the preferred measure of location (central tendency).

A median value minimizes the impact of extreme observations but extreme observations possibly play a critical role in summarizing the data. A significant question arises: Do extreme values belong with the collected data or do they represent some sort of contamination? Or, more simply, is a mean that reflects these values or median that minimizes their impact the appropriate summary? Observations entirely unrelated to the variable under study can result from a failure of the method of measurement or a failure to record the observation correctly or numerous other possibilities. Such observations are called *outliers*. "Out and out" outliers distort calculations based on the sampled data and should be eliminated from the data set. Whether an extreme observation is an outlier, however, is frequently not obvious and is generally a subjective decision, making the choice between a mean and a median difficult. Often scientific reports contain both values.

Mode

The *mode* is that value which occurs most frequently in a sample of observations. The mode of the numbers 1, 4, 5, 4, 8, 4, 9, 4 is 4. Unlike the mean and the median, a set of observations can have more than one mode. When the collected values have a single mode, however, the data are said to be *unimodal*. The mode for the body weight data of the five-year-old children is 43.5 lbs (Table 1.1). The mode is a relatively meaningless and infrequently used summary measure, except in introductory statistics texts.

Two properties of the sample mean value

Statistical methods have two components: the fundamental statistical concept underlying the method and a series of details that relate to why the method works. In the following, substantial effort is made to present enough details so that the "big-picture" becomes clearly visible. To paraphrase Yogi Berra, "Statistics is 90 percent mental. The other half is details."

Two such details necessary to understand fully the properties of the sample mean value are:

1. Adding a constant value c to each observation x_i produces a new set of observations $(x_i + c)$. The mean of these new observations is the original mean increased by c; that is, the new mean value is $\bar{x} + c$ (Box 1.1).

Box 1.1. The Mean of $x_i + c = $?

The mean of the observations $(x_1 + c, x_2 + c, \cdots, x_n + c)$ is

$$\frac{1}{n}\sum_{i=1}^{n}(x_i + c) = \frac{1}{n}\left(\sum_{i=1}^{n}x_i + \sum_{i=1}^{n}c\right) = \frac{1}{n}\left(\sum_{i=1}^{n}x_i + nc\right)$$

$$= \frac{1}{n}\sum_{i=1}^{n}x_i + \frac{1}{n}nc = \bar{x} + c.$$

Note that: $\sum_{i=1}^{n}c = c + c + \cdots + c = nc.$

The rules and properties of the summation notation $\sum$ are discussed in Appendix B.1.

Suppose that the scales used to weigh the 80 five-year-olds (Table 1.1) consistently overstated their weights by two pounds. If the value $c = 2$ lbs (a constant value) is subtracted from each of the 80 observed weights recorded in Table 1.1, the corrected sample mean of the 80 observations is 40.316 or, more simply, $\bar{x} - c = \bar{x} - 2.0 = 42.316 - 2.0 = 40.316$.

2. Multiplying each observation x_i by a constant value a produces a new set of observations ax_i. The mean of these new observations is the original mean multiplied by a factor a; that is, the new mean value is $a\bar{x}$ (Box 1.2).

Box 1.2. The Mean of $ax_i = ?$

The mean of the observations $(ax_1, ax_2, \cdots, ax_n)$ is

$$\frac{1}{n}\sum_{i=1}^{n} ax_i = a\frac{1}{n}\sum_{i=1}^{n} x_i = a\overline{x}$$

The body weights in Table 1.1 are measured in pounds and a new observation $ax_i = x_i/2.205$ is the body weight measured in kilograms, since one kilogram equals 2.205 pounds making $a = 1/2.205$. The mean value of the 80 five-year-olds in kilograms, therefore, becomes $a\overline{x} = \overline{x}/2.205 = 42.316/2.205 = 19.191$ kilograms.

Properties 1 and 2 are summarized by noting that the mean value of a sample of n observations $(ax_1 + c), (ax_2 + c), \cdots, (ax_n + c)$ is $a\overline{x} + c$.

Summary measures of dispersion

A mean value summarizes one property of a sample of observations. Another fundamental property is variability. A sample mean value does not usually reflect variability (a special case will be discussed in Chapter 4). For example, the mean of the four values 9, 10, 12, and 13 is

$$\overline{x} = \frac{9 + 10 + 12 + 13}{4} = 11$$

and the mean of 0, 10, 12, and 22 is

$$\overline{x} = \frac{0 + 10 + 12 + 22}{4} = 11.$$

The two sets of numbers obviously differ in variability, a fact not reflected by the mean or median values. Two common measures of variability are the range and the sample variance.

Range

The *range* is the difference between the largest and the smallest sampled values or

$$\text{range} = \text{maximum } x_i - \text{ minimum } x_i.$$

The range from the body weight data (Table 1.1) is $52.7 - 33.1 = 19.6$ lbs. A range identifies the difference between the extremes found in a sample of data but is not the best description of overall variability because it depends entirely on two observations out of the total sampled.

Sample variance

The sum of squared deviations of each observation x_i from the mean $\bar{x}$ divided by $(n-1)$ is called the *sample variance* (denoted S_X^2). In symbols, the process of calculating a sample variance is described by

$$S_X^2 = \frac{(x_1 - \bar{x})^2 + (x_2 - \bar{x})^2 + (x_3 - \bar{x})^2 + \cdots + (x_n - \bar{x})^2}{n-1}$$

$$= \frac{1}{n-1}\left[\sum_{i=1}^{n}(x_i - \bar{x})^2\right].$$

The sample variance is a common and effective summary of the variability among the collected observations.

The sum of squared deviations, sometimes called the *total sum of squares*, is divided by $(n-1)$, not n, for reasons discussed later (Chapter 8). If the total sum of squares were divided by n, it would be the mean of the squared deviations. The sum of deviations from the mean (not squared) fails to reflect variability because this sum is always zero (Box 1.3), as mentioned. The fundamental importance of the sample variance becomes clear in the following chapters (starting particularly in Chapter 4).

Box 1.3. Sum of Deviations from the Mean Value

$$\sum_{i=1}^{n}(x_i - \bar{x}) = \sum_{i=1}^{n}x_i - \sum_{i=1}^{n}\bar{x} = \sum_{i=1}^{n}x_i - n\bar{x} = \sum_{i=1}^{n}x_i - n\left[\frac{\sum_{i=1}^{n}x_i}{n}\right]$$

$$= \sum_{i=1}^{n}x_i - \sum_{i=1}^{n}x_i = 0$$

A sample variance of zero occurs only when all observations are identical (no variability). Otherwise, it is a positive number that increases as the degree of variability among sampled observations increases. A large value of S_X^2 occurs when at least some of the observed values differ substantially from the mean value. Conversely, a small variance occurs when extreme values are rare and most of the observations are generally close to the mean value $\bar{x}$. The mean value identifies a "typical" value and the sample variance indicates how well this "typical" value reflects the sampled data. The sample variance S_X^2 is frequently the key to assessing the effectiveness of a statistical summary, such as $\bar{x}$ (Chapters 5 and 6), to identify the properties of an entire set of observations.

Sample standard deviation

The *sample standard deviation* is defined as the square root of the sample variance or

$$S_X = \sqrt{S_X^2} = \sqrt{\frac{1}{n-1}\sum_{i=1}^{n}(x_i - \bar{x})^2}.$$

This seemly redundant measure of variability also plays a key role in later discussions. One immediate feature of the sample standard deviation is that it is expressed in the same units as the measurements summarized. If the observations are measured in pounds, for example, then the units of standard deviation are also in pounds. In contrast, the units associated with the sample variance are the squared units of the original measurement [for example, (pounds)^2].

The sample variance from the 80 body weights (Table 1.1) is

$$S_X^2 = \frac{(33.1 - 42.316)^2 + \cdots + (52.7 - 42.316)^2}{79}$$

$$= \frac{1}{79}\left[\sum_{i=1}^{80}(x_i - 42.316)^2\right] = 19.010 \text{ lbs}^2$$

and the sample standard deviation is $S_X = \sqrt{19.010} = 4.360$ lbs.

Two properties of the sample variance

More details:

1. Adding a constant value c to each observation x_i produces a new set of observations $(x_i + c)$ but does not change the sample variance or

$$S_{X+c}^2 = S_X^2. \quad \text{See Box 1.4.}$$

Box 1.4. $S^2_{X+c} = ?$

The variance of the observations $(x_1 + c, x_2 + c, \cdots, x_n + c)$ is

$$S^2_{X+c} = \frac{1}{n-1} \sum_{i=1}^{n} [(x_i + c) - (\bar{x} + c)]^2 = \frac{1}{n-1} \sum_{i=1}^{n} (x_i + c - \bar{x} - c)^2$$

$$= \frac{1}{n-1} \sum_{i=1}^{n} (x_i - \bar{x})^2 = S^2_X.$$

---

2. Multiplying each observation x_i by a constant value a produces a new set of observations ax_i and multiplies the original sample variance by a factor a^2 or

$$S^2_{aX} = a^2 S^2_X. \quad \text{See Box 1.5.}$$

Box 1.5. $S^2_{aX} = ?$

The variance of the observations $(ax_1, ax_2, \cdots, ax_n)$ is

$$S^2_{aX} = \frac{1}{n-1} \sum_{i=1}^{n} (ax_i - a\bar{x})^2 = \frac{1}{n-1} \sum_{i=1}^{n} [a(x_i - \bar{x})]^2$$

$$= a^2 \frac{1}{n-1} \sum_{i=1}^{n} (x_i - \bar{x})^2 = a^2 S^2_X.$$

Properties 1 and 2 are summarized by noting that the sample variance of the transformed values $(ax_1+c), (ax_2+c), \cdots, (ax_n+c)$ is a^2 times the original sample variance or

$$S^2_{aX+c} = a^2 S^2_X.$$

The sample standard deviation of the transformed values $(ax_1 + c), (ax_2 + c), \cdots, (ax_n + c)$ is a times the original sample standard deviation, or

$$S_{aX+c} = \sqrt{S^2_{aX+c}} = \sqrt{a^2 S^2_X} = aS_X.$$

If the 80 sampled body weights of five-year-old males measured in pounds are converted to kilograms, then each new weight x_i^* would be $x_i/2.205$

(again, $a = 1/2.205$) making the sample variance

$$S_{X*}^2 = a^2 S_X^2 = S_X^2/(2.205)^2 = 19.010/4.862 = 3.910 \text{ kilograms}^2.$$

The sample standard deviation is $S_{X*} = \sqrt{3.910} = 1.977$ kilograms or $S_{X*} = aS_X = 4.360/2.205 = 1.977$ kilograms.

EXAMPLE

When the mean value $\bar{x} = 42.316$ is subtracted from each child's observed body weight ($x_i^* = x_i - 42.316$ where $c = 42.316$), the mean value of the new observations is zero ($\bar{x}^* = \bar{x} - c = 42.316 - 42.316 = 0.0$) but the sample variance is unchanged ($S_{X*}^2 = S_{X+c}^2 = S_{X-\bar{x}}^2 = S_X^2 = 19.101$ where $c = \bar{x} = 42.316$). However, if the sample mean is subtracted from each body weight and each observation is also divided by the sample standard deviation ($x_i^* = (x_i - 42.316)/4.360$ where again $c = 42.316$ and $a = 1/4.360$), then the mean of the new 80 observations x_i^* remains 0.0 but the sample variance becomes 1.0. In symbols,

$$S_{X*}^2 = S_{aX+c}^2 = S_{\frac{1}{S_X}(X-\bar{x})}^2 = \left[\frac{1}{S_X}\right]^2 S_{X-\bar{x}}^2 = \left[\frac{1}{S_X}\right]^2 S_X^2 = 1$$

when $c = \bar{x}$ and $a = \frac{1}{S_X}$. ∎

Two alternate forms for the sample variance, sometimes called *computational expressions*, that make its calculation somewhat easier are:

$$(1) \quad S_X^2 = \frac{1}{n-1}\left[\sum_{i=1}^{n} x_i^2 - n\bar{x}^2\right] \quad \text{see Box 1.6.}$$

and

$$(2) \quad S_X^2 = \frac{1}{n-1}\left[\sum_{i=1}^{n} x_i^2 - \frac{\left(\sum_{i=1}^{n} x_i\right)^2}{n}\right]. \quad \text{See Box 1.6.}$$

Note that the sum $\sum_{i=1}^{n} x_i^2$ is not the same as $(\sum_{i=1}^{n} x_i)^2$. The symbol $\sum x_i^2$ represents the process of squaring the sample values first and then summing the resulting squared values; where the symbol $(\sum x_i)^2$ represents the process of summing the values first and then squaring the resulting sum. A few calculators and certainly computers produce the sample variance and standard deviation automatically, making shortcut formulas unnecessary. These computational expressions, nevertheless, have applications in other contexts.

Box 1.6. Equivalence of Computational Expressions

Note that:
$$(x_1 - \overline{x})^2 = (x_1 - \overline{x})(x_1 - \overline{x}) = x_1^2 - 2\overline{x}x_1 + \overline{x}^2$$
$$(x_2 - \overline{x})^2 = (x_2 - \overline{x})(x_2 - \overline{x}) = x_2^2 - 2\overline{x}x_2 + \overline{x}^2$$
$$(x_3 - \overline{x})^2 = (x_3 - \overline{x})(x_3 - \overline{x}) = x_3^2 - 2\overline{x}x_3 + \overline{x}^2$$
$$\underline{\quad} \qquad \underline{\quad} \qquad \underline{\quad}$$
$$\underline{\quad} \qquad \underline{\quad} \qquad \underline{\quad}$$
$$\underline{\quad} \qquad \underline{\quad} \qquad \underline{\quad}$$
$$(x_n - \overline{x})^2 = (x_n - \overline{x})(x_n - \overline{x}) = x_n^2 - 2\overline{x}x_n + \overline{x}^2.$$

Adding the n numbers in each column yields*

$$\sum(x_i - \overline{x})^2 = \sum x_i^2 - 2\overline{x}\sum x_i + n\overline{x}^2$$
$$= \sum x_i^2 - 2n\overline{x}^2 + n\overline{x}^2$$
$$= \sum x_i^2 - n\overline{x}^2 \qquad \text{expression (1) when divided by } n - 1$$
$$= \sum x_i^2 - n(\sum x_i / n)^2$$
$$= \sum x_i^2 - (\sum x_i)^2 / n \qquad \text{expression (2) when divided by } n - 1.$$

*From this point on, the symbol $\sum_{i=1}^{n}$ will be written more simply as $\sum$ for a sample of n observations.

The sample mean and sample variance are fundamental summary descriptions of sampled data. For some data sets these two values tell the "whole story" (Chapter 4—normal distribution). For others, these two summary values are useful but do not indicate other important features of the collected data. Two sets of observations with the same mean values and the same variances can differ in other respects. For example, the "shape" of the distribution of the sampled values is generally not reflected by the sample mean or variance and is the subject of a following section (graphical display of data).

An extreme view of variability was stated by Francis Galton (b. 1822). He wrote, "It is difficult to understand why statisticians commonly limit their enquires to Averages and do not revel in more comprehensive views. Their souls seem as dull to the charm of variety as that of the native of one of our flat countries, whose retrospect of Switzerland was that, if its mountains could be thrown into its lakes, two nuisances would be gotten rid of at once." A partial response to this criticism is to include a measure of variability whenever a sample mean is considered.

Weighted average

A *weighted average* is yet another kind of mean value. As before, it is a summary of the collected data but each observation has an associated weight. Using these weights allows different observations to have different influences on the calculated mean value. By a strategic choice of weights, a weighted average becomes an important and frequently used statistical tool.

A weighted average is formed by multiplying each observation by its corresponding weight, summing these products and dividing the resulting sum by the sum of the weights. In symbols, a weighted average (weights are denoted w_i) of n observations (again denoted x_i) is

$$weighted\ average = \frac{w_1 x_1 + w_2 x_2 + \cdots + w_n x_n}{w_1 + w_2 + \cdots + w_n} = \frac{\sum w_i x_i}{\sum w_i}.$$

The sample mean value ($\bar{x}$) is a special kind of weighted average where the n weights are equal ($w_i = 1$ or $1/n$ or any constant).

EXAMPLE

From the Table 1.1, mean of the five-year-old males who weigh less than 40 pounds (26 observations) is $\bar{x}_1 = 37.558$ and the mean of the five-year-old children who weigh 40 pounds or more (54 observations) is $\bar{x}_2 = 44.607$. One might be tempted to combine these two mean values to estimate the overall mean of the 80 body weights, where $(37.558 + 44.607)/2 = 41.083$ pounds. This approach does not produce the previously calculated mean value ($\bar{x} = 42.316$). Choosing weights equal to the number of five-year-old boys in each group, however, produces the previous mean body weight ($w_1 = 26$ and $w_2 = 54$). The weighted average is

$$weighted\ average = \frac{w_1 \bar{x}_1 + w_2 \bar{x}_2}{w_1 + w_2} = \frac{26(37.558) + 54(44.607)}{26 + 54} = 42.316,$$

which is identical to the mean value based on all 80 observations. ∎

EXAMPLE

Consider the college admissions data (adapted from an actual case) given in the following table:

Field	Males			Females			Weights
	Applied	Admitted	%	Applied	Admitted	%	
science	80	48	60.0	10	7	70.0	90
professional	60	35	58.3	5	3	60.0	65
social sciences	30	12	40.0	60	30	50.0	90
liberal arts	100	20	20.0	100	25	25.0	200
Total	270	115	42.6	175	65	37.1	445

Overall (bottom row), it appears that males are admitted more frequently than females based on these college admissions data (42.6% versus 37.1%). Comparing the percentages within each of the four academic groups shows the opposite pattern. Higher percentages of females are admitted in all four categories. The apparent contradiction occurs because two rates, rate of application and the rate of admission, are mixed together in a complex fashion.

A weighted average disentangles the different influences of these rates, producing a clear summary of the overall male/female admission pattern. The mean percentage (a weighted average) of males admitted (using the total number of applicants as weights) is

$$\overline{P}_{males} = \frac{90(60.0) + 65(58.3) + 90(40.0) + 200(20.0)}{90 + 65 + 90 + 200} = \frac{16790}{445} = 37.73\%$$

and similarly for females, the mean percentage admitted is

$$\overline{P}_{females} = \frac{90(70.0) + 65(60.0) + 90(50.0) + 200(25.0)}{90 + 65 + 90 + 200} = \frac{19700}{445} = 44.27\%$$

where the percent admitted for both males and females is weighted by the total number of applications in each field ($w_1 = 90$, $w_2 = 65$, $w_3 = 90$, and $w_4 = 200$—last column in the table). The weighted averages show that overall males are less frequently admitted than females (37.7% versus 44.3%). The weighted averages reflect more clearly the male/female admission rates because they are calculated as if the same number of males and females applied for admission (weights = total applicants) producing a comparison influenced only by differences in the admission patterns. ∎

Grouped data

It is often necessary and almost always convenient to summarize a large number of observations in a compact form, called a *frequency table*. A frequency table is crafted by classifying observations into a small number of carefully constructed categories, to separate the "forest from the trees."

To illustrate the utility of a frequency table, consider the most famous transcendental number *pi* (π) calculated to 2000 places,

3.14159265358979323846264338327950288419716939937510582097494459230781640628620899862803482534211706798214808651328230664709384460955058223172535940812848111745028410270193852110555964462294895493038196442881097566593344612847564823378678316527120190914564856692346034861045432664821339360726024914127372458700660631558817488152092096282925409171536436789259036001133053054882046652138414695194151160943305727036575959195309218611738193261179310511854807446237996274956735188575272489122793818301194912983367336244065664308602139494639522473719070217986094370277053921717629317675238467481846766940513200056812714526356082778577134275778960917363717872146844090122495343014654958537105079227968925892354201995611212902196086403441815981362977477130996051870721134999999837297804995105973173281609631859502445945534690830264252230825334468503526193118817101000313783875288658753320838142061717766914730359825349042875546873115956286388235378759375195778185778053217122680661300192787661119590921642019893809525720106548586327886593615338182796823030195203530185296899577362259941389124972177528347913151557485724245415069595082953311686172785588907509838175463746493931925506040092770167113900984882401285836160356370766010471018194295559619894676783744944825537977472726847104047534646208046684259069491293313677028989152104752162056966024058038150193511253382430035587640247496473263914199272604269922796782354781636009341721641219924586315030286182974555706749838505494588586926995690927210797509302955321165344987202755960236480665499119881834797753566369807426542527862551818417574672890977772793800081647060016145249192173217214772350141441973568548161361157352552133475741849468438523323907394143334547762416862518983569485562099921922218427255025425688767179049460165346680498862723279178608578438382796797668145410095388378636095068006422512520511739298489608412848862694560424196528502221066118630674427862203919494504712371378696095636437191728747646575739624138908658326459958133904780275901

One of the properties of a transcendental number is that no pattern exists among the digits that follow the decimal point. If no pattern exists, then each of the 10 digits should be about equally frequent. It is difficult or even impossible to get an idea of the distribution of the digits of the number π by inspecting the 2000 values without a systematic approach. When the distribution of the digits is summarized in a table, it is easily seen that each digit occurs, more or less, with the same frequency.

Such a frequency table is

Digit	0	1	2	3	4	5	6	7	8	9	Total
Frequency	181	213	207	189	195	205	200	197	202	211	2000

Details again:

The notation for a frequency table with k categories used to classify n observations is

Interval or category	Category midpoint	Category frequency	Relative frequency	Cumulative frequency	Relative cumulative frequency
L_i to L_{i+1}	y_i	f_i	f_i/n	F_i	F_i/n
L_1 to L_2	y_1	f_1	f_1/n	$F_1 = f_1$	F_1/n
L_2 to L_3	y_2	f_2	f_2/n	$F_2 = f_1 + f_2$	F_2/n
L_3 to L_4	y_3	f_3	f_3/n	$F_3 = f_1 + f_2 + f_3$	F_3/n
$\vdots$	$\vdots$	$\vdots$	$\vdots$	$\vdots$	$\vdots$
L_k to L_{k+1}	y_k	f_k	f_k/n	$F_k = f_1 + f_2 + \cdots + f_k = n$	$F_k/n = 1.0$
Total	—	n	1.0	—**	—**

**The sum of this column has no useful interpretation and depends on the choices for the interval limits.

The following defines the components of a frequency table:

Interval limits (denoted L_i and L_{i+1}) represent the lower and upper bounds of the ith-category.

Mid-point (denoted y_i) is defined as the exact center of the ith-category and $y_i = (L_i + L_{i+1})/2$.

Frequency (denoted f_i) is defined as the number of observations contained in the ith-category.

Relative frequency (denoted f_i/n) is defined as the proportion of observations contained in the ith-category. The relative frequency multiplied by 100 is the *percentage* $(100 \times [f_i/n] = \%)$ contained in the ith-category.

Cumulative frequency (denoted F_i) is defined as the total number of observations up to and contained in the ith-category.

Relative cumulative frequency (denoted F_i/n) is defined as the proportion of observations up to and contained in the ith-category.

TABLE 1.2: Body weights (in pounds) of 80 five-year-old white males.

Interval or category	Category midpoint	Category frequency	Relative frequency	Cumulative frequency	Relative cumulative frequency
L_i to L_{i+1}	y_i	f_i	f_i/n	F_i	F_i/n
less than 33 lbs	—	0	0.000	0	0.000
33 to 36 lbs	34.5	6	0.075	6	0.075
36 to 39 lbs	37.5	12	0.150	18	0.225
39 to 42 lbs	40.5	20	0.250	38	0.475
42 to 45 lbs	43.5	19	0.238	57	0.713
45 to 48 lbs	46.5	15	0.188	72	0.900
48 to 51 lbs	49.5	6	0.075	78	0.975
51 to 54 lbs	52.5	2	0.025	80	1.000
54 or more lbs	—	0	0.000	80	1.000
Total	—	80	1.000	—	—

The body weight data from Table 1.1 summarized in a frequency table are given in Table 1.2.

The choice of the interval bounds L_i requires a bit of care. The categories that establish a table must be *mutually exclusive* and are usually *exhaustive*. These two properties of a table require that no observation simultaneously belongs in more than one category (mutually exclusive) and a category exists for every observation (exhaustive). When a table does not have mutually exclusive categories, it is not of much use, as the following illustrates:

days in a year	365
weekends	104
days left in the year	261
days spent sleeping	121
days left in the year	140
summer	98
days left in the year	42
vacations	20
days left in the year	22
illness	12
days left in the year	10

If this table is to be believed, it explains why time "flies."

Calculations from a table

Occasionally it is necessary to calculate the sample mean, median, and variance from a table. A certain amount of accuracy is lost by grouping observations into categories but in most cases (especially for large data sets classified into a table with many categories) accurate estimates can be reconstructed without the actual observations. Values of the mean and variance estimated from counts contained in a table (denoted $\bar{y}$ and S_Y^2) are found by making the assumption that the value of the midpoint of each interval (denoted y_i) adequately represents all observations in that interval. For example, it is assumed that all 19 observations in the weight interval 42 to 45 pounds (Table 1.2) are represented accurately by the single midpoint value, namely $y_4 = (L_4 + L_5)/2 = (42 + 45)/2 = 43.5$ lbs. For narrow intervals, this assumption is rarely misleading.

Keeping in mind that y_i represents the midpoint of the ith-interval in a frequency table and not a specific sample observation, summary values can be calculated from a table. The number of midpoints (y-values) equals the number of intervals in the table and the mean value calculated from the table counts (f_i) becomes

$$\bar{y} = \frac{f_1 y_1 + f_2 y_2 + \cdots + f_k y_k}{f_1 + f_2 + \cdots + f_k} = \frac{\sum_{i=1}^k f_i y_i}{\sum_{i=1}^k f_i} = \frac{1}{n}\left[\sum_{i=1}^k f_i y_i\right].$$

The total number of counts $\sum_{i=1}^k f_i = n$ where k represents the number of categories. The reconstructed sample mean $\bar{y}$ is an application of a weighted average; each midpoint y_i is weighted by its corresponding interval frequency f_i (weights $= w_i = f_i$). Using the data on body weights of five-year-old males classified in Table 1.2, the sample mean is

$$\bar{y} = \frac{6(34.5) + 12(37.5) + 20(40.5) + \cdots + 2(52.5)}{6 + 12 + 20 + \cdots + 2} = \frac{3393}{80} = 42.413.$$

The sample variance calculated from tabled data, similarly using the k midpoints, is

$$S_Y^2 = \frac{f_1(y_1 - \bar{y})^2 + f_2(y_2 - \bar{y})^2 + \cdots + f_k(y_k - \bar{y})^2}{n - 1} = \frac{1}{n - 1}\sum_{i=1}^k f_i(y_i - \bar{y})^2.$$

The calculation of the sample standard deviation for grouped data is not different from ungrouped data and

$$S_Y = \sqrt{S_Y^2}, \text{ as before.}$$

Again from the counts in Table 1.2, the sample variance based on the $k = 7$ midpoints y_i is

$$S_Y^2 = \frac{6(34.5 - 42.413)^2 + \cdots + 2(52.5 - 42.413)^2}{80 - 1}$$

$$= \frac{1516.388}{79} = 19.195 \text{ lbs}^2$$

and the standard deviation is

$$S_Y = \sqrt{19.195} = 4.381 \text{ lbs.}$$

A median value calculated from a table is given by the expression

$$M_{0.5}^* = L + \left[\frac{n/2 - F}{f} \right] \times w$$

where,

L = the lower limit of the interval containing the median value,
F = the cumulative frequency up to L,
w = the width of the interval containing the median value, and
f = the frequency in the interval containing the median value.

A median from grouped data is reconstructed from a table by equating two "distances" (Figure 1.2). The difference between the estimated median value $(M_{0.5}^*)$ and the lower limit of the interval containing the median (L) relative to the interval width (w) is equated to the difference between the middle observation $(n/2)$ and the cumulative frequency up to L (F) relative to the interval frequency (f). In symbols,

$$\frac{M_{0.5}^* - L}{w} = \frac{n/2 - F}{f}$$

and solving for $M_{0.5}^*$ gives an estimated median from data contained in a table. The process is schematically displayed in Figure 1.2.

Using the body weight data in Table 1.2 illustrates the calculation of a median from grouped data. The median value is contained in the interval 42 to 45 pounds because the relative cumulative frequency of 0.5 is between the relative cumulative frequencies 0.475 and 0.713 making

$$L = 42, \quad F = 38, \quad f = 19, \quad w = 3 \quad \text{and} \quad n/2 = 80/2 = 40.$$

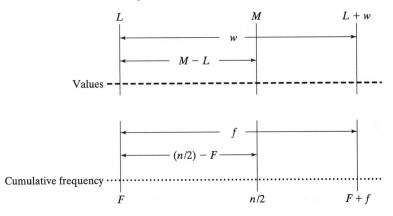

FIGURE 1.2: Schematic representation of the process of calculating a median from grouped data.

The estimated median is

$$\frac{M_{0.5}^* - 42}{3} = \frac{40 - 38}{19}$$

or

$$M_{0.5}^* = 42 + \left[\frac{40 - 38}{19}\right] \times 3 = 42 + 0.316 = 42.316 \text{ lbs.}$$

The expression for the median value $M_{0.5}^*$ is an application of a widely used technique called *linear interpolation*.

For the weights of the five-year-old children, the sample mean, median, variance, and standard deviation calculated for both ungrouped and grouped data are:

		Ungrouped (Table 1.1)		Grouped (Table 1.2)
sample sizes	n	80	$\sum f_i$	80
number of categories	—	—	k	7
means	$\bar{x}$	42.32	$\bar{y}$	42.41
sample variances	S_X^2	19.01	S_Y^2	19.20
standard deviations	S_X	4.36	S_Y	4.38
medians	$M_{0.5}$	42.15	$M_{0.5}^*$	42.32

The assumption that the midpoint of each interval accurately represents the weights of all five-year-olds within that interval works well. The sample summary values based on the entire data set (ungrouped data) are similar to those calculated from the table (grouped data). Of course, it is not usually possible to make this comparison because the original observations are typically not available when the individual observations are summarized in a table. Or, when the data are available, no reason exists to reconstruct the less accurate summary values from a table. This example also illustrates that summary values such as the midpoints y_i can accurately represent a large number of values in a useful way.

GRAPHIC REPRESENTATION

Introduction

Statistical graphics, as the name suggests, combines statistical and graphical techniques and, when well designed, the results are more than the sum of the parts. Plots, charts, graphs, or other visual displays are a kind of statistical analysis. For example, graphical methods display as a whole the location, the variability, and the shape of the distribution of a collection of data. The following three graphical techniques are just a few of the numerous ways observations can be displayed to identify visually the properties of sampled data.

It is said far too often that "a picture is worth a thousand words." More to the point, Will Rogers (b. 1879) noted that, "You must not tell a thing, you must illustrate it. We learn through the eye and not the noggin."

Histogram

A *histogram* displays in a single picture such properties of the observed values as the mean, the variability, any extreme values as well as the general shape of the distribution. The least complicated histogram is constructed from frequency table data with interval widths equal to one unit ($L_{i+1} - L_i = 1$ unit). Construction consists of creating a sequence of rectangles with widths equal to one unit and heights equal to the frequency or relative frequency (f_i or f_i/n) in each table category. The number of rectangles equals the number of categories. These rectangles are placed on a horizontal scale (Figure 1.3) at the corresponding category limits (L_i, L_{i+1}). Figure 1.3 displays the histogram created from the body weights of the 80 five-year-old children (Table 1.1) with all intervals equal to one pound (categories) and all rectangle heights equal to the frequency of the individuals in each category. For example, there are 10 children (rectangle height = 10) in the weight category 39 to 40 pounds (rectangle width = 1 lb—see Figure 1.3). The total area enclosed by the series of such rectangles equals the sample size n (heights = frequencies = f_i) or equals 1.0 (heights = relative frequencies = f_i/n). A histogram indicates where the observations are concentrated ("hills") and where they are not ("valleys").

A slight complication arises when the interval widths chosen to display the data are not in single units. When interval widths of other than one unit (for example, $L_{i+1} - L_i = c$) are convenient, the rectangle heights are no longer made equal to the frequency or relative frequency. The heights are made equal to f_i/c or $f_i/(cn)$. The choice creates rectangles with areas equal to the frequency or

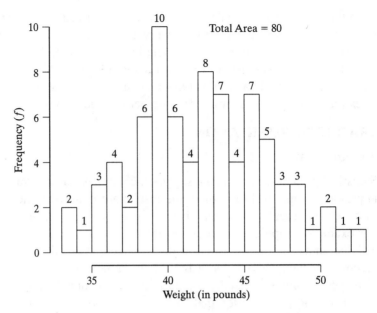

FIGURE 1.3: Frequency histogram of body weights of 80 five-year-old white males.

the relative frequency of the sampled observations within each interval (width × height = rectangle area = $c \times f_i/c = f_i$ or $c \times f_i/(nc) = f_i/n$—see Figure 1.4).

The histogram in Figure 1.4 displays the distribution of the body weight data constructed from relative frequencies (Table 1.2) with interval widths of three pounds ($L_{i+1} - L_i = c = 3$ lbs). The area of each rectangle equals the relative frequency making area (not height) the primary feature of a histogram plot. For example, the interval containing five-year-olds who weigh between 39 and 42 pounds has an area of 0.25 (height = 0.25/3 making the area = width × height = $3(0.25/3) = 3(0.0833) = 0.25$). The relative frequency histogram is designed so that the total area equals 1.0.

When the total area enclosed by the histogram equals 1.0, the area directly displays relative cumulative frequency. For example, the proportion of five-year-old boys who weigh less than 36 pounds is 0.075 or the proportion who weigh less than 39 pounds is $0.075 + 0.150 = 0.225$ or the proportion who weigh less than 45 pounds is $0.075 + 0.150 + 0.250 + 0.238 = 0.713$. In each case, the relative cumulative frequencies (0.075, 0.225, and 0.713) correspond to the proportion of the area to the left of the respective weights of 36 lbs, 39 lbs, and 45 lbs, located on the horizontal axis. A histogram is a picture of relative cumulative frequencies.

Relative frequency polygon

A relative frequency polygon is constructed by connecting points placed at the midpoint of each interval ($y_i = (L_i + L_{i+1})/2$) at a height proportional to the

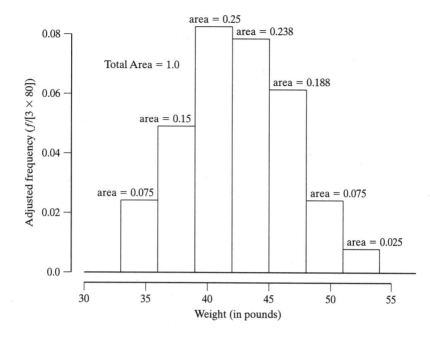

FIGURE 1.4: Relative frequency histogram of body weights of 80 five-year-old white males.

relative frequency of the observations in that interval. This approach is equivalent to connecting the midpoints at the top of the rectangles of a relative frequency histogram. The polygon is usually completed by assuming zero frequency in the "intervals" just before the first interval and just after the last interval containing data. As with a histogram, a relative frequency polygon is designed to have a total enclosed area equal to 1.0. This smoother graphic representation of the data is not very different from a histogram but more realistically displays the distribution of a continuous variable by removing the discontinuous jumps associated with the interval limits. Again, the body weight data illustrate (Figure 1.5 using the data from Table 1.2).

Parallel to the relative frequency histogram, the total area enclosed by the relative frequency polygon to the left of a specific point represents approximately the proportion of observations that are less than or equal to that point (approximate relative cumulative frequency) and equals the relative cumulative frequency (F_i/n) exactly when an interval endpoint L_i is the chosen point. Similarly, the area under the relative frequency polygon between two chosen points equals approximately the proportion of the observations that fall between the two selected values (relative cumulative frequency between two points). If two interval endpoints are chosen, then again the area between the two values corresponds exactly to the proportion of observations between the selected points.

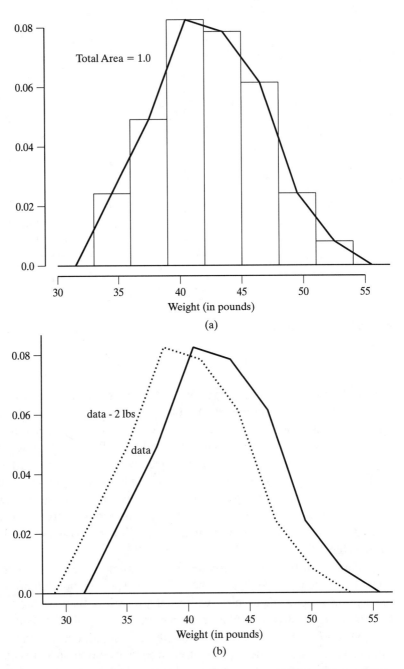

FIGURE 1.5: (a) The relative frequency polygon of body weights of 80 five-year-old white males. (b) Two relative frequency polygons displaying body weights of 80 five-year-old white males.

Examples from Figure 1.5 and Table 1.2 are:

>   proportion less than 42 lbs = 0.475 (exact),
>   proportion less than 50 lbs = 0.95 (approximate),
>   proportion more than 39 lbs and less than 48 lbs = 0.675 (exact),
>   proportion more than 35 lbs and less than 45 lbs = 0.66 (approximate), and
>   proportion more than 33 lbs and less than 54 lbs = 1.00 (exact).

A mechanical advantage of a polygon over a histogram is that two or more distributions can be easily compared. For example, comparing the previous body weight data with the same observations each decreased by two pounds $(x_i - 2)$. Notice that the mean is shifted exactly 2 pounds to the left but the variability (shape) is unaffected (Boxes 1.1 and 1.4).

Relative cumulative frequency polygon

A relative cumulative frequency polygon is another kind of visual display of data. It is constructed by connecting the points plotted at the upper endpoint of each interval from a frequency table with a height equal to the relative cumulative frequency associated with that interval. In symbols, the plotted points are (horizontal = L_{i+1}, vertical = F_i/n). These points are then connected with a single line starting at zero and ending at one. The height (vertical axis) of this line is approximately the proportion of observations less than or equal to the corresponding point on the horizontal axis. Again, this proportion is exactly the relative cumulative frequency when the point chosen corresponds to one of the endpoints (L_i) used to construct the polygon. The relative cumulative frequency polygon and the relative frequency polygon address the same question from different perspectives: What proportion of the sampled observations is less than or equal to a selected value? Figure 1.6, again constructed from the body weight data in Table 1.2, illustrates.

The numbers on the plot are the relative cumulative frequencies (height = F_i/n; the last column in Table 1.2). Examples from Figure 1.6 are:

>   proportion less than 34 lbs = 0.025 (approximate),
>   proportion less than 39 lbs = 0.225 (exact),
>   proportion less than 48 lbs = 0.900 (exact), and
>   proportion less than 50 lbs = 0.95 (approximate).

A relative cumulative frequency polygon displays the same values displayed by a relative frequency histogram or polygon. For example, the proportion of five-year-old boys who weigh less than 39 lbs read directly from the vertical axis of the relative cumulative frequency polygon is also the area to the left of 39 lbs read directly from a relative frequency histogram or polygon. In both cases, the proportion is 0.225. The relative cumulative frequency polygon is an important graphical description of observed data and is a key element in statistical analysis in general (Chapter 4).

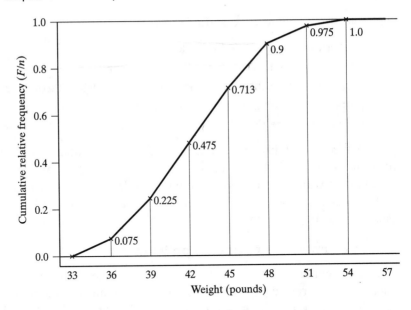

FIGURE 1.6: The relative cumulative frequency polygon of body weights of 80 five-year-old white males.

Percentiles

The Pth percentile is the point that divides a sample of ordered observations into two pieces; P-percent below and $(100 - P)$-percent above the selected point (denoted M_P). The 50th percentile is the median ($M_{0.5}$). In other words, the median is that value for which the relative cumulative frequency is 0.5. The 90th percentile from the body weight data of five-year-old white males is $M_{0.9} = 48.0$ lbs. Thus, 90% (72 out of 80 observations) of the weights are below 48.0 lbs and 10% (8 out of 80 observations) are above 48.0 lbs. A relative cumulative frequency polygon is a visual display of percentiles. Specific percentiles are found by reading the relative cumulative frequency polygon "backwards." A value is selected on the vertical axis ($P = 100$ times the relative cumulative frequency or $100 \times F_i/n$) and the corresponding percentile is located on the horizontal axis, which is then the Pth percentile and has the value denoted by $M_{P/100}$. Examples from Figure 1.6, using again the data in Table 1.2, are:

the 7.5th percentile $= M_{0.075} = 36$ lbs (exact),

the 10th percentile $= M_{0.1} = 36.5$ lbs (approximate),

the 50th percentile $= M_{0.5} =$ median $= 42.2$ lbs (approximate),

the 80th percentile $= M_{0.8} = 46.4$ lbs (approximate),

the 90th percentile $= M_{0.9} = 48$ lbs (exact), and

the 97.5th percentile $= M_{0.975} = 51$ lbs (exact).

A measure of sample variability used occasionally is the *interquartile range* (sometimes abbreviated as IQR). This statistical summary is defined as the difference between the 75th and the 25th percentiles ($IQR = M_{0.75} - M_{0.25}$). Specifically, for the body weight data (Figure 1.6), the approximate 25th percentile $= M_{0.25} = 39.3$ lbs and the approximate 75th percentile $= M_{0.75} = 45.6$ lbs, making the interquartile range $45.6 - 39.3 = 6.3$ lbs. The interquartile range reflects variability as the spread of the middle 50% of the observations. Like the median value, this measure of variation is relatively unaffected by extreme values.

A data set is frequently described effectively with five summary values (the minimum value, $M_{0.25}$, $M_{0.5}$, $M_{0.75}$, and the maximum value). For the data on five-year-old males, these values are:

minimum	25th percentile	50th percentile	75th percentile	maximum
$M_0 = 33.1$	$M_{0.25} = 39.3$	$M_{0.5} = 42.2$	$M_{0.75} = 45.6$	$M_{1.0} = 52.7$

The five summaries can be calculated from the sampled observations but are also readily obtained from a histogram or a polygon display of data.

The relative frequency histogram, polygon, and cumulative polygon are different displays of the same issue, namely area. Area is made geometrically equivalent to relative cumulative frequency displaying visually many of the properties of the collected data. The importance of viewing relative cumulative frequency as area becomes even clearer when the concept of a probability distribution is introduced (Chapters 3 and 4).

This chapter contains just a few of the huge variety of techniques referred to as descriptive statistics. The choice of a descriptive summary frequently depends on the focus of the investigator as well as the subject matter under study. For example, an executive of a large corporation could choose to report the same phenomenon as (1) a 2% return on sales or (2) a 12% decrease in sales over last year or (3) 30% return on investments or (4) an increase in profits of 40% during the last decade or (5) a 20 million dollar profit. The choice largely depends on the impression he or she wishes to convey. The availability of a large number of descriptive statistics allows a wide range of choices for expressing different features of the sampled data and led British statesman Benjamin Disraeli to state, "there are lies, damned lies and statistics." Author Rex Stout expressed the same uneasiness with statistical summaries when he wrote, "there are two kinds of statistics, the kind you look up and the kind you make up." Others have said, "statistics do not lie, but statisticians do." Regardless of what the critics say, descriptive statistics remain a critical part of the process of identifying, understanding, and communicating the properties of data.

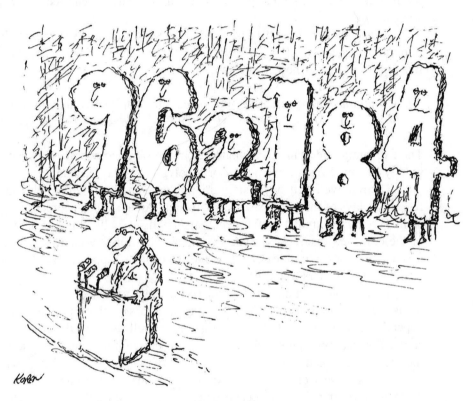

"Tonight, we're going to let the statistics speak for themselves."

PROBLEM SET 1

The length of time a person spends waiting in a physician's office for an appointment can be a frustrating experience. The results* below are the responses of internists from two multispecialty group practices to the following question: "When patients arrive for midmorning or midafternoon appointments, how long do they generally have to wait before they are seen by you?" A sample of the responses in minutes is:

Group practice A	Group practice B
9	23
20	9
7	17
24	26
13	21
29	10
35	8
5	16
0	14
28	26

1. Compute the mean, median, and standard deviation of the internists' responses from both kinds of group practices.
2. If you had to make an appointment and wanted some assurance that you would not spend more than 30 minutes waiting in the office, which would you choose? Why?

The age distribution of 400 homosexual/bisexual men who are antibody positive to the AIDS virus, HIV positive, is given below. These data are from a larger random sample of men selected from census tracts in a specific neighborhood in San Francisco. Following are the untabulated ages of these 400 men.

3. Describe how the following frequency table was prepared. Check several of the intervals to see if you get the same frequency.

Frequency distribution of ages (at last birthday) of 400 HIV positive men, San Francisco

Reported age limits	Frequency (f_i)	cf_i	
20–24	2	2	.005
25–29	85	87	.2175
30–34	135	222	.555
35–39	91	313	.7825
40–44	57	370	.925
45–49	20	390	.975
50–54	10	400	1.0
Total	400		

*Adapted from: Parker, A.W.: *Relationships of Organization Characteristics in Multi-specialty Group Practices to Primary Care Performance.*

Ages (last birthday) of 400 HIV positive men, San Francisco									
49	40	28	31	27	27	32	34	27	32
42	36	28	32	33	40	28	25	47	40
28	38	35	32	23	39	31	26	31	31
40	51	32	29	30	28	34	29	34	36
42	38	37	28	27	28	38	38	40	33
52	37	45	35	39	28	33	30	40	37
37	32	33	32	28	49	31	30	33	29
37	33	41	44	37	29	31	54	36	34
40	38	47	42	42	36	37	28	35	32
30	36	28	28	30	28	34	28	34	37
41	33	30	38	42	41	49	43	38	38
40	30	33	35	26	47	42	49	40	36
37	30	50	44	33	28	37	29	34	38
34	50	38	47	29	35	38	34	38	32
38	27	37	34	29	32	34	41	40	39
36	28	33	33	44	31	36	25	42	38
31	37	32	28	43	35	26	29	34	38
26	30	39	30	30	36	36	32	29	35
35	40	50	28	50	32	29	37	32	26
32	34	25	40	44	49	31	26	26	34
40	34	44	33	34	37	28	29	25	24
42	42	43	35	34	34	31	41	40	25
41	28	34	38	26	29	35	37	32	39
38	30	35	36	49	34	29	27	41	35
30	41	40	39	28	39	29	29	32	27
27	27	34	38	36	37	30	47	30	33
29	31	32	39	31	34	31	39	29	29
27	44	33	30	43	26	34	33	40	44
34	39	39	33	42	37	52	34	26	29
52	40	40	32	31	30	28	30	35	33
37	33	30	33	32	45	32	35	27	48
34	39	27	30	31	30	33	30	43	31
46	41	37	44	26	36	39	29	33	32
30	34	32	49	30	39	46	37	31	39
33	29	34	44	33	39	32	42	48	34
28	36	25	30	30	27	27	37	26	31
27	34	48	36	35	35	33	29	32	31
29	30	25	30	43	30	43	28	37	47
31	29	33	42	37	33	34	28	42	34
33	27	36	35	35	41	31	52	32	27

4. Since age is typically reported as the number of completed years, what are the actual limits of the second interval? What is its midpoint?

5. Compute the mean, median, and standard deviation using the frequency distribution in this table.

6. Plot a relative frequency histogram and relative frequency polygon for the data.
7. Plot a relative cumulative frequency polygon and estimate the 25th percentile $(M_{0.25})$, the 50th percentile $(M_{0.50})$, and the 75th percentile $(M_{0.75})$ from the plot.
8. What is the relationship between the 50th percentile in (7) and median in (5)?
9. Estimate the interquartile range. What percent of the total frequency is contained within this range?
10. Find the mean, median, and standard deviation of the ages of these patients when they are three years older. Justify your answer.

Since 1973 Medicare has financed an end-stage renal disease program. The cost is estimated at \$3 billion for 1998 for patients on dialysis or transplants.*
    Given the data below on Medicare end-stage renal disease patients:

11. Plot the relative frequency polygons of dialysis and transplant age distributions on the same graph.
12. Write a brief statement (25 words or less) comparing these two distributions.

Age (in years)	Dialysis frequency	f/cn	Functioning transplants frequency	f/cn
0–14	756	.009	664	.034
15–24	3113	.035	2162	.110
25–34	8373	.095	5276	.269
35–44	11670	.132	5424	.277
45–54	14686	.166	3764	.192
55–64	22141	.250	2022	.103
65–74	19495	.220	290	.015
75–84	8276	.094	8	.00025
Total	88510		19610	
mean age	55.0		38.3 years	

Select the correct answer:

13. $\bar{x} + 2 > 2$ | always true   sometimes true   never true
14. $\bar{x} < S_X$ | always true   sometimes true   never true
15. $\sum (x_i - \bar{x}) < 3$ | always true   sometimes true   never true
16. $\bar{x} - median = 0$ | always true   sometimes true   never true
17. $S^2_{X+c} > S^2_X$ | always true   sometimes true   never true
18. $S^2_X - 5 \geq 0$ | always true   sometimes true   never true
19. $S^2_{aX} \leq S^2_X$ | always true   sometimes true   never true
20. $\bar{x} \times 3 > \bar{x}$ | always true   sometimes true   never true

---

*Source: Eggers, P.W. "Effect of Transplantation on the Medicare End-Stage Renal Disease Program." *New England Journal of Medicine*.

CHAPTER 2

Probability

In his book on probability, entitled "How to Take a Chance,"[3] Darrell Huff states that, "Probability theory is the underpinning of the modern world. Current research in both the physical sciences and social sciences cannot be understood without it .... By ignoring, or failing to grasp, the laws of chance we hurt ourselves in many ways." It is less dramatic but definitely true that probabilities are part of everyday life: in weather reports: "There is a 70 percent chance of rain tomorrow;" in medical prognoses, "A patient has a 50 percent chance of surviving five years;" in state lotteries, "The probability of winning the super payoff is 1 in 41 million." A confusing use of probability comes from the moviemaker Samuel Goldwyn when he replied, "[That is] a definite maybe."

Probability also plays an important role in statistical theory and methods. It links summary values calculated from data, such as a mean value (Chapter 1), to rigorous inferences about the sampled population (topics of Chapter 5 and beyond). A few basic concepts of probability are a prerequisite for understanding the analysis of sample data.

Fundamental definition

A surprising property of the study of probability is that it can be developed at almost any level of sophistication, from simple to extremely complex. For the following, the approach is designed for a first course in statistics, at the cost of some slightly fuzzy and mathematically weak arguments.

A DEFINITION OF A PROBABILITY   The *probability of occurrence for an event labeled A* ("the probability of A" for short) is defined as the ratio of the number of events where event A occurs to the total number of possible events that could occur. More precisely, suppose that a random "experiment" consists of a number of mutually exclusive and equally likely events (denoted n) and a specific number of these events are of special interest (denoted $n[A]$). Then, the probability of the occurrence of these special events is defined as the ratio of the two counts $n[A]$ and n where

$$\text{probability of event } A = P(A) = \frac{n[A]}{n}.$$

The probability of an event can be represented in a variety of equivalent ways. For example,

$$P(a\ white\ ball\ is\ selected\ from\ an\ urn\ containing\ 25\ balls)$$
$$= P(a\ white\ ball\ is\ selected) = P(white\ ball)$$
$$= P(white) = P(W) = n[W]/n.$$

The meaning of *mutually exclusive* events is straightforward. It means that the occurrence of any one event precludes the occurrence of another. Event A is mutually exclusive of event B, if event A occurs, then event B cannot occur and conversely, if event B occurs, then event A cannot occur. Tossing a coin once yields two mutually exclusive events—either heads or tails occurs—never both. If the event A is drawing a king on the first draw from a deck of normal playing cards and event B is drawing a queen on the first draw, then events A and B are mutually exclusive events since drawing a king (event A) precludes drawing a queen (event B) and similarly drawing a queen precludes drawing a king. If the event A is drawing a king from a normal deck of playing cards on the first draw and event B is drawing a club on the first draw, then A and B are not mutually exclusive events since both events can occur simultaneously, drawing the king of clubs. It is frequently said that, "you cannot have your cake and eat it too," which is just a more poetic way of indicating that two events are mutually exclusive.

The term *equally likely* events means equally probable events. If A and B represent two events, then they are equally likely only when $P(A) = P(B)$. The simple definition of probability used here, therefore, involves a degree of circular reasoning since it requires events to be equally probable to define probability. Furthermore, it is easy to visualize events that are not equally likely. To avoid circular reasoning and to deal with events that are not equally likely, alternative definitions of probability are used. These more general definitions are frequently preferred, especially in a mathematical context. The slightly flawed but simple definition of probability, however, provides an adequate basis for understanding the role of probability in the applications of the statistical methods discussed in following chapters.

In his book, *The Basics of Winning Lotto/Lottery*, Professor Jones writes,

There are two schools of thought regarding how to play numbers that seem to be drawn randomly. You either play the ones that come up the most or the ones that are overdue to come up. To beat the lottery, I suggest that you play numbers that show a high frequency rather than a low frequency of occurrence."

This is useless advice since the numbers selected in a lottery are mutually exclusive (the selection of a specific number precludes the selecting of any other number on each draw) and equally likely (by state law and common sense, all numbers have the same probability of being selected on each draw), picking so called "hot" and "cold" numbers is nonsense. Ironically, a strategy based on this bad advice does not affect the probability of winning, because the probability that a "hot" or "cold" number occurs is identical to the probability that any other lottery number occurs. If this were not the case, hundreds or, perhaps, thousands of people would win the lottery every week.

Probabilities from big to small to very small

probability = 0.75 (3/4)
   P(at least one heads in two tosses of a coin), P(living beyond age 65)
probability = 0.50 (1/2)
   P(heads in one toss of a coin), P(male birth)
probability = 0.10 (1/10)
   P(one heads in six tosses of a coin), P(having a traffic accident in one year)
probability = 0.01 (1/100)
   P(one heads in ten tosses of a coin), P(IRS audit), P(birth of twins)
probability = 0.001 (1/1000)
   P(no heads in ten tosses of a coin), P(birth of triplets), P(full-house)
probability = 0.000001 (1/1,000,000)
   P(no heads in twenty tosses of a coin), P(birth of quadruplets), P(royal flush)
probability = 0.00000001 (1/100,000,000)
   P(no heads in twenty-six tosses of a coin), P(all clubs in a bridge hand),
   P(for life, 5000 dollars/week from Publishers Clearing House)
probability = 0.0000000000000001 ($1/10^{16}$)
   P(no heads in fifty-three tosses of a coin), P(guessing the number on a VISA card correctly).

Illustrative examples

The following examples illustrate the notion of a random "experiment" and the corresponding structure:

EXAMPLE

When a fair coin is tossed to choose randomly between two alternatives, what is the probability of heads? The random "experiment" is *tossing a fair coin once* with possible outcomes heads or tails. The two possible outcomes are mutually exclusive and equally likely. The total number of outcomes that can occur is $n = 2$. Suppose the event A of interest is heads occurs, then the number of events where event A occurs is $n[A] = 1$ making the probability of heads $P(A) = n[A]/n = 1/2$. ∎

EXAMPLE

When tossing a fair coin twice, what is the probability of two heads? The random "experiment" is *tossing a fair coin twice*. All mutually exclusive and equally likely events are: heads then heads (*HH*), heads then tails (*HT*), tails then heads (*TH*), and tails then tails (*TT*). Suppose event A is heads, then heads (*HH*) occurs. The total number of mutually exclusive and equally likely events is $n = 4$. The number of events where event A occurs is $n[A] = 1$. Therefore, the probability $P(A) = P(heads\ then\ heads) = P(HH) = n[HH]/n = 1/4$. Suppose event B is a tail and a head occurs in two tosses (*TH* or *HT*). The probability of a heads/tails combination is $P(B) = P(heads\ then\ tails$ or $tails\ then\ heads) = P(TH$ or $HT) = n[B]/n = 2/4 = 1/2$. ∎

EXAMPLE

As part of a study of birth defects,[4] 320 birth certificates from a series of small villages in France were reviewed. There were 176 male and 144 female births over 10 years. A *certificate is drawn at random* from the village records (the random "experiment"). What is the probability that the certificate drawn belongs to a male (denoted M)? The total number of equally likely and mutually exclusive events is $n = 320$ and number of male birth certificates is $n[M] = 176$. Therefore, the probability of selecting a male's birth certificate is

$$P(male) = P(M) = \frac{n[M]}{n} = \frac{176}{320} = 0.55.$$

Similarly, the probability of drawing a female's birth certificate is

$$P(female) = P(F) = \frac{n[F]}{n} = \frac{144}{320} = 0.45. \qquad ∎$$

EXAMPLE

An ordinary bridge deck consists of 52 cards. A card is selected at random (the random "experiment") creating 52 mutually exclusive and equally likely events ($n = 52$). If the event A is *the card drawn is an ace*, then the probability of event A is $P(A) = 4/52 = 1/13$ ($n[A] = 4$). If the event B is *the card drawn is a club*, then the probability of event B is $P(B) = 13/52 = 1/4$ ($n[B] = 13$). If the event C is *the card drawn is the ace of clubs,* then the probability of event C is $P(C) = 1/52$ ($n[C] = 1$). This last probability is not the probability of drawing an ace or a club (probability $= 16/52$; to be discussed). ∎

EIGHT RULES OF PROBABILITY

Possible values of a probability

The number of events where event A occurs is never less than zero and never greater than the total number of possible events. In symbols,

$$0 \leq n[A] \leq n,$$

and dividing by n gives

$$\frac{0}{n} \leq \frac{n[A]}{n} \leq \frac{n}{n} \qquad \text{or} \qquad 0 \leq P(A) \leq 1. \qquad\qquad \textit{rule 1}$$

In words, the value of a probability is always a zero or a one or a number between zero and one.

Aside: Expressions involving symbols such as $<$ or $\leq$ are called *inequalities*. For example, $M \leq N$ is read "M is less than or equal to N." Both sides of an inequality can be divided or multiplied by the same positive number without affecting the validity of the expression. For example, for $5 < 10$, then $1 < 2$ or $10 < 20$ or $55 < 110$. Dividing or multiplying by a negative number reverses the inequality. For example, for $5 < 10$, then $-5 > -10$ or $-1 > -2$ or $-10 > -20$ or $-55 > -110$ and identically, $-10 < -5$ or $-2 < -1$ or $-20 < -10$ or $-110 < -55$.

Sure event and impossible event

A sure event is an event that always occurs. If S represents the sure event, then $n[S] = n$ and

$$P(S) = \frac{n[S]}{n} = \frac{n}{n} = 1.$$

It is occasionally suggested that if you are going to bet on a sure thing, remember to keep enough money for bus fare.

An impossible event is an event that never occurs. If I represents the impossible event, then $n[I] = 0$ and

$$P(I) = \frac{n[I]}{n} = \frac{0}{n} = 0.$$

Winning the lottery is an extremely rare event if you buy a ticket and is the impossible event if you don't buy a ticket.

Complementary event

The total number of events in a random "experiment" always divides into two mutually exclusive possibilities: the event occurs or the event does not occur.

The nonoccurrence of event A (denoted $\overline{A}$ and read "not" A) is called the *complementary event*. Therefore, it follows that for n mutually exclusive events

$$n[A] + n[\overline{A}] = n$$

where $n[\overline{A}]$ is the number of events where A does not occur.

When tossing a coin once, tails occurs (event T) is the complement of heads occurs (event H). If a coin is tossed twice, then the complement of the event that two heads occurs (event HH) is the event that at least one tail occurs (events HT or TH or TT—all the other events). For the study of birth defects, selecting a male birth certificate (event M) is the complement of selecting a female birth certificate (event F).

The definition of the probability of the complementary event $\overline{A}$ is in principle no different from the definition of $P(A)$. The probability of $\overline{A}$ is

$$P(\overline{A}) = \frac{n[\overline{A}]}{n}.$$

Additionally, whatever event A may be, $n[A] + n[\overline{A}] = n$ and

$$\frac{n[A]}{n} + \frac{n[\overline{A}]}{n} = P(A) + P(\overline{A}) = 1.$$

The probability of the complementary event $\overline{A}$ is, therefore, simply related to the probability of event A because

$$P(\overline{A}) = 1 - P(A). \qquad \qquad rule\ 2$$

For the birth certificate example, the total possible number of events that can occur is $n = 320$ and $n[F] + n[M] = n$ or $144 + 176 = 320$. The probability of randomly selecting a female birth certificate is

$$P(F) = 1 - P(M) \quad \text{or} \quad \frac{144}{320} = 1 - \frac{176}{320} \quad \text{or} \quad 0.45 = 1 - 0.55$$

because events M and F are complementary events $(P(M) + P(F) = 1)$.

The probability that at least one tail occurs in two tosses of a coin is

$$P(at\ least\ one\ tail) = P(TT\ or\ TH\ or\ HT) = P(\overline{HH}) = 1 - P(two\ heads)$$

$$= 1 - P(HH) = 1 - \frac{1}{4} = \frac{3}{4}.$$

The event "two heads (HH)" is the complementary event to "at least one tail (TT, TH, HT)." The total number of possible events that can occur is

$n[\overline{HH}] + n[HH] = 3 + 1 = 4$ and, therefore, $P(at\ least\ one\ tails) + P(two\ heads) = P(\overline{HH}) + P(HH) = 3/4 + 1/4 = 1$, making $P(\overline{HH}) = 1 - P(HH) = 1 - 1/4 = 3/4$.

Aside: Another measure of probability is called the *odds*. The odds are defined as the ratio of the probability of an event divided by the probability of the complementary event. In symbols, for event A, with probability of occurring represented by $P(A)$, the odds are

$$odds\ of\ A = \frac{P(A)}{P(\overline{A})} = \frac{P(A)}{1 - P(A)}.$$

Because $P(two\ heads\ in\ two\ tosses) = 1/4$, the odds of two heads occurring in two tosses are 1/4 divided by 3/4 or 1 to 3 (1/3).

The odds are a peculiar measure of probability used primarily to express probability in gambling but are also found in epidemiological applications. In addition, odds are even peculiar in the English language. The odds are a single entity but treated usually as a plural noun. The popularity of the odds in gambling comes from the fact that the odds directly express the payoff. If the probability of winning is 1/4, then the odds are (1/4)/(3/4) or 1 to 3. That is, if one dollar is bet, then the payoff is three dollars when both players expect to win the same amount of money (a fair game). The back of the California superlotto ticket reads in very small print that the odds of winning are "1 to 41,419,353," which is actually the probability of winning. The odds are 1 to 41,419,352 but the lottery is not a fair game and the payoff is considerably less than 41.4 million dollars. From another perspective, a fictional character from a Damon Runyon short story stated that, "All life is six to five against [odds = 5/6]." In less colorful language, the probability of a good outcome is 5/11.

COMPOSITE EVENTS

The basic definition of probability applies to a single or elementary event. A more sophisticated probability involving two or more events is called a *composite event*. Suppose A and B represent two elementary events. Two possible composite events are "A and B" occurs and "A or B" occurs.

Composite event "A and B"

The composite event "A and B" (AB, for short) occurs when both elementary events A and B occur simultaneously. The event AB is also referred to as the *intersection* of the two events A and B. The basic definition of probability applies equally to a composite event. Consider a random "experiment" with n mutually exclusive and equally likely composite events. When $n[AB]$ represents the number of times the composite event AB occurs, the probability of event AB is, as before,

$$P(AB) = \frac{n[AB]}{n}.$$

For a person chosen at random from 500 married couples, suppose A represents the event that a husband is selected and $\overline{A}$ represents the complementary event that a wife is selected. Additionally, suppose B represents the event that an individual with symptoms of arthritis is selected and $\overline{B}$ represents the complementary event that an individual who has no symptoms of arthritis is selected. Four different composite events occur with respect to these two elementary events. They are:

1. a male who has arthritis is selected (denoted AB),
2. a male who does not have arthritis is selected (denoted $A\overline{B}$),
3. a female who has arthritis is selected (denoted $\overline{A}B$) and
4. a female who does not have arthritis is selected (denoted $\overline{A}\,\overline{B}$).

These four composite events are mutually exclusive; no person belongs to more than one of the four groups. Furthermore, these four events are *exhaustive* since no other joint occurrence is possible. A population of 500 married couples classified by sex and the present/absence of arthritis is given in Table 2.1.

When an individual is selected at random from this population, what is the probability that the selected individual is a male with arthritis? The composite event of interest is represented as AB (a male with arthritis). A total of $n = 1000$ mutually exclusive and equally likely events can occur (individuals) and $n[AB] = 40$ events are males with arthritis.

The probability of the event AB, applying the basic definition, is

$$P(AB) = \frac{n[AB]}{n} = \frac{40}{1000}.$$

TABLE 2.1: One thousand individuals classified by sex and the presence or absence of arthritis displayed in a 2 by 2 table.

	A = male	$\overline{A}$ = female	Total
B = arthritis	40	20	60
$\overline{B}$ = no arthritis	460	480	940
Total	500	500	1000

The probabilities of the other three composite events calculated the same way are: $P(A\overline{B}) = 460/1000$, $P(\overline{A}B) = 20/1000$ and $P(\overline{A}\,\overline{B}) = 480/1000$. Since the four events are mutually exclusive and make up the only four possible composite events (exhaustive), the sum of their probabilities equals one. In symbols,

$$n[AB] + n[A\overline{B}] + n[\overline{A}B] + n[\overline{A}\,\overline{B}] = n \qquad \text{or} \qquad 40 + 460 + 20 + 480 = 1000,$$

and

$$P(AB) + P(A\overline{B}) + P(\overline{A}B) + P(\overline{A}\,\overline{B}) = \frac{40}{1000} + \frac{460}{1000} + \frac{20}{1000} + \frac{480}{1000} = 1.$$

The probability that a person selected from the 1000 individuals belongs to one of the four categories (Table 2.1) is the sure event, probability $= 1$.

These four composite probabilities can be represented visually in terms of two circles called a *Venn diagram* named after John Venn (b. 1834), the originator (Figure 2.1).

The square represents all possible events and is constructed to have an area equal to one. The area of the larger circle (labeled A) equals the probability that event A occurs ($P(A) = 500/1000$). The area of the smaller circle (labeled B) equals the probability that event B occurs ($P(B) = 60/1000$). The diagonally lined area equals the probability that the composite event $A\overline{B}$ occurs ($P(A\overline{B}) = 460/1000$); the horizontally lined area equals the probability that the composite event $\overline{A}B$ occurs ($P(\overline{A}B) = 20/1000$), the area outside the two circles equals the probability that the composite event $\overline{A}\,\overline{B}$ occurs ($P(\overline{A}\,\overline{B}) = 480/1000$) and finally the cross-hatched area equals the probability that the composite event AB occurs ($P(AB) = 40/1000$). A Venn diagram is a visual display of a 2 by 2 table and provides a geometric explanation of the reason that the event "A and B" is sometimes called the intersection of the elementary events A and B.

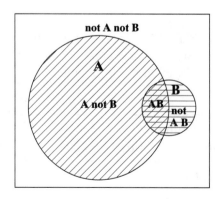

FIGURE 2.1: A Venn diagram.

The probability of event A expressed in a sometimes useful form is

$$P(A) = P(AB) + P(A\overline{B}).\qquad rule\ 3$$

Since $n[A] = n[AB] + n[A\overline{B}]$, the expression for $P(A)$ follows directly from the 2 by 2 table (Table 2.1). In words, the event A occurs in either of two mutually exclusive ways; A occurs and B occurs or A occurs and B does not occur. There are no other ways event A can occur. For example, a male (A) has arthritis (AB) or does not have arthritis $(A\overline{B})$. Also, $P(B) = P(AB) + P(\overline{A}B)$, for the same reason—a person with arthritis is either a male or a female.

The Venn diagram (Figure 2.1) displays the geometry of rule 3. From Table 2.1, the probability of selecting a person with arthritis is the probability of selecting a male with arthritis $(P(AB) = 40/1000)$ plus the probability of selecting a female with arthritis $(P(\overline{A}B) = 20/1000)$. In symbols,

$$n[B] = n[AB] + n[\overline{A}B]\qquad \text{or}\qquad 60 = 40 + 20$$

giving

$$P(B) = P(AB) + P(\overline{A}B) = \frac{40}{1000} + \frac{20}{1000} = \frac{60}{1000},$$

which also can be calculated directly $(n[B]/n = 60/1000)$.

Another view of rule 3 comes from considering each row or column of Table 2.1. For example, the number of males with arthritis (40) plus the number of males without arthritis (460) is the total number of males (500) or $n[AB] + n[A\overline{B}] = n[A]$ or, specifically, $40 + 460 = 500$ (first column). The total of the first column labeled A (males) is simply the sum of its two components. The associated probabilities follow the same pattern, so that $P(AB) + P(A\overline{B}) = 40/1000 + 460/1000 = 500/1000 = P(A)$. The decomposition of a single event into a series of composite events is a property of tables in general.

Conditional probability

A *conditional probability*, as the name suggests, is a probability calculated under specific conditions. The conditional probability that event B occurs when event A has already occurred is denoted as $P(B\,|\,A)$. The vertical line "|" between B and A indicates that the event to the right of the vertical line (event A) is a condition potentially influencing the probability of the event to the left (event B). The expression "$B\,|\,A$" is read "event B, given that event A has occurred." For example, if event $A = \{male\}$ and event $B = \{arthritis\}$, then the conditional probability that a randomly selected person has arthritis given that the person is a male is represented as $P(B\,|\,A) = P(arthritis\,|\,male)$.

A conditional probability is the ratio of the probability of the composite event AB to the probability of the event A or

$$P(B \mid A) = \frac{P(AB)}{P(A)}. \qquad \textit{rule 4}$$

Again applying the basic definition of probability, a conditional probability is the number of events of interest divided by the total number of mutually exclusive and equally likely events that can occur. In symbols,

$$P(B \mid A) = \frac{n[AB]}{n[A]}.$$

The total number of possible events now being considered is not all n events but $n[A]$ events because the condition states that event A has already occurred. Only events AB and $A\overline{B}$ are considered, because the condition requires that only events where event A has occurred are relevant. The number of these events that result in event B is $n[AB]$, making

$$P(B \mid A) = \frac{n[AB]}{n[AB] + n[A\overline{B}]} = \frac{n[AB]}{n[A]} = \frac{n[AB]/n}{n[A]/n} = \frac{P(AB)}{P(A)}.$$

All events that involve the event "not A" $(\overline{A})$ are not relevant and are ignored, namely the events $\overline{A}B$ and $\overline{A}\,\overline{B}$.

From the previous example (Table 2.1), the conditional probability $P(B \mid A) = P(arthritis \mid male)$ is the probability that an individual picked at random from the males has arthritis. There are $n[A] = 500$ males and among them $n[AB] = 40$ have arthritis and $n[A\overline{B}] = 460$ do not. The condition requires that only these 500 specific individuals are relevant (males), making the conditional probability

$$P(arthritis \mid male) = P(B \mid A) = \frac{n[AB]}{n[A]} = \frac{40}{40 + 460} = \frac{40}{500} = 0.08$$

or, using the expression $P(B \mid A) = P(AB)/P(A)$,

$$P(arthritis \mid male) = \frac{P(arthritis \; and \; male)}{P(male)} = \frac{40/1000}{500/1000} = \frac{40}{500} = 0.08.$$

All events involving females (event $\overline{A}$) are not relevant ($n[\overline{A}] = n[\overline{A}B] + n[\overline{A}\,\overline{B}] = 20 + 480 = 500$ individuals).

Conditional probabilities can be displayed using a Venn diagram (Figure 2.2). For the conditional probability $P(B \mid A)$, only one circle is needed because event A has occurred making the rest of the Venn diagram unnecessary (the parts labeled $\overline{A}B$ and $\overline{A}\,\overline{B}$ in Figure 2.1). The geometry of rule 3 requires

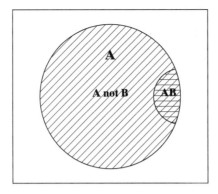

FIGURE 2.2: A Venn diagram representation of the conditional probability $P(B \mid A)$.

that area AB plus area $A\overline{B}$ add to the total area A. The probability $P(B \mid A)$ is the ratio of the area labeled AB to the total area of the entire circle labeled A.

The conditional probability $P(B \mid A)$ generally differs from the conditional probability $P(A \mid B)$. The conditional probability that a male has arthritis is $P(B \mid A) = 40/500 = 0.08$ (first column in Table 2.1), while the conditional probability that a person with arthritis is a male is $P(A \mid B) = 40/60 = 0.67$ (first row in Table 2.1). The conditional probability $P(B \mid A)$ equals the probability $P(A \mid B)$ only when $P(A) = P(B)$ (to be discussed). Care must be taken to identify which of the two elementary events A or B is the condition (it is not always obvious) since confusing $P(A \mid B)$ and $P(B \mid A)$ usually leads to the wrong conclusion.

EXAMPLE

In an article published in a California medical journal, the author reported on 400 suicide deaths in a specific California county during a five-year period, with the conclusion:

> Sixty-six percent of the group were males. . . . In both sexes approximately 50 percent of the suicides were married and 16 percent were either divorced or separated at the time of death. Widows constituted 15 percent of the [female] suicides but the comparable figure in widowers was only 5 percent [of the male suicides], suggesting that males better tolerate the loss of their marital partners.

The study is conditional on suicide. The data consist of 400 suicide deaths and all calculations necessarily refer only to individuals who committed suicide. The event suicide has occurred and those who did not commit suicide are not part of the study. The author's conclusion, however, states that

$$P(male\ suicide \mid widow) < P(female\ suicide \mid widower)$$

which may or may not be true but these probabilities cannot be calculated from the study data without information about those individuals who did not commit suicide. The two conditional probabilities reported in the article are

$$P(widow \,|\, female\ suicide) = 0.15 \text{ and } P(widower \,|\, male\ suicide) = 0.05.$$

These two conditional probabilities tell us something about the likelihood of widowhood status among suicide deaths but little about the probability of suicidal behavior among those who have lost their marital partner. To repeat, $P(B \,|\, A)$ is generally different from $P(A \,|\, B)$. ∎

EXAMPLE

It was reported that a visitor to New York City (NYC) was more likely to have a heart attack than a NYC resident (*Newsweek*, 1998). In terms of conditional probabilities, then

$$P(heart\ attack \,|\, visitor) > P(heart\ attack \,|\, NYC\ resident).$$

The report is not based on a comparison of these two conditional probabilities because it is not possible to count visitors to New York City who did not have a heart attack. It is necessary to know this number to calculate the probability of a heart attack among NYC visitors. More likely the comparison is between conditional probabilities $P(visitor \,|\, heart\ attack)$ and $P(NYC\ resident \,|\, heart\ attack)$ calculated from the more easily obtained medical records, namely records from all those people hospitalized because of a heart attack. These two conditional probabilities do not reflect directly the risk of a heart attack but rather indicate the likelihood that a NYC visitor and a NYC resident are among those individuals who had a heart attack. The conditional event is a heart attack, not visitor status. ∎

Independence

Two events A and B are *independent* when the conditional probability of event B given A has occurred equals the probability of event B. In symbols, two events A and B are independent, when

$$P(B \,|\, A) = P(B). \qquad rule\ 5$$

Independence requires that the occurrence of event B is not influenced by the occurrence of event A. Incidentally, if B is independent of A, then B is independent of $\overline{A}$ or

$$\text{if } P(B \,|\, A) = P(B), \text{ then } P(B \,|\, \overline{A}) = P(B).$$

When two events are independent, the probability of event B is unchanged whether event A occurred or did not occur. For example, the probability of tossing a fair coin and heads occurs is 1/2 regardless of whether heads or tails occurred on the previous toss. That is,

$$P(heads \mid heads \ on \ the \ previous \ toss) = P(heads) = \tfrac{1}{2}$$

and

$$P(heads \mid tails \ on \ the \ previous \ toss) = P(heads) = \tfrac{1}{2}$$

when the outcomes of tossing a coin are independent events.

EXAMPLE

The probability of "coming into substantial wealth" is the same regardless of the message contained in your fortune cookie or $P(wealth \mid message) = P(wealth)$. The two events are independent.   ∎

In more general terms, independence means that knowledge about the occurrence of one event produces no information about the likelihood of the occurrence of another event.

Independence is a symmetric relationship; if event B is independent of event A, then event A is independent of event B. In symbols,

$$\text{if } P(B \mid A) = P(B), \quad \text{then } P(A \mid B) = P(A).$$

A direct way to ascertain whether event B and event A are independent is to compare the probabilities $P(B \mid A)$ and $P(B)$. If the two probabilities are equal, events A and B are independent; otherwise they are not. For example, if again event $A = \{male\}$ and event $B = \{arthritis\}$, then using the values from Table 2.1 gives

$$P(B \mid A) = P(arthritis \mid male) = \frac{40}{500} = 0.08 \quad \text{and}$$

$$P(B) = P(arthritis) = \frac{60}{1000} = 0.06.$$

Since the two probabilities differ, arthritis is not independent of sex among married couples. Knowing that an individual is a male (event A) increases the probability that the person has arthritis from $60/1000 = 0.06$ to $40/500 = 0.08$, which occurs because the two events are related.

EXAMPLE

Consider the nine numbers {1, 2, 3, 4, 5, 6, 7, 8, and 9}. A number is picked at random. Suppose X represents selecting a number between 2 and 6 or event $X = \{3 \text{ or } 4 \text{ or } 5\}$ and Y represents selecting a number between 4 and 8 or event $Y = \{5 \text{ or } 6 \text{ or } 7\}$. Some probabilities are:

$$P(X) = \tfrac{3}{9} = \tfrac{1}{3}, \quad P(Y) = \tfrac{3}{9} = \tfrac{1}{3}, \quad P(Y \mid X) = \tfrac{1}{3} \quad \text{and} \quad P(X \mid Y) = \tfrac{1}{3}.$$

The events X and Y are independent since $P(Y \mid X) = P(Y)$. Also note that $P(Y \mid \overline{X}) = P(Y) = 1/3$.

The relevant probabilities are easily calculated from a 2 by 2 table where

	Y	$\overline{Y}$	Total
X	1	2	3
$\overline{X}$	2	4	6
Total	3	6	9

∎

If X represents selecting a number less than 6 or event $X = \{1 \text{ or } 2 \text{ or } 3 \text{ or } 4 \text{ or } 5\}$ and the Y again represents selecting a number between 4 and 8 or event $Y = \{5 \text{ or } 6 \text{ or } 7\}$, then $P(X) = 5/9$ and $P(X \mid Y) = 1/3$ showing that events X and Y are not independent. Knowing that the number selected is a 5 or 6 or 7 (event Y) reduces the probability of selecting a number less than 6 (event X) from 5/9 to $3/9 = 1/3$.

Multiplication theorem

The probability of the composite event AB equals the product of the probability of event A multiplied by the conditional probability of event B given event A has occurred or

$$P(AB) = P(A) \times P(B \mid A). \qquad rule \ 6 \quad \text{See Box 2.1.}$$

Box 2.1. Multiplication Theorem

$$P(AB) = \frac{n[AB]}{n} = \frac{n[A]}{n} \times \frac{n[AB]}{n[A]}$$
$$= P(A) \times P(B \mid A)$$

For example, Table 2.1 shows directly that

$$P(\textit{male and arthritis}) = P(AB) = \frac{40}{1000}$$

or alternatively

$$P(\textit{male and arthritis}) = P(\textit{male}) \times P(\textit{arthritis} \mid \textit{male})$$

$$= \frac{500}{1000} \times \frac{40}{500} = \frac{40}{1000},$$

illustrating the multiplication theorem. The multiplication theorem hardly differs from the definition of conditional probability.

The multiplication theorem applies regardless of whether or not events A and B are independent. When elementary events A and B are independent, however, the multiplication theorem simplifies and

$$P(AB) = P(A)P(B \mid A) = P(A) \times P(B).$$

That is, when $P(B \mid A) = P(B)$, then $P(A)P(B \mid A) = P(A)P(B)$ giving $P(AB) = P(A)P(B)$.

EXAMPLE

Suppose A represents the event that a randomly selected person has an AB blood type and suppose B represents the event that a randomly selected person has an Rh-negative blood type where $P(A) = P(AB\text{-}type) = 0.02$ and $P(B) = P(Rh\text{-}negative) = 0.15$. The probability that a randomly selected person has both AB and Rh-negative blood type is (assuming blood types are independent)

$$P(AB\text{-}type \text{ and } Rh\text{-}negative) = P(AB\text{-}type) \times (Rh\text{-}negative)$$

$$= (0.02)(0.15) = 0.003. \qquad \blacksquare$$

EXAMPLE

To win the California lottery superlotto payoff, you must correctly pick five numbers from a list of 47 possible values [$P(\textit{five matches}) = 1/1{,}533{,}939$] and, furthermore, correctly select a single "mega" number from 27 possible values [$P(\textit{mega match}) = 1/27$]. Since the "mega" number is selected independently, the probability of matching all six lottery numbers is $P(\textit{win}) = P(\textit{six matches}) = P(\textit{five matches and a mega match}) = P(\textit{five matches}) \times P(\textit{mega match}) = (1/1{,}533{,}939) \times (1/27) = 1/41{,}416{,}353. \qquad \blacksquare$

When n elementary events (denoted A_1, A_2, $\cdots$, A_n) are independent, the probability of the composite event $\{A_1$ and A_2 and $\cdots$ and $A_n\}$ is

$$P(A_1 \text{ and } A_2 \text{ and } \cdots \text{ and } A_n) = P(A_1 A_2 \cdots A_n)$$
$$= P(A_1) \times P(A_2) \times \cdots \times P(A_n).$$

Thus, the probability of the joint occurrence of n independent events equals the product of their elementary probabilities.

EXAMPLE

Suppose that the probability of being left-handed is 0.10. Then, what is the probability that four independently selected individuals are left-handed?

$$P(\textit{four left-handed individuals}) = P(L_1 \text{ and } L_2 \text{ and } L_3 \text{ and } L_4)$$
$$= (0.1)(0.1)(0.1)(0.1) = 0.0001$$

where L_i represents the event of independently being a left-handed person. It is not an unlikely event, however, that four of the last six presidents were left-handed.[5] They certainly have many characteristics in common and someone noticed that one of these characteristics was left-handedness.   ■

EXAMPLE

Suppose the probability of being diagnosed with colon cancer is 10 per 100,000 individuals who are at risk for the disease [$P(\textit{colon cancer})$ $=$ $P(C)$ $=$ $10/100{,}000$ $=$ 0.0001]. What is the probability no cases will be diagnosed in a community of 20,000 people? The probability of not being diagnosed with colon cancer is $P(\textit{disease--free})$ $=$ $P(\overline{C})$ $=$ $1 - P(C)$ $=$ $1 - 0.0001$ $=$ 0.9999. Assuming each diagnosis of colon cancer is independent of any other diagnosis of colon cancer in this community, the probability of observing no cases is

$$P(\textit{no cases are diagnosed}) = P(\overline{C}_1 \text{ and } \overline{C}_2 \text{ and } \cdots \text{ and } \overline{C}_{20{,}000})$$
$$= P(\overline{C}_1)P(\overline{C}_2) \cdots P(\overline{C}_{20{,}000})$$
$$= (0.9999)(0.9999) \cdots (0.9999)$$
$$= (0.9999)^{20{,}000} = 0.135.$$

The probability of at least one diagnosed colon cancer case among the 20,000 individuals is

$$P(\textit{at least one case is diagnosed}) = 1 - 0.135 = 0.865.   ■$$

The Malcolm Collins case (a true crime story)

A woman was robbed in an alley in San Pedro, a city near Los Angeles, California.[6] The police called to the scene of the crime gathered the following description of the perpetrator. He was described as an African-American man who drove a yellow car. A girl was reported riding in his car who had blond hair worn in a ponytail. Witnesses said that the couple appeared to be interracial. Additionally, it was stated that the perpetrator had both a mustache and a beard. Malcolm Collins, who was found to fit all six characteristics, was arrested and tried for the crime. The heart of the prosecutor's case was the claim that finding a person with the same six characteristics who had not committed the crime was exceeding unlikely ("beyond a reasonable doubt"). To bolster this contention, a mathematician from a nearby college was asked to compute the probability that a random person would match all six characteristics. Using the following probabilities:

yellow car	1/10	girl with blond hair	1/3
black man with a beard	1/10	girl with a ponytail	1/10
man with a mustache	1/4	interracial couple	1/1000

the college professor produced an answer by multiplying these probabilities (i.e. $(1/10)(1/3)(1/10) \cdots (1/1000) = 1/12$ million). He then testified that the likelihood the police had arrested an innocent man who matched all six characteristics by chance alone was 1 in 12 million. The jury agreed with the prosecutor that the likelihood of matching by chance was beyond a reasonable doubt and convicted Mr. Collins.

Malcolm Collins served three years in jail until his case was reviewed by the California Supreme Court. In overruling his conviction, the court made three points:

1. The court record contained no evidence to support the probabilities used in the calculation [where did these elementary probabilities come from?]. The court labeled them as having "dubious origin."
2. No evidence was introduced to support the multiplying of the probabilities that requires independence [who says blond hair and a ponytail are independent events?].
3. There remains a substantial probability that the couple who committed the crime did not possess the characteristics [witnesses can be wrong or lie or the guilty couple could have been disguised].

Additionally,

4. The probability that a person who matches the characteristics is innocent was confused with the probability of an innocent (random) person matching the characteristics. That is, the conditional probability $P(innocent \mid match)$ was confused with $P(match \mid innocent) = 1/12$ million. Presumably,

Malcolm Collins would not have been arrested unless he matched all six characteristics. In fact, any defendant in this case would have all six characteristics because only matching individuals would come to trial. The relevant probability of innocence is, therefore, conditional on matching the six characteristics reported by the witnesses, which is not 1 in 12 million.

In its decision the court wrote, "mathematics, a veritable sorcerer in our computer society, while assisting the trier of fact in the search for truth, must not cast a spell over him."

Bayes' rule

Bayes' rule makes it possible to calculate $P(B \mid A)$ from $P(A \mid B)$ using $P(A)$ and $P(B)$. Bayes' rule states

$$P(B \mid A) = \frac{P(A \mid B)P(B)}{P(A)}. \qquad rule\ 7$$

A conditional probability is

$$P(B \mid A) = \frac{P(AB)}{P(A)} \qquad \text{(definition of conditional probability, rule 4)}$$

and

$$P(AB) = P(A \mid B)P(B), \qquad \text{(multiplication theorem, rule 6)}$$

then replacing $P(AB)$ in the conditional probability with $P(A \mid B)P(B)$ gives Bayes' rule

$$P(B \mid A) = \frac{P(A \mid B)P(B)}{P(A)}.$$

A more complicated but frequently useful version of Bayes' rule is

$$P(B \mid A) = \frac{P(A \mid B)P(B)}{P(A)} = \frac{P(A \mid B)P(B)}{P(A \mid B)P(B) + P(A \mid \overline{B})P(\overline{B})}$$

since

$$P(A) = P(AB) + P(A\overline{B}) = P(A \mid B)P(B) + P(A \mid \overline{B})P(\overline{B})$$

applying rules 3 and 6.

Returning to the suicide/widowhood example, the $P(suicide \mid widow)$ and $P(suicide \mid widower)$ can be calculated with Bayes' rule. Four additional probabilities, however, are necessary. They are

$$P(\textit{female suicide}) = 0.00086, \quad P(\textit{widow}) = 0.096,$$

$$P(\textit{male suicide}) = 0.0018 \quad \text{and} \quad P(\textit{widower}) = 0.022.$$

Using Bayes' rule,

$$P(\textit{female suicide} \mid \textit{widow}) = \frac{P(\textit{widow} \mid \textit{female suicide}) P(\textit{female suicide})}{P(\textit{widow})}$$

$$= \frac{(0.15)(0.00086)}{0.096} = 0.0013$$

and

$$P(\textit{male suicide} \mid \textit{widower}) = \frac{P(\textit{widower} \mid \textit{male suicide}) P(\textit{male suicide})}{P(\textit{widower})}$$

$$= \frac{(0.05)(0.0018)}{0.022} = 0.0040.$$

These two conditional probabilities indicate that a widower is about three times more likely to commit suicide than a widow, which is essentially the reverse of the earlier conclusions based on the "backwards" conditional probabilities.

Perhaps the clearest way to sort out conditional probabilities is to construct a 2 by 2 table. For the widowhood and suicide calculations, the 2 by 2 table displaying the widow data (females) is

	Widow	Nonwidow	Total
suicide	20	116	136
nonsuicide	15,146	142,857	158,003
Total	15,166	142,973	158,139

The first row of the table is the data from the suicide study and, as before, $P(\textit{widow} \mid \textit{suicide}) = 20/136 = 0.15$. Additionally, it is clear that the $P(\textit{suicide} \mid \textit{widow})$ cannot be calculated from this row alone. The second row of the table comes from U.S. census counts and vital records of the county where the study was conducted and were not part of the original study. Using these additional data, the likelihood of suicide among widows calculated directly from the table is $P(\textit{suicide} \mid \textit{widow}) = 20/15,166 = 0.0013$ (first column).

For the widower and suicide calculations, the parallel 2 by 2 table for the widower data (males) is

	Widower	Nonwidower	Total
suicide	13	251	264
nonsuicide	3,212	146,524	149,736
Total	3,225	146,775	150,000

These data also reproduce exactly the probability achieved using Bayes' rule where $P(suicide \mid widower) = 13/3,225 = 0.0040$ (first column).

EXAMPLE

Circumstantial evidence—an application of Bayes' rule

In certain situations it can be determined that the probability a woman is a carrier for a specific genetic disease is 1/2 (such as specific kinds of hemophilia and muscular dystrophy—the details are in most introductory human genetics texts). The probability that she will pass this genetic disease to a son is also 1/2. This disease cannot be passed from father to son. If a mother has a normal son, what is the probability that she is a carrier for this disease? In terms of a conditional probability the question is, $P(mother\ is\ a\ carrier \mid a\ normal\ son) = ?$ The birth of a normal son adds evidence, but certainly not conclusive evidence, that the mother is not a carrier of the disease gene. The probability she is a carrier is reduced, but by how much?

Bayes' rule provides a way to assess the impact of this circumstantial evidence. The relevant and known probabilities are:

$$P(mother\ is\ a\ carrier) = 1/2,$$

$$P(mother\ is\ not\ a\ carrier) = 1/2,$$

$$P(normal\ son \mid mother\ is\ a\ carrier) = 1/2$$

and

$$P(normal\ son \mid mother\ is\ not\ a\ carrier) = 1.$$

The probability of a normal son may be decomposed (rules 3 and 6) as follows:

$$P(normal\ son) = P(normal\ son\ \text{and}\ mother\ is\ a\ carrier)$$
$$+ P(normal\ son\ \text{and}\ mother\ is\ not\ a\ carrier)$$
$$= P(normal\ son \mid mother\ is\ a\ carrier)P(mother\ is\ a\ carrier)$$
$$+ P(normal\ son \mid mother\ is\ not\ a\ carrier)$$
$$P(mother\ is\ not\ a\ carrier).$$

Thus, from the four previous probabilities

$$P(normal\ son) = (1/2)(1/2) + (1.0)(1/2) = 3/4.$$

Bayes' rule now gives the probability that a woman is a carrier when she has one normal son as

$$P(mother\ is\ a\ carrier \mid a\ normal\ son)$$
$$= \frac{P(normal\ son \mid mother\ is\ a\ carrier)P(mother\ is\ a\ carrier)}{P(normal\ son)}$$
$$= \frac{(1/2)(1/2)}{3/4} = \frac{1}{3}.$$

The circumstantial evidence provided by the birth of a normal son reduces the probability that the mother in fact carries the disease gene from 1/2 to 1/3. Of course, the birth of an affected son is conclusive evidence that the mother is a carrier.

Notice particularly the use of the multiplication theorem to calculate the probabilities $P(normal\ son$ and $mother\ is\ a\ carrier)$ and $P(normal\ son$ and $mother\ is\ not\ a\ carrier)$. Decomposition of the probability of a composite event $P(AB)$ into $P(A \mid B)P(B)$ is frequently useful when $P(A \mid B)$ and $P(B)$ are calculated easily and $P(AB)$ is not.

Using Bayes' rule, the same logic, and a bit more manipulation produces the general expression

$$P(mother\ is\ a\ carrier \mid k\ normal\ sons) = 1 - \frac{1}{1 + (\frac{1}{2})^k}.$$

This application of Bayes' rule shows in concrete terms that the birth of each normal son (as k increases) makes it less and less likely the mother carries the disease-causing gene. For example,

$$P(mother\ is\ a\ carrier \mid five\ normal\ sons) = 1 - \frac{32}{33} = \frac{1}{33}.$$

This genetic example illustrates the fundamental significance of Bayes' rule. In a rigorous way, it becomes possible to "update" a probability based on additional information. From the example, the initial probability that the mother is a carrier is 1/2 but new evidence (the birth of a normal son) allows the original probability to be revised (from 1/2 to 1/3). Subsequent births of normal sons further reduces this probability. Thomas Bayes' (b. 1702) fundamental contribution to probability theory, not recognized in his lifetime, provided the first mathematical understanding of circumstantial evidence. ∎

EXAMPLE

Laboratory Testing—another application of Bayes' rule

Laboratory tests, by and large, give accurate and useful results. Of course, the possibility of an error always exists. Exploring a hypothetical laboratory test for marijuana use illustrates the issues surrounding the accuracy of laboratory testing in general. The symbols used are:

$$M = \text{user of marijuana} \quad \text{and} \quad \overline{M} = \text{nonuser of marijuana,}$$

"+test" = a positive test for marijuana use   and

"−test" = a negative test for marijuana use.

Testing 1000 known users and 1000 known nonusers of marijuana produces the hypothetical data:

Laboratory test results (hypothetical)

	User (M)	Nonuser ($\overline{M}$)	Total
positive (+test)	950	100	1050
negative (−test)	50	900	950
Total tested	1000	1000	2000

From the laboratory test results: the probability of a positive test among the known users of marijuana is $P(+test \mid M) = 950/1000 = 0.95$ (called *sensitivity*—column 1) and the probability of a negative test among the known marijuana nonusers is $P(-test \mid \overline{M}) = 900/1000 = 0.90$ (called *specificity*—column 2).

Among those who tested positive, a person who is a nonuser is called a *false positive*. The probability of a false positive is represented by $P(\overline{M} \mid +test)$ and Bayes' rule gives

$$P(\text{false positive}) = P(\overline{M} \mid +test) = \frac{P(+test \mid \overline{M})P(\overline{M})}{P(+test)}.$$

Suppose, one among every ten individuals uses marijuana, $P(M) = 0.10$, then

$$P(+test) = P(+test \text{ and } M) + P(+test \text{ and } \overline{M})$$

$$= P(+test \mid M)P(M) + P(+test \mid \overline{M})P(\overline{M})$$

$$= (950/1000)(1/10) + (100/1000)(9/10) = 0.185$$

and, applying Bayes' rule,

$$P(\text{false positive}) = P(\overline{M} \mid +test) = \frac{(100/1000)(9/10)}{0.185} = 0.486.$$

Among the positive tests for marijuana use, about half are nonusers. This calculation demonstrates that the accuracy of a laboratory test depends not only on sensitivity (0.95) and specificity (0.90) but also on the prevalence of marijuana use (0.10). Other values of $P(M)$ produce the following probabilities of a false positive test:

$P(M)$	$P(+test)$	$P(\overline{M} \mid +test)$
0.50	0.525	0.095
0.10	0.185	0.486
0.05	0.143	0.667
0.005	0.104	0.954
0.0005	0.100	0.995

As prevalence of marijuana users decreases, the probability of a false positive increases. At the most extreme, when no one is a marijuana user [$P(M) = 0$], the probability of a false positive must be one because all positive tests are then an error.

One might ask, why not calculate the probability of a false positive test directly from the 2000 people tested to evaluate the effectiveness of the laboratory procedure? The answer is that the probability of a positive test ($1050/2000 = 0.525$ in the example) is substantially influenced by the arbitrary numbers of users and nonusers selected to be tested (1000 in the example) and, therefore, does not reflect the actual probability of a positive test [$P(+test) = 0.185$ in the example].

If the individuals tested were exactly a representative sample, then the numbers of individuals in the 2 by 2 table would look like

Laboratory test results (again hypothetical)

	User (M)	Nonuser ($\overline{M}$)	Total
positive (+test)	95	90	185
negative (−test)	5	810	815
Total tested	100	900	1000

In this case, the probability of a false positive is $P(\overline{M} \mid +test) = 90/185 = 0.486$, calculated directly from the table. These kinds of representative data, however, are difficult to collect accurately and are rarely available. But, using more easily collected data and Bayes' theorem produces the same results. ∎

Composite event "A or B"

When the probability of rain on Saturday is 1/2 and the probability of rain on Sunday is also 1/2, the probability of rain on the weekend is not a sure thing

$(1/2 + 1/2 = 1)$. The following theorem and examples indicate when adding elementary probabilities give the correct probability associated with a series of events.

The composite event "*A* or *B*" occurs when one of three mutually exclusive composite events occurs, namely event *A* occurs and not event *B* $(A\overline{B})$ or event *B* occurs and not event *A* $(\overline{A}B)$ or both events *A* and *B* occur (AB). That is, rain occurs during the weekend if it rains only on Saturday or if it rains only on Sunday or if it rains on both days. The event "*A* or *B*" is sometimes referred to as the *union* of the two events *A* and *B*. In the context of probability, "or" means "and/or" and is called the nonexclusive "or."

EXAMPLE

Suppose the following probabilities apply to a winter day:

$$P(\textit{the car will not start}) = P(A) = 0.10 \text{ and}$$

$$P(\textit{it snowed during the night}) = P(B) = 0.20,$$

then, what is the probability of not getting to work on time? or $P(\textit{not getting to work on time}) = P(A \text{ or } B) =?$ Being late to work is the composite event *A* or *B*. ∎

Addition theorem

The probability $P(A \text{ or } B)$ expressed in terms of the probabilities $P(A)$, $P(B)$, and $P(AB)$ is

$$P(A \text{ or } B) = P(A) + P(B) - P(AB). \qquad \textit{rule 8} \quad \text{See Box 2.2.}$$

To calculate the probability of the composite event $P(A \text{ or } B)$, the sum $P(A) + P(B)$ is too large because $P(AB)$ is contained in both $P(A)$ and $P(B)$ when $P(AB) \neq 0$. Subtracting $P(AB)$ from $P(A) + P(B)$ gives $P(A) + P(B) - P(AB)$ which equals $P(A \text{ or } B)$, called the *addition theorem*.

Box 2.2. Addition Theorem

$$P(A \text{ or } B) = \frac{n[A \text{ or } B]}{n} = \frac{n[A\overline{B}] + n[\overline{A}B] + n[AB]}{n} \quad \text{and}$$

$$n[A] = n[AB] + n[A\overline{B}] \qquad \text{or} \qquad n[A\overline{B}] = n[A] - n[AB]$$

$$n[B] = n[AB] + n[\overline{A}B] \qquad \text{or} \qquad n[\overline{A}B] = n[B] - n[AB]$$

Box 2.2. Addition Theorem (*continued*)

then

$$P(A \text{ or } B) = \frac{(n[A] - n[AB]) + (n[B] - n[AB]) + n[AB]}{n} \quad \text{or}$$

$$P(A \text{ or } B) = P(A) - P(AB) + P(B) - P(AB) + P(AB)$$

$$= P(A) + P(B) - P(AB).$$

A Venn diagram illustrating the addition theorem is

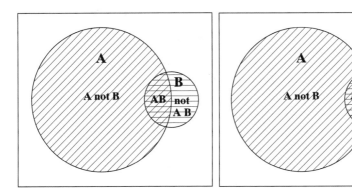

Like the intersection of two events, the geometry of the Venn diagram indicates why the composite event A or B is referred to as the union of events A and B. It also clearly displays the fact that the composite event AB is contained in event A and is also contained in event B (right side).

EXAMPLE

Suppose that event A is selecting an ace from a deck of 52 cards and event B is selecting a club, then $P(A) + P(B) = 4/52 + 13/52 = 17/52$ is not the probability of the composite ace or club (event A or B), because the ace of clubs (event AB) is counted twice (once as an ace and once as a club). The direct sum of these two probabilities is too large. But, $P(ace \text{ or } club) = P(A \text{ or } B) = P(A) + P(B) - P(AB) = 4/52 + 13/52 - 1/52 = 16/52$, which can be directly calculated (3 *aces* + 12 *clubs* + 1 *ace of clubs* = 16 cards). ∎

The composite events associated with the two elementary events A and B displayed in a 2 by 2 table are

	A	$\overline{A}$	Total
B	$P(AB)$	$P(\overline{A}B)$	$P(B)$
$\overline{B}$	$P(A\overline{B})$	$P(\overline{A}\,\overline{B})$	$P(\overline{B})$
Total	$P(A)$	$P(\overline{A})$	1

Applied to the deck of cards example, then

	$A = ace$	$\overline{A} = nonace$	Total
$B = club$	1/52	12/52	13/52
$\overline{B} = nonclub$	3/52	36/52	39/52
Total	4/52	48/52	1

Directly form the table, $P(ace \text{ or } club) = P(A \text{ or } B) = P(AB) + P(\overline{A}B) + P(A\overline{B}) = 1/52 + 12/52 + 3/52 = 16/52.$

A corollary to the addition theorem is

$$P(A \text{ or } B) = 1 - P(\overline{A}\,\overline{B})$$

since $P(AB) + P(\overline{A}B) + P(A\overline{B}) + P(\overline{A}\,\overline{B}) = 1$ and $P(AB) + P(\overline{A}B) + P(A\overline{B}) = P(A \text{ or } B)$, then

$$P(A \text{ or } B) + P(\overline{A}\,\overline{B}) = 1 \quad \text{and} \quad P(A \text{ or } B) = 1 - P(\overline{A}\,\overline{B}).$$

Again, $P(ace \text{ or } club) = 1 - P(nonace \text{ and } nonclub) = 1 - 36/52 = 16/52.$

In the case of not getting to work on time, assuming independence, the joint probability that the car starts (event $\overline{A}$) and snow does not occur (event $\overline{B}$) is

$$P(getting \text{ } to \text{ } work \text{ } on \text{ } time) = P(\overline{A}\,\overline{B}) = P(\overline{A}) \times P(\overline{B})$$

$$= (0.9)(0.8) = 0.72$$

since $P(\overline{A}) = 1 - P(A) = 0.9$ and $P(\overline{B}) = 1 - P(B) = 0.8$. Then, $P(A \text{ or } B) = 1 - P(\overline{A}\,\overline{B}) = 1 - (0.9)(0.8) = 1 - 0.72 = 0.28$ is the probability of arriving late to work. Again assuming the independence of events A and B, the same probability calculated from the addition theorem is

$$P(A \text{ or } B) = P(A) + P(B) - P(AB) = P(A) + P(B) - P(A)P(B)$$

and

$$P(late) = 0.1 + 0.2 - (0.1)(0.2) = 0.3 - 0.02 = 0.28.$$

A 2 by 2 table displays all the possibilities that can occur where

	A = car fails	$\overline{A}$ = car runs	Total
B = snow	0.02 (late)	0.18 (late)	0.20
$\overline{B}$ = no snow	0.08 (late)	0.72 (not late)	0.80
Total	0.10	0.90	1

and $P(A$ or $B) = 0.10 + 0.20 - 0.02 = 0.02 + 0.18 + 0.08 = 1 - 0.72 = 0.28$, again. Represented by a Venn diagram,

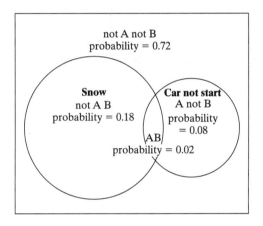

EXAMPLE

Consider again the nine numbers {1, 2, 3, 4, 5, 6, 7, 8, and 9}. A number is picked at random. Suppose X represents selecting a value less than 6 or event $X = \{1, 2, 3, 4,$ or $5\}$ and suppose Y represents selecting a value between 3 and 7 or event $Y = \{4, 5,$ or $6\}$. Some probabilities are:

$$P(X) = 5/9, \quad P(Y) = 3/9, \quad P(XY) = 2/9, \quad P(X\overline{Y}) = 3/9$$
$$P(\overline{X}Y) = 1/9, \quad P(\overline{X}\,\overline{Y}) = 3/9 \qquad \text{and} \qquad P(X \text{ or } Y) = 6/9.$$

Specifically, $P(X$ or $Y) = P(X) + P(Y) - P(XY) = 5/9 + 3/9 - 2/9 = 6/9$ or $P(X$ or $Y) = P(\overline{X}Y) + P(X\overline{Y}) + P(XY) = 1/9 + 3/9 + 2/9 = 6/9$ or $P(X$ or $Y) = 1 - P(\overline{X}\,\overline{Y}) = 1 - 3/9 = 6/9$. Again, these probabilities are readily found from a 2 by 2 table where

	Y	$\overline{Y}$	Total
X	2	3	5
$\overline{X}$	1	3	4
Total	3	6	9

If again event $X = \{1, 2, 3, 4, \text{or } 5\}$ and Y represents selecting a value greater than 3 or event $Y = \{4, 5, 6, 7, 8, \text{or } 9\}$, as above then $P(X) = 5/9$, $P(Y) = 6/9$ and $P(XY) = 2/9$ and $P(X \text{ or } Y) = 5/9 + 6/9 - 2/9 = 1$ showing that picking a number less than 6 or greater than 3 includes all numbers from 1 to 9, the sure event. ∎

A special case, vital to many applications, occurs when events A and B are mutually exclusive, which requires that $P(AB) = 0$. Because the occurrence of event A precludes the occurrence of event B, the joint occurrence of A and B is impossible. The Venn diagram looks like this.

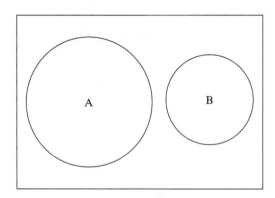

For mutually exclusive elementary events A and B, a special case of the addition theorem becomes

$$P(A \text{ or } B) = P(A) + P(B)$$

because $P(AB) = 0$.

In general, for the mutually exclusive elementary events (denoted $A_1, A_2, \cdots, A_n$), then

$$P(A_1 \text{ or } A_2 \text{ or } \cdots \text{ or } A_n) = P(A_1) + P(A_2) + \cdots + P(A_n).$$

The probability of a composite event (union) made up of n mutually exclusive events equals the sum of their elementary probabilities. If these n mutually exclusive events are additionally exhaustive (include all possible events), then

$$P(A_1 \text{ or } A_2 \text{ or } \cdots \text{ or } A_n) = P(A_1) + P(A_2) + \cdots + P(A_n) = 1.$$

EXAMPLE

The probability of rolling a single die and observing a number less than or equal to 4 is

$$P(face\ equals\ 1\ or\ 2\ or\ 3\ or\ 4) = P(face = 1) + P(face = 2)$$
$$+ P(face = 3) + P(face = 4)$$
$$= \frac{1}{6} + \frac{1}{6} + \frac{1}{6} + \frac{1}{6} = \frac{4}{6}.$$

Each of the four events is mutually exclusive of the other three events because the occurrence of any specific face (number) excludes the occurrence of any other face (number). Additionally,

$$P(face\ equals\ 1\ or\ 2\ or\ 3\ or\ 4\ or\ 5\ or\ 6) = P(face = 1) + P(face = 2)$$
$$+ \cdots + P(face = 6)$$
$$= \frac{1}{6} + \frac{1}{6} + \frac{1}{6} + \frac{1}{6} + \frac{1}{6} + \frac{1}{6} = 1 \quad ■$$

EXAMPLE

Consider again the nine numbers {1, 2, 3, 4, 5, 6, 7, 8, and 9}. A number is picked at random. Suppose X represents selecting a value less than 5 or event $X = \{1, 2, 3,\ or\ 4\}$ and suppose Y represents selecting a value greater than 6 or event $Y = \{7, 8,\ or\ 9\}$. No single number is both less than 5 and greater than 6, making the events X and Y mutually exclusive. In symbols, $P(XY) = 0$. Some probabilities are:

$$P(X) = 4/9, \quad P(Y) = 3/9, \quad P(XY) = 0, \quad P(\overline{X}\,\overline{Y}) = 2/9 \quad \text{and}$$

$P(X\ or\ Y) = 7/9.$

Specifically, $P(X\ or\ Y) = P(X) + P(Y) = 4/9 + 3/9 = 7/9$. Once again, a 2 by 2 table clearly displays the frequencies of the four possible outcomes where

	Y	$\overline{Y}$	Total
X	0	4	4
$\overline{X}$	3	2	5
Total	3	6	9

■

FOUR PROBABILITY PROBLEMS

EXAMPLE

A quiz show pits two contestants against each other where four questions are asked of each participant. The contestant with the most correct answers wins. Say person A will always get two questions correct, $P(A = 2) = 1$. Additionally, suppose that person B will get one question correct with probability 0.8 and four questions correct with probability 0.2, $P(B = 1) = 0.8$ and $P(B = 4) = 0.2$. Person A will beat person B with probability 0.8 because

$$P(A \ beats \ B) = P(A = 2 \ and \ B = 1) = P(A = 2) \times P(B = 1)$$
$$= 1.0(0.8) = 0.8$$

assuming that the answers are independent. Say a third person C enters the competition and this person gets no answers correct with probability 0.5 and three answers correct with probability also 0.5, $P(C = 0) = P(C = 3) = 0.5$. Now, because the three possible outcomes where B wins are mutually exclusive, person B beats person C with probability 0.6 or

$$P(B \ beats \ C) = P(B = 1 \ and \ C = 0) + P(B = 4 \ and \ C = 0)$$
$$+ P(B = 4 \ and \ C = 3)$$
$$= 0.8(0.5) + 0.2(0.5) + 0.2(0.5) = 0.6$$

again assuming that the answers are independent.

These probabilities indicate that it is likely that person A beats person B (0.8) and likely that person B beats person C (0.6). The conventional wisdom is that it is then rather likely that person A will beat person C. However,

$$P(A \ beats \ C) = P(A = 2 \ and \ C = 0)$$
$$= P(A = 2)P(C = 0) = 1.0(0.5) = 0.5$$

showing no difference between contestants A and C. This simple, perhaps simplistic, quiz show example indicates that "upset" victories may be more frequent than thought. ∎

EXAMPLE

Monsieur Chevalier de Mèrè and his dice games.

A French nobleman named Antoine Gombaud who was also known as the Chevalier de Mèrè (b. 1654) became famous by incorrectly applying probability theory. He played a dice game where he tossed a die four times. He bet even money that he could roll at least one six in four tosses. Clearly unaware of the addition theorem, he thought the probability of winning was $1/6 + 1/6 + 1/6 + 1/6 = 4(1/6) = 4/6$ (the events are not mutually exclusive). In the long run, he won more often than he lost. Monsieur Chevalier de Mèrè grew bored with this game or, perhaps, his friends grew tired of losing, so he changed the rules. He bet that he could roll at least one pair of sixes when he tossed a pair of dice 24 times. Still unaware of the addition theorem, he thought the probability of winning was $24(1/36) = 4/6$. Playing under these new rules, however, Chevalier de Mèrè lost more frequently than he won. Unable to understand his losses, he asked a famous mathematician named Blaise Pascal to calculate the probabilities associated with these two games. This event was perhaps the first formal application of probability theory to a real-world problem.

Solution: Suppose A represents the event that at least one six occurs in four tosses (a win). The complementary event $\overline{A}$ is that no sixes occur in four tosses (a loss). Postulating that the die is fair and the tosses are independent, the probability that one toss produces a "nonsix" is 5/6 making the probability of all "nonsixes" in four tosses $P(loss) = P(\overline{A}) = (5/6)(5/6)(5/6)(5/6) = (5/6)^4$. Therefore, the probability of the complementary event that at least one six occurs in four tosses is

$$P(win) = P(A) = 1 - P(\overline{A}) = 1 - (5/6)^4 = 0.518.$$

Chevalier de Mèrè won this game more frequently than he lost, $P(win) > 0.5$.

Playing the second game, the probability of not rolling a pair of sixes with two dice is 35/36 and not rolling a pair of sixes in 24 independent tosses of a pair of dice is then $P(loss) = (35/36)^{24}$. Therefore, the probability of the complementary event of at least one pair of sixes or the probability of winning is

$$P(win) = P(A) = 1 - P(loss) = 1 - P(\overline{A}) = 1 - (35/36)^{24} = 0.491.$$

Chevalier de Mèrè lost this game more frequently than he won, $P(win) < 0.5$.

One should be suspicious of this frequently told story because it is unlikely that Monsieur Chevalier de Mèrè could detect empirically the difference between these two games ($0.516 \approx 0.491$), even if he played them for most of his life. ∎

EXAMPLE

A famous birthday problem.

One occasionally hears the following conversation,

person 1: "My birthday is June 8th."
person 2: "Wow, what a coincidence! My birthday is on the same day!"

This is indeed a coincidence. The probability of two people matching a specific date is $1/365 = 0.003$.

A related but different problem is:

How likely is it that two or more individuals in a group have the same birthday (same day and same month)?

This probability certainly depends on the number of people in the group. If 366 people are considered, the probability that at least two people have the same birthday is one.

Again, it is easier to compute the probability of the complementary event that among a specific number of individuals no one has the same birthday. Subtracting the probability of not matching birthdays from one gives the probability of at least two birthdays occurring on the same day (the complementary event). In general, for a group with k members,

$$P(\textit{not matching birthdays} \mid k \textit{ members}) = \frac{365}{365} \times \frac{364}{365} \times \frac{363}{365} \times \cdots \times \frac{366-k}{365}$$

and

$$P(\textit{matching birthdays} \mid k \textit{ members}) = 1 - P(\textit{not matching birthdays} \mid k \textit{ members}).$$

For some selected group sizes (k), the following table gives the same-day probabilities:

Group size (k)	P(not matching birthdays | k)	P(matching birthdays | k)
2	$(365/365)(364/365) = 0.997$	0.003
3	$(365/365)(364/365)(363/365) = 0.992$	0.008
4	$(365/365)(364/365)\cdots(362/365) = 0.984$	0.016
5	$(365/365)(364/365)\cdots(361/365) = 0.973$	0.027
10	$(365/365)(364/365)\cdots(356/365) = 0.883$	0.117
20	$(365/365)(364/365)\cdots(346/365) = 0.589$	0.411
30	$(365/365)(364/365)\cdots(336/365) = 0.294$	0.706
50	$(365/365)(364/365)\cdots(316/365) = 0.030$	0.970

The probability that at least two individuals in a group of 23 individuals will have the same birthday is close to one-half (0.507). So it is not all that surprising that one hears occasionally of individuals with the same birthday.

This birthday problem demonstrates an unappreciated fact. The likelihood of a coincidence depends on the number of people involved. Two birthdays occurring on the same day is more probable (0.5) when 23 people are considered. Two events each with probability of 1 in a billion ($1/10^9$) are likely to occur simultaneously (again, with probability 0.5) when 37,234 people are involved. Therefore, it is probable that this "extremely unlikely coincidence" will be observed even in a small town.   ■

EXAMPLE

We're watching "Let's Make a Deal"—a famous TV game show starring Monty Hall.[7]

Monty Hall:	One of the three boxes labeled A, B, and C contains the keys to that new sports car. The other two are empty. If you choose the box containing the keys, you win the car.
Contestant:	GASP!!!
Monty Hall:	Select one of these boxes.
Contestant:	I'll take box B.
Monty Hall:	Now box A and box C are on the table and here is box B (contestant grips box B tightly). It is possible the car keys are in that box. I'll give you $100 for the box.
Contestant:	No, thank you.
Monty Hall:	How about $200?
Contestant:	No!
Audience:	NO!!!
Monty Hall:	Remember that the probability of your box containing the keys to the car is 1/3 and the probability of your box being empty is 2/3. I'll give you $500.
Audience:	NO!!!!!
Contestant:	No, I think I'll keep this box.
Monty Hall:	I'll do you a favor and open one of the remaining boxes on the table (he opens box A). It's empty! (Audience: Applause) Now either box C or your box B contains the car keys. Since there are two boxes left, the probability of your box containing the keys is now 1/2. I'll give you $1000 cash for your box.

WAIT!!!

Is Monty Hall right? The contestant knows that at least one of the boxes on the table is empty. He now knows that box A was empty. Does this knowledge change his probability of having the box containing the keys from 1/3 to 1/2? At least one of the boxes on the table had to be empty. Has Monty done the contestant a favor by showing him which box was empty? Is the probability of winning the car 1/2 or 1/3?

Contestant:	I'll trade you my box B for the box C on the table.
Monty Hall:	That's weird!!

Solution: The computation of the contestant's probability of winning is left to the reader.   ■

Factorials, permutations, combinations, and arrangements

The next few pages are devoted to a review of four mathematical tools: factorials, permutations, combinations, and arrangements. These tools provide efficient ways to calculate probabilities, particularly probabilities that involve large numbers of events. Frequently, it is not possible nor is it necessary to produce an exhaustive list of all possible events (n) and count the number of events that constitute a specific subset ($n[A]$). It is often easier to calculate the relevant numbers of events. For example, what is the probability of a perfect bridge hand? The event A is {*Ace*, 2, 3, 4, 5, 6, 7, 8, 9, 10, *Jack, Queen*, and *King*} all of the same suit dealt from a 52-card deck so $n[A] = 4$. But it is an impossible task to enumerate all possible different 13-card hands ($n = ?$). Using the appropriate mathematical tool, however, the total number of equally likely and mutually exclusive 13-card hands can be calculated (in fact, $n = 6.35 \times 10^{11}$). Then, applying the basic definition of probability, the probability of a perfect hand is $P(A) = n[A]/n = 4/(6.35 \times 10^{11})$.

Factorials

For a positive integer n, the product of the consecutive integers from 1 to n is called the *factorial of n*. Symbolically, the factorial of n is written as $n!$, which represents the multiplication process

$$n! = n(n - 1)(n - 2) \cdots 1.$$

Five examples are:

$$1! = 1, 2! = 2 \cdot 1 = 2, 3! = 3 \cdot 2 \cdot 1 = 6, 4! = 4 \cdot 3 \cdot 2 \cdot 1 = 24 \text{ and}$$

$$10! = 10 \cdot 9 \cdot 8 \cdot 7 \cdot 6 \cdot 5 \cdot 4 \cdot 3 \cdot 2 \cdot 1 = 3,628,800.$$

Three properties of factorials are:

1. $n! = n(n - 1)!$;

   for example, $5! = 5 \cdot 4 \cdot 3 \cdot 2 \cdot 1 = 5(4!) = 5(24) = 120$ or $10! = 10(9!) = 10(362,880) = 3,628,800$,

2. $0! = 1$. Since $n! = n(n - 1)!$ or $n!/n = (n - 1)!$, then $n = 1$ yields $1!/1 = (1 - 1)!$ or $1 = 0!$.

   The fact that $0! = 1$, a not very intuitive property, results from a general mathematical definition of a factorial and a complete discussion is left to a mathematics text.

3. $n! = [n(n-1)(n-2)\cdots(n-k+1)](n-k)!$;

for example, $n = 5$, $k = 2$, then $5! = [5\cdot4](5-2)! = [5\cdot4](3!) = (20)(6) = 120$.

EXAMPLE

For $n = 6$ and five values of k, then

n	k	Factorial
6	1	$[6](6-1)! = [6](5!) = (6)(120) = 720$
6	2	$[6\cdot5](6-2)! = [6\cdot5](4!) = (30)(24) = 720$
6	3	$[6\cdot5\cdot4](6-3)! = [6\cdot5\cdot4](3!) = (120)(6) = 720$
6	4	$[6\cdot5\cdot4\cdot3](6-4)! = [6\cdot5\cdot4\cdot3](2!) = (360)(2) = 720$
6	5	$[6\cdot5\cdot4\cdot3\cdot2](6-5)! = [6\cdot5\cdot4\cdot3\cdot2](1!) = (720)(1) = 720$

Permutations

A permutation is a specific ordering of a set of distinct objects. If A, B, and C represent three distinct objects, then there are $3! = 3\cdot2\cdot1 = 6$ different orderings or permutations. They are: ABC, ACB, BAC, BCA, CAB, and CBA. In general, the *number of permutations of* n distinct objects (denoted P^n) is $n!$ or, in symbols,

$$P^n = n!.$$

There are n ways to choose the first of n distinct objects and $n-1$ ways to choose a second distinct object making a total of $n(n-1)$ distinct pairs where each pair is a permutation. For example, if $n = 3$, then the $(3)(2) =$ six pairs are AB, BA, AC, CA, BC, and CB. There are $n-2$ ways of choosing a third distinct object and, therefore, $[n(n-1)](n-2)$ total permutations of three distinct objects and $[n(n-1)(n-2)](n-3)$ is the number of permutations of four distinct objects and so forth, until the last distinct object is chosen making the total number of permutations $n(n-1)(n-2)\cdots1 = n!$.

EXAMPLE

The books of James Fenimore Cooper.

James Fenimore Cooper wrote five books referred to as the "Leatherstocking Tales." These five novels tell the story of the main character named Natty Bumppo (also know as Hawkeye, Leatherstocking, Pathfinder, or Deerslayer) from ages 25 to 82. They are:

Title	Published	Order 1	Age	Order 2
The Deerslayer	1841	5	21	1
The Last of the Mohicans	1826	2	38	2
The Pathfinder	1840	4	42	3
The Pioneers	1823	1	70	4
The Prairie	1827	3	82	5

Controversy exists in the literary world over the best order to read these books; in the order they were written (order 1) or in the chronological order of Leatherstocking's life (order 2). When the volumes are in order by Leatherstocking's age, the books are also in alphabetical order. Is this specific ordering chance or is Cooper perhaps obscurely communicating his preference? When titles are chosen at random, there are $5 \times 4 \times 3 \times 2 \times 1 = 120$ possible permutations and only one is in alphabetical order, so the probability that these books' titles are in alphabetical order by chance alone is $1/120 = 0.008$. Of course, we could take Mark Twain's advice and not read them at all (suggested in his essay "The Literary Crimes of James Fenimore Cooper"). ∎

The number of permutations of k objects selected from n distinct objects (denoted P_k^n) is

$$P_k^n = [n(n-1)\cdots(n-k+1)] = [n(n-1)\cdots(n-k+1)]\frac{(n-k)!}{(n-k)!}$$

$$= \frac{n!}{(n-k)!}.$$

EXAMPLE

Consider the five letters A, B, C, D, E, and three letters are selected ($n = 5$ and $k = 3$). There are 60 different permutations of these three letters. Each permutation can be viewed as a set of possible occupants of three cells in a table. Since five possible letters can occupy the first cell, four possible letters can occupy of the second cell, and three letters can occupy the third cell, the total number of possible distinct permutations is

$$P_3^5 = [5 \cdot 4 \cdot 3] = [5 \cdot 4 \cdot 3]\frac{2!}{2!} = \frac{5!}{2!} = \frac{120}{2} = 60.$$

Thus, there are 60 permutations of three letters when they are selected from five distinct letters. Some examples of the 60 permutations are: ABC, CAB, ACD, CDE, EDC, BDC,···, and ECD. There are no repeated letters in each set of three but each set forms a distinct permutation (for example, {ABC} ≠ {CAB}). ∎

Combinations

To count the number of permutations among a set of distinct objects, the order of the objects is critical. As noted, ABC is different from CAB. A *combination* is a set of distinct objects, like a permutation, but the order of the objects is not relevant and is ignored. For example, ABC is considered the same as CBA ({ABC} = {CAB}). The set {A, B, C} forms 3! = 6 permutations but is only one combination of three letters. In selecting three letters from the set of five {A, B, C, D, E}, there are a total of 60 permutations, but only 10 combinations. They are:

$$ABC, ABD, ABE, ACD, ACE,$$

$$ADE, BCD, BCE, BDE, \text{and } CDE.$$

Each of the 10 combinations has 3! possible orderings. Therefore, the total number of permutations (60) is 3! times the number of combinations (10) or $60 = 3! \times 10$. Conversely, the number of combinations is the number of permutations divided by 3! or $60/3! = 10$.

EXAMPLE

If $n = 4$ distinct objects A, B, C, D and $k = 3$ are selected, then an array of all possible permutations is

$$
\begin{array}{cccccc}
ABC & ACB & BAC & BCA & CAB & CBA \\
ABD & ADB & BAD & BDA & DAB & DBA \\
ACD & ADC & CAD & CDA & DAC & DCA \\
BCD & BDC & CBD & CDB & DBC & DCB
\end{array}
$$

Each row is six permutations (3!) of a single combination. The total number of permutations is the number of rows (4) times the number of columns (6), a total of $6 \times 4 = 24$. In short, $4 \times 6 = 4 \times 3! = 24$. In addition, the number of combinations is the total permutations divided by the number of columns; thus, $24/6 = 24/3! = 4!/3! = 4$ combinations.   ∎

In general, the number of combinations of k objects selected from n, denoted traditionally as $\binom{n}{k}$, equals the number of permutations of k objects selected from n distinct objects (P_k^n) divided by $k!$. In symbols,

$$\binom{n}{k} = \frac{P_k^n}{k!} = \frac{n!}{(n-k)!}\frac{1}{k!} \qquad \text{See Box 2.3.}$$

Box 2.3. Justification of $\binom{n}{k} = \frac{n!}{(n-k)!k!}$

---

total number of permutations = (number of combinations) × (number of possible permutations of each combination) or

$$P_k^n = \binom{n}{k}k! \quad \text{or} \quad \frac{n!}{(n-k)!} = \binom{n}{k}k!$$

Therefore, the number of combinations is $\binom{n}{k} = n!/(n-k)!k!$.

The number of combinations of $(n-k)$ objects selected from n distinct objects also equals $\binom{n}{k}$ or

$$\binom{n}{n-k} = \frac{n!}{k!(n-k)!} = \binom{n}{k}.$$

For every set of k objects selected, there is a set of $n-k$ objects not selected. For example, again when $n = 5$ and $k = 3$, selecting ABC, leaves DE; selecting ACE, leaves BD, and selecting ADE, leaves BC, and so on, making $\binom{5}{3} = \binom{5}{2} = 10$. Specifically,

selected:	ABC	ABD	ABE	ACD	ACE	ADE	BCD
not selected:	DE	CE	CD	BE	BD	BC	AE

selected:	BCE	BDE	CDE
not selected:	AD	AC	AB.

For small values of n and k the quantity $\binom{n}{k}$ is easily calculated. Values of $\binom{n}{k}$ for $n = 1, 2, \cdots, 12$, and $k = 0, 1, \cdots, 8$ are given in Table 2.2. Historically, considerable time has been spent studying the patterns in Table 2.2, particularly the patterns among the diagonal values.

EXAMPLE

The total number of different five-card hands dealt from a 52-card deck (poker):

$$\binom{52}{5} = \frac{52!}{47!5!} = 2,598,960. \qquad \blacksquare$$

TABLE 2.2: Values of $\binom{n}{k}$ for $n = 1, 2, \cdots, 12$, sometimes called *binomial coefficients*.

	$k=0$	$k=1$	$k=2$	$k=3$	$k=4$	$k=5$	$k=6$	$k=7$	$k=8$	Total*
$n=1$	1	1	—	—	—	—	—	—	—	2
$n=2$	1	2	1	—	—	—	—	—	—	4
$n=3$	1	3	3	1	—	—	—	—	—	8
$n=4$	1	4	6	4	1	—	—	—	—	16
$n=5$	1	5	10	10	5	1	—	—	—	32
$n=6$	1	6	15	20	15	6	1	—	—	64
$n=7$	1	7	21	35	35	21	7	1	—	128
$n=8$	1	8	28	56	70	56	28	8	1	256
$n=9$	1	9	36	84	126	126	84	36	9	512**
$n=10$	1	10	45	120	210	252	210	120	45	1024**
$n=11$	1	11	55	165	330	462	462	330	165	2048**
$n=12$	1	12	66	220	495	792	924	792	495	4096**

*The total is 2^n.

**The remainder of table is not shown for $k \geq 9$ but can be found since the rows are symmetrical, that is, $\binom{n}{k} = \binom{n}{n-k}$. For example, in row 10, $\binom{10}{9} = \binom{10}{1} = 10$.

EXAMPLE

The total number of different 13-card hands dealt from a 52 card deck (bridge):

$$\binom{52}{13} = \frac{52!}{39!13!} = 6.35 \times 10^{11}.$$ ∎

EXAMPLE

The total number of different triple-decker ice cream cones from 31 flavors:

$$\binom{31}{3} = \frac{31!}{28!3!} = 4,495.$$ ∎

In all three examples, the order of the distinct objects is not considered. Four aces beats a full-house regardless of the order in which the cards are dealt.

Arrangements

Consider a group of n objects, where k objects are alike (represented by x's) and the remaining $n - k$ objects are also alike (represented by o's) but different from the x's. How many different *arrangements* (distinguishable orderings) can be made from these n objects? The answer is $\binom{n}{k}$.

EXAMPLE

When $n = 5(x, x, x, o, o)$, $k = 3(x, x, x)$, and $n - k = 2(o, o)$, the total number of arrangements is $\binom{5}{3} = 10$. The 10 different arrangements are:

$$xxooo, xxoxo, xxoox, xoxxo, xoxox, xooxx,$$

$$oxxxo, oxxox, oxoxx, \text{ and } ooxxx. \qquad \blacksquare$$

To verify that the number of arrangements equals the number of combinations, consider five positions $(1, 2, 3, 4, 5)$. Each arrangement is equivalent to selecting three (distinct) positions out of the five possible and assigning them to the three x's, leaving two positions for the two o's. If positions 1, 2, and 3 are selected, then the ordering is $xxxoo$, if the positions 3, 4, and 5 are selected, the ordering is $ooxxx$ and if positions 1, 3, and 5 are selected, then the ordering is $xoxox$ and so forth. For $n = 5$ and $k = 3$, the three possible positions for the x-values are: (1,2,3), (1,2,4), (1,2,5), (1,3,4), (1,3,5), (1,4,5), (2,3,4), (2,3,5), (2,4,5), (3,4,5), and, necessarily, the two positions remaining for the o-values are: (4,5), (3,5), (3,4), (2,5), (2,4), (2,3), (1,5), (1,4), (1,3), (1,2). Displayed in a table, all 10 arrangements are:

	Arrangements					Positions	
	1	2	3	4	5	x's	o's
1.	x	x	x	o	o	(1,2,3)	(4,5)
2.	x	x	o	x	o	(1,2,4)	(3,5)
3.	x	x	o	o	x	(1,2,5)	(3,4)
4.	x	o	x	x	o	(1,3,4)	(2,5)
5.	x	o	x	o	x	(1,3,5)	(2,4)
6.	x	o	o	x	x	(1,4,5)	(2,3)
7.	o	x	x	x	o	(2,3,4)	(1,5)
8.	o	x	x	o	x	(2,3,5)	(1,4)
9.	o	x	o	x	x	(2,4,5)	(1,3)
10.	o	o	x	x	x	(3,4,5)	(1,2)

The number of ways three distinct positions without regard to order, therefore, can be selected from five is identical to the number of ways three objects of one kind and two objects of another kind can be placed in different arrangements. That is, $\binom{5}{3} = 10$.

In general, the number of different arrangements of k objects of one kind and $n - k$ objects of another kind is the number of different positions for the k objects of one kind (order is not relevant), namely $\binom{n}{k}$.

EXAMPLE

How many ways can families of four be composed when there are two boys and two girls?—answer: $\binom{4}{2} = 6$. ∎

EXAMPLE

How many arrangements can be made out of the words "toot" or "deeded"?—answers: $\binom{4}{2} = 6$ and $\binom{6}{3} = 20$. ∎

EXAMPLE

When a team plays seven games and wins four, how many distinct ways can this occur?—answer: $\binom{7}{4} = 35$. ∎

EXAMPLE

How many ways can three heads and five tails occur when a coin is tossed eight times?—answer: $\binom{8}{3} = \binom{8}{5} = 56$. ∎

Another view of the number of arrangements that can be made from n objects of which k are of one kind and $n - k$ are of another kind is illustrated below.

> There are $n!$ distinct permutations if all objects are distinct. This number is too large when k and $n - k$ objects are not distinct because, unlike distinct objects, permuting the order of identical objects does not change the arrangement. The $n!$ permutations are too large by factors $k!$ and $(n - k)!$, which are the number of permutations that would occur if the objects were distinct. Therefore, the total number of permutations reduced by the factor $k!(n - k)!$ is $n!/[(n - k)!k!] = \binom{n}{k}$ and is again the number of distinct arrangements.

A last example: Sampling with replacement.

This last example illustrates seven statistical/mathematical tools from this chapter that reappear in the following chapters, namely sampling, independence, arrangements, mutually exclusive events, the addition theorem, and a series of exhaustive events.

Consider a special deck of cards used in a child's game made up of five red cards (denoted R) and four black cards (denoted B). Suppose five cards are drawn one at a time, each card is replaced after noting its color and the deck of nine cards is shuffled before the next card is drawn, technically called *sampling with replacement*. What is the probability of drawing five times and observing two black cards and, necessarily, three red cards? The probability of drawing a black card is the same on each draw and is 4/9. Similarly, for the red cards, the probability of drawing a red card on each draw is 5/9. These probabilities remain constant because each card is selected from a deck that always contains five red cards and four black cards. In addition, the deck is shuffled after each draw making each selection an independent event.

Consider the specific outcome of selecting a black, then a red, then a black, then a red, and finally a red card (BRBRR). The probability of this event is $P(BRBRR) = (4/9)(5/9)(4/9)(5/9)(5/9) = (4/9)^2(5/9)^3 = 0.0339$, because each selection is independent. How many ways can two black and three red cards be drawn? A list of all possible distinct and mutually exclusive sets of five selections where two black and three red cards occur is: RRRBB, RRBRB, RRBBR, RBRRB, RBRBR, RBBRR, BRRRB, BRRBR, BRBRR, BBRRR. There are $\binom{5}{2} = 10$ different arrangements (mutually exclusive possibilities) and each arrangement has the same probability of occurring (0.0339). Therefore, when sampling with replacement, the probability of observing two black cards and necessarily three red cards among the five cards selected is $0.0339+0.0339\cdots+$ $0.0339 = 10(0.0339) = 10(4/9)^2(5/9)^3 = \binom{5}{2}(4/9)^2(5/9)^3 = 0.339$ (addition theorem applied to 10 mutually exclusive events).

More generally, the probability of drawing k black cards and $5-k$ red cards when the five cards are sampled independently with replacement is

$$P(k\ black\ cards) = P(X = k) = \binom{5}{k}\left(\frac{4}{9}\right)^k\left(\frac{5}{9}\right)^{5-k}$$

because, there are:

1. $\binom{5}{k}$ different mutually exclusive arrangements of k black cards and $5-k$ red cards, and

2. each arrangement has the same probability, namely $\left(\frac{4}{9}\right)^k\left(\frac{5}{9}\right)^{5-k}$.

For all six possible outcomes, then

Outcomes	k	Symbol	Calculation	Probability
no black cards	0	$P(X=0)$	$\binom{5}{0}(4/9)^0(5/9)^5 = 1(0.0529)$	0.053
one black card	1	$P(X=1)$	$\binom{5}{1}(4/9)^1(5/9)^4 = 5(0.0423)$	0.212
two black cards	2	$P(X=2)$	$\binom{5}{2}(4/9)^2(5/9)^3 = 10(0.0339)$	0.339
three black cards	3	$P(X=3)$	$\binom{5}{3}(4/9)^3(5/9)^2 = 10(0.0271)$	0.271
four black cards	4	$P(X=4)$	$\binom{5}{4}(4/9)^4(5/9)^1 = 5(0.0217)$	0.108
five black cards	5	$P(X=5)$	$\binom{5}{5}(4/9)^5(5/9)^0 = 1(0.0173)$	0.017

These six events are mutually exclusive and exhaustive so the six probabilities add to one. Because $a^0 = 1$, then $(4/9)^0 = (5/9)^0 = 1$. The fact that $a^0 = 1$

makes sense when viewed from the perspective that $1 = a^m/a^m = a^{(m-m)} = a^0$. Also, $\binom{5}{0} = \binom{5}{5} = \frac{5!}{5!0!} = 1$, because $0! = 1$.

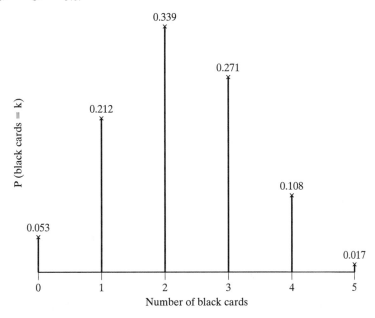

Summary of the eight rules of probability

Rule	Description	Expression
1	range	$0 \leq P(A) \leq 1$
2	complementary probability	$P(\overline{A}) = 1 - P(A)$
3	decomposition of a probability	$P(A) = P(AB) + P(A\overline{B})$
4	conditional probability	$P(B \mid A) = P(AB)/P(A)$
5	independence	$P(B \mid A) = P(B)$ or $P(AB) = P(A)P(B)$
6	multiplication rule	$P(AB) = P(B \mid A)P(A)$
7	Bayes' rule	$P(B \mid A) = P(A \mid B)P(B)/P(A)$
8	addition rule	$P(A \text{ or } B) = P(A) + P(B) - P(AB)$

The famous French mathematician Emile Borel (b. 1871) questioned, "Can there be laws of chance? The answer, it would seem should be negative, since chance is in fact defined as the characteristic of the phenomena which would follow no law, phenomena whose causes are too complex to permit prediction." Metaphysics aside, rules 1 to 8 are essential elements in the following chapters where probability is a major part of the application of statistical reasoning to the analysis of data.

MONOPOLY PROBABILITIES

(probability of landing on each square)

	Property	Probability		Property	Probability
1.	Mediterranean	0.0238	23.	Indiana	0.0305
2.	Community Chest	0.0211	24.	Illinois	0.0355
3.	Baltic	0.0242	25.	B. and O. Railroad	0.0343
4.	Income Tax	0.0260	26.	Atlantic	0.0301
5.	Reading Railroad	0.0332	27.	Ventnor	0.0299
6.	Oriental	0.0253	28.	Water Works	0.0315
7.	Chance	0.0097	29.	Marvin Gardens	0.0289
8.	Vermont	0.0257	30.	Go to Jail	—
9.	Connecticut	0.0257	31.	Pacific	0.0299
10.	Just Visiting	0.0254	32.	North Carolina	0.0293
11.	St. Charles Place	0.0303	33.	Community Chest	0.0264
12.	Electric Company	0.0310	34.	Pennsylvania	0.0279
13.	States	0.0258	35.	Short Line Railroad	0.0272
14.	Virginia	0.0288	36.	Chance	0.0097
15.	Pennsylvania Railroad	0.0313	37.	Park Place	0.0244
16.	St. James Place	0.0318	38.	Luxury Tax	0.0244
17.	Community Chest	0.0272	39.	Boardwalk	0.0295
18.	Tennessee	0.0335	40.	Go	0.0346
19.	New York	0.0334		Jail probabilities	
20.	Free parking	0.0355		Sent to jail	0.0444
21.	Kentucky	0.0310		In jail one turn	0.0370
22.	Chance	0.0124		In jail two turns	0.0308

PROBLEM SET 2

Use the following data to decide whether political party affiliation is related to sex:

	Democrat	Republican	Independent	Total
females	250	300	50	600
males	250	100	50	400
Total	500	400	100	1000

Find the following:

1. $P(Democrat) = ?$
2. $P(Republican) = ?$
3. $P(Independent) = ?$
4. $P(Republican$ and $male) = ?$
5. $P(Independent$ and $male) = ?$
6. $P(Independent$ and $female = ?$
7. $P(female$ and $Republican) = ?$

8. $P(Republican \mid male) = ?$
9. $P(Republican \mid female) = ?$
10. $P(male \mid Democrat) = ?$
11. $P(female \mid Democrat) = ?$
12. $P(female \mid Republican) = ?$
13. $P(Democrat \mid not\ Independent) = ?$
14. $P(Republican \mid not\ Independent) = ?$

Is party affiliation likely related to sex? Why or why not?

Two fair dice are tossed:

15. What is the probability of a sum of six? a sum of five?
16. What is the probability of doubles?
17. What is the probability of a sum of six or doubles?
18. What is the probability of a sum of six and doubles?
19. What is the probability of a sum of five or doubles?
20. What is the probability of a sum of five and doubles?
21. In the simplest form of Mendelian inheritance, a physical characteristic of a plant or animal is determined by a single pair of genes. The color of seeds from sweet pea plants is an example. Letting y and g represent yellow and green genes, seeds will be green if the plant has the color-gene pair (g, g); it will be yellow if the plant has color-gene pair (y, y) or (y, g). In view of this last combination, yellow is said to be dominant to green. Progeny get one gene from each parent plant and are equally likely to get either gene. When two (y, g)-plants are crossed, what is the probability that a yellow seed will be the result? What is the probability that a yellow seed will be (y, y)?
22. What is wrong with the following argument? "If two coins are tossed, then there are three possible outcomes: (1) 2 heads, (2) 1 head and 1 tail, (3) 2 tails. Hence the probability of two heads is 1/3."
23. Suppose that 25 percent of a forest consists of trees of species A, 40% of species B, and 35% of species C. What is the probability that a tree selected at random will be of species A? What is the probability that the tree selected will not be of species A? If it is known that the tree is not of species A, what is the probability that it will be of species B?
24. In an experiment with a mosquito insecticide, it is found that 80% are killed during the initial application, but those that survive develop a resistance. The percentage of the survivors killed in any later application is half that of the immediately preceding application; i.e., 40% of the survivors of the first application would succumb to the

second application, while only 20% of the survivors of two applications would be killed by a third application, etc. Consider each application independent of any other application.

Find the probability (a) that a mosquito will survive 5 applications; (b) that a mosquito will survive 5 applications, given that it has survived the first 2 applications.

25. A club has 90 members. Fifty are lawyers and 50 are liars. Everyone is either a lawyer or a liar. What is the probability that a randomly selected member is both a lawyer and a liar? What is the probability that a randomly selected member is a lawyer but not a liar? What is the probability that a lawyer is not a liar?

26. Monozygotic twins (identical) and dizygotic twins (fraternal) occur with the following probabilities: $P(MZ) = 0.3$ and $P(DZ) = 1 - P(MZ) = 0.7$.
What are the following probabilities for twin births:

$$P(MM \mid MZ), P(MF \mid MZ) \text{ and } P(FF \mid MZ)$$

$$P(MM \mid DZ), P(MF \mid DZ) \text{ and } P(FF \mid DZ)$$

where MM = male/male pair, MF = male/female pair, and FF = female/female pair, and $P(\text{male}) = P(\text{female}) = 0.5$?
What are the following probabilities for twin births:

$$P(MM), P(FF), \text{ and } P(MF)?$$

What are these three probabilities for two consecutive independent singleton (non-twin) births?

27. A hotel has 10 rooms in a row on one floor. The clerk assigns guests to these rooms at random. If the rooms are all empty and two guests arrive, what is the probability that they will have adjoining rooms?

28. There are three coins in a bag. One has two heads. Another has one head and one tail. The third coin has two tails. You reach in the bag and randomly take one coin. Without looking at it, you toss it and it lands heads up. What's the probability it's the 2-headed coin?

29. Like the puzzles in the Sunday comics, match the terms with their definitions:

_____	equally likely	(a) $P(A \mid B) = P(AB)/P(B)$
_____	mutually exclusive	(b) $P(A \text{ or } B) = P(A) + P(B) - P(AB)$
_____	conditional probability	(c) $P(A \mid B) = P(A)$
_____	exhaustive	(d) $P(A) = P(B)$
_____	Bayes' rule	(e) $P(AB) = P(B \mid A)P(A)$
_____	multiplication rule	(f) $P(AB) = 0$
_____	independence	(g) $P(A \mid B) = P(B \mid A)P(A)/P(B)$
_____	addition theorem	(h) $P(A_1) + P(A_2) + P(A_3) = 1$

A fair coin is tossed independently five times [$P(heads) = P(tails) = 0.5$].

Compute:

30. probability of all heads,
31. probability of no heads,
32. probability of at least one heads,

720

33. probability of more heads than tails, and
34. probability of less than three heads.

Eight decks of 52 playing cards are shuffled and the top card on each deck is turned up.

35. What is the probability all eight are face cards (King, Queen, and Jack)?
36. What is the probability all eight are face cards of the same suit (all hearts, diamonds, spades, or clubs)?
37. What is the probability of exactly four face cards among the 8 cards turned up?
38. Calculate the probabilities of $0, 1, 2, \cdots, 8$ face cards among the eight decks.
39. An automobile license plate consists of three numbers followed by three letters of the alphabet. How many license plates are possible if (a) repetition is allowed; (b) no repetition is allowed; (c) no repetition is allowed and the three numbers are in ascending order?

Suppose that license plates are given out in random fashion. Mr. and Ms. Brown (a two-car family) went to get automobile license plates. (d) If repetition is allowed, what is the probability that their plates would end with the same letter? (e) Begin with the same digit? (f) Begin with the same digit and end with the same letter?

Suppose Mr. Brown went to get his automobile license after Ms. Brown had already gotten hers. (g) What is the probability that Mr. Brown's automobile license would have the same ending letter as Ms. Brown's? (h) Same beginning number?

Life tables for the United States males and females are given below. They are constructed by estimating the probability of death, q_x, for each age interval. Applying this probability to survivors of the previous interval beginning with l_0 of 100,000 persons, the number who died and survived each age interval is calculated. The number dying in each interval, d_x and surviving l_x, yield the total number of years lived in the interval L_x and total years lived beyond age x, T_x. The average years lived beyond age x is $\hat{e}_x = T_x/l_x$. This average at age 0, $\hat{e}_0$, is an often used single summary of the overall mortality pattern.

ABRIDGED LIFE TABLE BY SEX: UNITED STATES

males

Interval	$q(x)$	$d(x)$	$l(x)$	$L(x)$	$T(x)$	$e(x)$
0–1	0.0120	1196	100000	99402	7115680	71.2
1–5	0.0023	226	98804	394764	7016278	71.0
5–10	0.0014	140	98578	492540	6621514	67.2
10–15	0.0017	169	98438	491768	6128974	62.3
15–20	0.0057	560	98269	489945	5637206	57.4
20–25	0.0082	802	97709	486540	5147261	52.7
25–30	0.0083	807	96907	482518	4660721	48.1
30–35	0.0094	908	96100	478230	4178204	43.5
35–40	0.0118	1121	95192	473158	3699974	38.9
40–45	0.0166	1560	94071	466455	3226816	34.3
45–50	0.0254	2347	92511	456688	2760361	29.8
50–55	0.0409	3688	90164	441600	2303674	25.5

Interval	$q(x)$	$d(x)$	$l(x)$	$L(x)$	$T(x)$	$e(x)$
55–60	0.0651	5631	86476	418302	1862074	21.5
60–65	0.0985	7965	80845	384312	1443771	17.9
65–70	0.1429	10414	72880	338365	1059458	14.5
70–75	0.2135	13338	62466	278985	721094	11.5
75–80	0.3044	14955	49128	208252	442108	9.0
80–85	0.4315	14744	34173	134005	233856	6.8
85+	1.0000	19429	19429	99851	99851	5.1

females

Interval	$q(x)$	$d(x)$	$l(x)$	$L(x)$	$T(x)$	$e(x)$
0–1	0.0094	935	100000	99532	7663625	76.6
1–5	0.0017	173	99065	395914	7564092	76.4
5–10	0.0011	105	98892	494198	7168178	72.5
10–15	0.0010	100	98787	493685	6673981	67.6
15–20	0.0023	229	98687	492862	6180296	62.6
20–25	0.0026	260	98458	491640	5687434	57.8
25–30	0.0030	294	98198	490255	5195794	52.9
30–35	0.0039	385	97904	488558	4705538	48.1
35–40	0.0055	540	97519	486245	4216981	43.2
40–45	0.0087	842	96979	482790	3730736	38.5
45–50	0.0142	1364	96137	477275	3247946	33.8
50–55	0.0229	2169	94773	468442	2770671	29.2
55–60	0.0355	3287	92604	454802	2302228	24.9
60–65	0.0547	4883	89317	434378	1847426	20.7
65–70	0.0805	6801	84434	405168	1413048	16.7
70–75	0.1230	9545	77633	364302	1007881	13.0
75–80	0.1875	12768	68088	308520	643578	9.5
80–85	0.2993	16557	55320	235208	335058	6.1
85+	1.0000	38763	38763	99851	99851	2.6

Notation for the life table is:

$q(x)$ = probability of dying in the age interval x

$d(x)$ = number who died in age interval x

$l(x)$ = number alive at the beginning of age interval x

$L(x)$ = total person-years lived in age interval x

$T(x)$ = total person-years lived beyond age x

$e(x)$ = average years lived beyond age x

and

$x = 0, 1, 5, 10, 15, \ldots, 80$, and 85^{+}.

Find the probability for each of the following events:

40. A newborn male (age 0) will die in the interval (0, 1).

41. A newborn male (age 0) will die in the interval (1, 5), if he survives the (0, 1) interval.

42. A newborn male (age 0) will die either in interval (0, 1) or in (1, 5).

43. A newborn male (age 0) will die before the 10th year.

44. A male will survive to age 25, if he survived to the 10th year.

Suppose event $A = \{$*the survival of a 60-year-old male to age 80 years*$\}$ and event $B = \{$*the survival of a 60-year-old female to age 80 years*$\}$.

Find the following probabilities assuming that events A and B are independent:

45. $P\{AB\}$ **46.** $P\{\overline{A}\,B\}$ **47.** $P\{\overline{A} \text{ or } B\}$ **48.** $P\{\overline{A}\,\overline{B}\}$ **49.** $P\{A \text{ or } B\}$.

Assume that in 5% of professional football games one or more field goals are missed, $p = P(one\ or\ more\ misses) = 0.05$. This result is occasionally interpreted to mean that there is no chance of completing a 20-game season without missing a field goal. (There are 4 preseason games and 16 regular season games.) Is this interpretation correct?

Suppose $p = 0.05$ represents the probability of missing at least one field goal in any single game. Assume the field goal attempts per game are independent events. Let X represent the number of games with missed field goals.

50. In the 4 preseason games, what are the possible values of X and what are the corresponding probabilities?

51. For the entire season of 20 games, what is the probability a kicker will not miss a single field goal (perfect record)? What is the probability he will not have a perfect season?

52. A bag contains 3 white and 2 black balls; another contains 2 white and 1 black ball. If a bag is chosen at random and then a ball selected from it, what is the probability of a white ball? If a white ball is selected, what is the probability it came from the first bag? If all the balls are combined into one bag and a ball is drawn, what is the probability of getting a white ball?

53. Suppose p_x represents the probability that an individual alive at time x will survive the interval $(x, x + 1)$ and let q_x be the corresponding probability of dying in the interval. Then, $p_x + q_x = 1$ (why or why not?).

Compute the probability that an individual alive at time $x = 0$ will die in the interval $(0, 3)$ and show that this probability equals $1 - p_0 p_1 p_2$.

54. Select the correct answer:

$P(A)/2 = 0.6$	always true	sometimes true	never true
$P(A\,|\,\overline{B}) + P(\overline{A}\,|\,\overline{B}) = 1$	always true	sometimes true	never true
$P(B\,|\,A) = P(A\,|\,B)$	always true	sometimes true	never true
$P(A) = P(B)$	always true	sometimes true	never true
$P(A\,|\,B) - P(A) = 0$	always true	sometimes true	never true
$P(A\,|\,B)P(B) = P(B\,|\,A)P(A)$	always true	sometimes true	never true
$P(\overline{A} \text{ or } B) = P(\overline{A}\,\overline{B})$	always true	sometimes true	never true
$P\{AB\}/P(B) = P(A)$	always true	sometimes true	never true

C H A P T E R   3

Random Variables

Surprisingly, the term *random* is not easy to define mathematically but has been long recognized as an important part of human activities. Sophocles (997) recommended, "Tis best to live random, as one may." More recently, the Rand Corporation (1950) produced a book entitled *A Million Random Digits with 100,000 Normal Deviates.* Today, many games, codes, and computer models depend on random numbers. Random is usually defined, somewhat unsatisfactorily, as a failure to find a pattern. Precisely defined or not, random is an integral part of the statistical analysis of data.

The concept of a variable, introduced in Chapter 1, can be extended and formalized to create the definition of a random variable and is the first topic of this chapter. A series of companion topics then directly follow once a formal definition is established: such as a probability distribution, the expectation of a random variable, the variance of a random variable, and the properties of a sample mean value.

Random variable

The term *random variable* is a formal and convenient way to describe a special kind of variable, which is the basis of most statistical analyses. The two defining properties of a discrete random variable (represented by capital letters such as X) are:

1. a random variable X takes on one of a series of numeric values (for example, $X = 0, 1, 2, \cdots, x, \cdots$), and
2. each occurrence of a random variable X has an associated probability (for example, $p_0, p_1, p_2, \cdots, p_x, \cdots$).

A capital letter is typically used as an abstract symbol for a random variable. For example, X could represent {*height of an individual*}. The quantity symbolized by X is not a number. The actual numeric value that the random variable assumes is denoted by the same lowercase letter. A specific height would be represented as x (for example, $x = 72$ inches). The value denoted by x is technically called the *realization of the random variable X* or more simply the observed value. This notation allows parsimonious expressions such as:

In symbols	In words
$X = x$	an individual's height equals a specific value x
$X > x$	an individual's height is greater than a specific value x
$P(X > x)$	the probability an individual's height is greater than a specific value x
$P(a < X < b)$	the probability an individual's height is greater than a and less than b

EXAMPLE

Toss a die once and observe the value that appears on the top face. The random variable X represents {*the number on the top face of a randomly tossed die*} with the possible realizations $x = 1, 2, 3, 4, 5,$ or 6 and has a specific probability of occurrence described in detail by

$$X = 1 \quad p_1 = P(X = 1) = 1/6 \qquad X = 4 \quad p_4 = P(X = 4) = 1/6$$
$$X = 2 \quad p_2 = P(X = 2) = 1/6 \qquad X = 5 \quad p_5 = P(X = 5) = 1/6$$
$$X = 3 \quad p_3 = P(X = 3) = 1/6 \qquad X = 6 \quad p_6 = P(X = 6) = 1/6.$$

Each realization of the random variable X has the same associated probability of 1/6. In symbols, $p_x = P(X = x) = 1/6$ for $x = 1, 2, 3, 4, 5,$ or 6. ∎

EXAMPLE

Consider a mating between two heterozygous individuals (Aa × Aa) and suppose the random variable measured is the number of A genes in an offspring. The random variable Y represents {*the number of A-genes*} with realizations $y = 0$, 1, or 2 and the associated probabilities are

$$\text{aa-offspring or } Y = 0 \text{ and } p_0 = P(Y = 0) = 1/4$$
$$\text{Aa-offspring or } Y = 1 \text{ and } p_1 = P(Y = 1) = 1/2, \text{ and}$$
$$\text{AA-offspring or } Y = 2 \text{ and } p_2 = P(Y = 2) = 1/4. \qquad ∎$$

EXAMPLE

Consider a population made up of 10 numbers where

$$population = \{1, 2, 2, 3, 3, 3, 4, 4, 4, 4\}.$$

A single randomly selected value is chosen from this population, then the random variable X represents {*the value of a random selection*} and the values p_x are:

X	$X = 1$	$X = 2$	$X = 3$	$X = 4$	Total
p_x	$p_1 = 0.1$	$p_2 = 0.2$	$p_3 = 0.3$	$p_4 = 0.4$	1.0

The probabilities associated with each outcome X are $p_x = P(X = x) = x/10$ where $x = 1$, 2, 3, or 4, defining all possible probabilities associated with the random variable X.   ■

EXAMPLE

Sampling with replacement from a special five-card deck made up of four black and five red cards (repeated from Chapter 2) produces a random variable. Specifically, the random variable X represents {*the number of black cards in a sample of five cards sampled with replacement from a deck of nine cards*} and the associated probabilities are $p_x = P(X = x) = \binom{5}{x}(4/9)^x(5/9)^{5-x}$ for $x = 0$, 1, 2, 3, 4, or 5 and again

X	$X = 0$	$X = 1$	$X = 2$	$X = 3$	$X = 4$	$X = 5$	Total
p_x	$p_0 = 0.053$	$p_1 = 0.212$	$p_2 = 0.339$	$p_3 = 0.271$	$p_4 = 0.108$	$p_5 = 0.017$	1.0

■

The set of probabilities p_x associated with all possible values of a random variable X is called the *probability distribution* of the random variable X. Each of the four previous examples illustrates a probability distribution. For these probability distributions, $\sum_{all\ x} p_x = 1.0$ and is a property of probability distributions in general when the p_x-values are probabilities from a set of mutually exclusive and exhaustive outcomes.

Probability theory postulates a theoretical structure and provides tools to characterize samples that might arise from a probability distribution (the rest of this chapter and Chapter 4). Statistics, on the other hand, are calculated from sample data selected from a probability distribution (population) and provides estimates of what the sampled structure might be, while at the same time giving an idea of the confidence that can be placed in these estimates. Probability theory argues from probability distributions to samples and, reversing the process, statistics argues from samples to probability distributions. In either case, it is imperative to keep in mind that two different entities exist—a probability distribution generated from nonstatistical and usually theoretical considerations and a collection of observations generated from values sampled from a probability distribution.

Measure of location—mean of a probability distribution

Parallel to a mean value ($\bar{x}$) calculated from sampled observations, a need exists to identify the location of a probability distribution. One such summary value is called the *expected value*. The expected value is the mean of a probability distribution, usually denoted $E(X)$ where X represents the variable under study. For a discrete random variable X, the expected value is defined as

$$E(X) = \frac{\sum\limits_{all\ x} w_x x}{\sum\limits_{all\ x} w_x} = \frac{\sum\limits_{all\ x} p_x x}{\sum\limits_{all\ x} p_x} = \sum\limits_{all\ x} p_x x \qquad \left(\sum\limits_{all\ x} w_x = \sum\limits_{all\ x} p_x = 1 \right)$$

where $w_x = p_x = P(X = x)$. The sums are taken over all possible values of x. The expected value $E(X)$ is a weighted average of all possible values of a random variable, each weighted by its probability of occurrence (weights $= w_x = p_x$). It is the mean of the probability distribution defined by the probabilities p_x. The expected value is also referred to as the *population mean*.

Note the similarity to the sample mean, which is also a weighted average (weights $= w_i = \hat{p}_i$), where

$$\bar{x} = \frac{\sum w_i x_i}{\sum w_i} = \sum \hat{p}_i x_i. \qquad \left(\text{again, } \sum w_i = \sum \hat{p}_i = 1\right).$$

The symbol $\hat{p}_i$ represents the estimated proportion or relative frequency ($\hat{p}_i = f_i/n$) of the occurrences of the value x_i in a sample of n values (Chapter 1). The circumflex added to the symbol p_i indicates that the value is calculated from sampled data. When all sample values x_i differ ($f_i = 1$), $w_i = \hat{p}_i = 1/n$, and $\bar{x} = \sum x_i/n$.

The expected value can be thought of as the idealized or infinite sample size measure of location associated with a probability distribution, the mean of the probability distribution. The probabilities p_x replace the sample proportions $\hat{p}_i$ and all possible values of x are considered rather than just those n values available from a sample. The expected value, therefore, is a fixed value determined entirely by the probabilities p_x (the probability distribution) and the outcomes of x. The sample mean, on the other hand, is calculated from observed values ($\hat{p}_i$ and x_i) and is determined by which values occur and which values do not occur in the sampled data. The sample mean is the mean of the distribution of a sample of data and the expected value is analogously the mean of a probability distribution, both indicating the center of gravity or location of a distribution of values.

EXAMPLE

To clarify the distinctions and similarities between the sample mean and the population mean (expected value) consider the following simple example. Suppose three coins are tossed at the same time a total of 20 times. The random variable X represents {*the number of heads among the three coins on each toss*} and the possible outcomes are $x = 0, 1, 2,$ or 3 heads. The number of heads recorded for $k = 20$ tosses of three coins ($x_i, i = 1, 2, 3, \cdots, k = 20$) are:

number of heads (x_{i_i}): 2 1 0 2 2 1 3 1 2 1 0 2 3 0 2 1 2 0 2 1

or displayed in a table

X is {*number of heads in three tosses*} possible results	$X = 0$ no heads	$X = 1$ one head	$X = 2$ two heads	$X = 3$ three heads	Total
Number of occurrences (f_i) relative frequency = $\hat{p}_i = f_i/k$	$f_0 = 4$ $\hat{p}_0 = 0.2$	$f_1 = 6$ $\hat{p}_1 = 0.3$	$f_2 = 8$ $\hat{p}_2 = 0.4$	$f_3 = 2$ $\hat{p}_3 = 0.1$	$k = 20$ 1.0

The mean number of heads per toss of three coins ($\overline{x} = \sum x_i/k$) calculated from this sample is

$$\overline{x} = \frac{2+1+0+2+2+1+3+\cdots+1+0+2+1}{20}$$
$$= \frac{0+0+0+0+1+1+1+\cdots+2+2+3+3}{20}$$
$$= \frac{4}{20}(0) + \frac{6}{20}(1) + \frac{8}{20}(2) + \frac{2}{20}(3)$$
$$= 0.2(0) + 0.3(1) + 0.4(2) + 0.1(3) = 1.4.$$

The sample mean 1.4 is a weighted average calculated from the distribution of observed values and is one of the many possible means that could have occurred when three coins are tossed 20 times. Another 20 tosses would yield another set of observations, creating another set of estimated $\hat{p}_i$-values and almost surely produces a different sample mean value. Because the observed values (x_i) vary from sample to sample, the $\hat{p}_i$ values vary, causing the sample means ($\overline{x}$) to vary from sample to sample. These sample mean values vary because different samples are made up of different observations, called *sampling variation.* ■

The expected value $E(X)$ is not subject to sampling variation and depends entirely on the components of the probability distribution. When three coins are tossed simultaneously, the probability distribution is (assuming independence of the tosses and the probability of heads is 1/2):

X is {number of heads in three tosses} possible results	$X = 0$ no heads	$X = 1$ one head	$X = 2$ two heads	$X = 3$ three heads	Total
Probability $= P(X = x) = p_x$	$p_0 = (1/2)^3$ $= 1/8$ $= 0.125$	$p_1 = 3(1/2)^3$ $= 3/8$ $= 0.375$	$p_2 = 3(1/2)^3$ $= 3/8$ $= 0.375$	$p_3 = (1/2)^3$ $= 1/8$ $= 0.125$	1.0 1.0 1.0

The population expected value is

$$E(X) = \sum_{all\ x} p_x x$$

$$= p_0 x_0 + p_1 x_1 + p_2 x_2 + p_3 x_3$$

$$= \frac{1}{8}(0) + \frac{3}{8}(1) + \frac{3}{8}(2) + \frac{1}{8}(3)$$

$$= 0.125(0) + 0.375(1) + 0.375(2) + 0.125(3) = 1.5.$$

Thus, the expected number of heads per toss of three coins calculated from the theoretical probability distribution is 1.5. The mean of the population $[E(X) = 1.5]$ does not vary because it is entirely determined by four values of X and the four corresponding probabilities p_x.

When three coins are tossed 20 times and the frequency of the results tabulated, it is natural that the relative frequencies reflect only loosely the underlying probabilities. For example, the sampled values $\hat{p}_i$ (0.2, 0.3, 0.4, or 0.1) clearly do not reflect accurately the theoretical values p_i (0.125, 0.375, 0.375, or 0.125). The lack of correspondence results because sampling variation produces sample values that are most variable when the number of observations involved is small. As the number of tosses increases, the influence of this sampling variation decreases. More specifically, as the number of tosses increases, the difference between data estimated proportions ($\hat{p}_i$) and the theoretical probabilities (p_i) decreases. To illustrate, Table 3.1 shows results from tossing three coins a large number of times (actually a computer simulation of tossing coins).

Figure 3.1 is a plot of the relationship between sample size and the observed proportion of heads from independent tosses of three coins. The horizontal axis displays the number of times the three coins are tossed (k) and the vertical axis displays the sample proportions of the four possible results ($\hat{p}_i$). The plot (Figure 3.1) clearly shows the expected property that the four proportions calculated from a sample are less and less likely to differ from their theoretical values (0.125, 0.375, 0.375, or 0.125) as the number of observations increases.

TABLE 3.1: The relationship between sample size (k = number of tosses of three coins) and the theoretical probabilities (p_x).

Proportion	$k = 10$	$k = 20$	$k = 50$	$k = 500$	$k = 1,000$	$k = 10,000$	Expected value
no heads ($\hat{p}_0$)	0.2	0.2	0.04	0.108	0.143	0.128	$p_0 = 0.125$
one heads ($\hat{p}_1$)	0.4	0.3	0.46	0.406	0.358	0.378	$p_1 = 0.375$
two heads ($\hat{p}_2$)	0.3	0.5	0.36	0.358	0.368	0.373	$p_2 = 0.375$
three heads ($\hat{p}_3$)	0.1	0.1	0.14	0.128	0.131	0.121	$p_3 = 0.125$

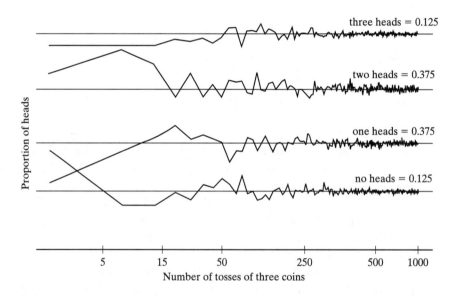

FIGURE 3.1: Plot of the results from tossing three coins k times where k ranges from 5 to 1000 tosses.

It follows that, as sample size increases, the increasingly more precise values of the relative frequencies produce a sample mean value that is increasingly more likely to reflect the mean of the sampled probability distribution (expected value). Table 3.2 illustrates this property using the relative frequencies from the previous computer coin tossing data (Table 3.1).

For example, $\bar{x} = \sum \hat{p}_i x_i = 0.04(0) + 0.46(1) + 0.36(2) + 0.14(3) = 1.600$ for $k = 50$.

TABLE 3.2: The relationship between sample size (k = number of tosses of three coins) and the expected value $E(X)$.

Sample mean	$k = 10$	$k = 20$	$k = 50$	$k = 500$	$k = 1,000$	$k = 10,000$	Expected value
$\bar{x}$	1.300	1.400	1.600	1.506	1.487	1.487	$E(X) = 1.500$

The probability that a sample mean differs from its expected value is largest for a sample of one observation and decreases for each observation added to the sample of data. The phenomenon that the probability of a difference between an estimate and its expected value decreases as the number of observations increases is at the center of statistics in general. Events that are random, capricious, and unanticipated, when observed for a large group, become systematic, stable, and predictable.

ANOTHER EXAMPLE

From the earlier illustration (Chapters 2 and 3) of drawing of red and black cards from a special deck of nine cards with replacement, the expected number of black cards is

$$E(X) = \sum_{all\ x} p_x x = p_0(0) + p_1(1) + p_2(2) + p_3(3) + p_4(4) + p_5(5)$$
$$= 0.053(0) + 0.212(1) + 0.339(2) + 0.271(3) + 0.108(4) + 0.017(5)$$
$$= 2.222.$$

Although no set of five cards contains 2.222 black cards, the expected value of 2.222 is the "average" number of black cards among the five cards drawn that would occur in the "long-run." Thus, after drawing hundreds or, perhaps, thousands of five-card sets, the mean number of black cards per set would be essentially equal to the expected value of 2.222. It is the mean ("balancing point") of the probability distribution even though the specific value is not a possible outcome. Incidentally, the expected number of red cards among the five cards drawn is $5 - 2.222 = 2.778$.   ∎

Two properties of the expected value of a probability distribution

Once again details:

1. If a constant value is added to a random variable producing a new random value $X + c$, then $E(X + c) = E(X) + c$ (Box 3.1) when c is a constant value (a nonrandom value).

Box 3.1. $E(X + c) = ?$

$$E(X + c) = \sum_{all\ x} p_x(x + c) = \sum_{all\ x} p_x x + c \sum_{all\ x} p_x = E(X) + c.$$

Note: $\sum_{all\ x} p_x = 1.0$ is a property of probability distributions when the p_x-values are probabilities from a set of mutually exclusive and exhaustive events.

The sample mean has a similar property. The mean value of the n observations $x_i + c$ is $\bar{x} + c$ (Chapter 1).

2. If a random variable is multiplied by a constant producing a new random value aX, then $E(aX) = aE(X)$ when a is a constant value (Box 3.2).

Box 3.2. $E(aX) = ?$

$$E(aX) = \sum_{all\ x} a p_x x = a \sum_{all\ x} p_x x = aE(X).$$

Again, the sample mean has a similar property. The mean value of the n observations ax_i is $a\bar{x}$ (Chapter 1). To summarize these two properties of the expected value, $E(aX + c) = aE(X) + c$.

The expected value $E(X)$ is a fixed quantity, as mentioned, and $\bar{x}$ is not. The sample mean $\bar{x}$, however, is an estimate of the expected value. It typically differs, at least to some extent, from the $E(X)$ because sampled values vary from sample to sample (subject to sampling variation). The extent of this variation and the relationship of $\bar{x}$ to $E(X)$ is a topic that is pursued further, particularly in Chapter 4.

Measure of dispersion—variance of a probability distribution

Perhaps the most fundamental characteristic of a probability distribution is its mean. An additionally important characteristic is its variability. As with the sample mean value, the expected value does not usually indicate the variability associated with a probability distribution.

The variance of the discrete random variable X (denoted σ_X^2), defined as

$$\sigma_X^2 = \sum_{all\ x} p_x [x - E(X)]^2,$$

measures the variability associated with a probability distribution. This measure of the variation is a weighted average of squared deviations of all possible observations of x from its expected value. The corresponding probabilities p_x serve as weights (again, weights $= w_x = p_x$). In some contexts the variance associated with a probability distribution is referred to as the *population variance*.

EXAMPLE

For example, for the previous coin tossing probability distribution, the population variance is

$$\sigma_X^2 = \sum_{all\ x} p_x[x - E(X)]^2 = 0.125(0 - 1.5)^2 + 0.375(1 - 1.5)^2$$

$$+ 0.375(2 - 1.5)^2 + 0.125(3 - 1.5)^2 = 0.75.$$

Like the expected value, the variance is a fixed quantity that depends only on the values of x (for example, 0, 1, 2, or 3) and the probabilities p_x (for example, 0.125, 0.375, 0.375, or 0.125). As the name population variance suggests, the variance of a probability distribution does not involve sampled observations. ■

The relationship just discussed between $\bar{x}$ and $E(X)$, similarly exists between the sample variance (S_X^2) and the variance of a random variable X (σ_X^2). The elements of the population variance have parallel elements in the expression for the sample variance (Chapter 1) where

$$S_X^2 = \sum \left[\frac{f_i}{n-1}\right](x_i - \bar{x})^2 \approx \sum \hat{p}_i(x_i - \bar{x})^2.$$

The quantity $f_i/(n-1)$ is approximately equal to the relative frequency $f_i/n = \hat{p}_i$ especially for a large sample size n and the sample mean $\bar{x}$ plays the same role as the expected value $E(X)$. The variance σ_X^2 calculated from a probability distribution has much the same interpretation as the variance S_X^2 calculated from a sample of data.

As with the relationship between $\bar{x}$ and $E(X)$, the estimated value S_X^2 is subject to sampling variation and the population variance σ_X^2 is not. Again, more precise relative frequencies produce an estimated sample variance that more precisely reflects the population variance. In other words, as the sample size increases, the sample estimate S_X^2 is less and less likely to differ from the population value σ_X^2. Table 3.3 based on the previous "tossing of three coins" data illustrates.

The standard deviation associated with the probability distribution of X is

$$\text{the square root of the variance of } X = \sqrt{\sigma_X^2} = \sigma_X.$$

The variance associated with the probability distribution generated by tossing three coins is $\sigma_X^2 = 0.75$, making the standard deviation $\sigma_X = \sqrt{0.75} = 0.866$.

TABLE 3.3: The relationship between sample size (k = number of tosses of three coins) and the population variance σ_X^2.

Sample variance	$k = 10$	$k = 20$	$k = 50$	$k = 500$	$k = 1,000$	$k = 10,000$	Population value
S_X^2	0.810	0.840	0.600	0.722	0.798	0.748	$\sigma_X^2 = 0.750$

For example, the sample variance $S_X^2 \approx 0.04(0 - 1.600)^2 + 0.46(1 - 1.600)^2 + 0.36(2 - 1.600)^2 + 0.14(3 - 1.600)^2 = 0.600$ for $k = 50$.

Two properties of the variance of a probability distribution

1. Adding a constant value to a random variable X does not affect the original population variance or $\sigma_{X+c}^2 = \sigma_X^2$ (Box 3.3).

Box 3.3. $\sigma_{X+c}^2 = ?$

$$\sigma_{X+c}^2 = \sum_{all\ x} p_x[x + c - E(X + c)]^2 = \sum_{all\ x} p_x[x - E(X)]^2 = \sigma_X^2$$

---

2. Multiplying a random variable X by a constant value multiplies the original population variance by a factor equal to the square of the constant or $\sigma_{aX}^2 = a^2\sigma_X^2$ (Box 3.4).

Box 3.4. $\sigma_{aX}^2 = ?$

$$\sigma_{aX}^2 = \sum_{all\ x} p_x[ax - aE(X)]^2 = \sum_{all\ x} p_x a^2[x - E(X)]^2$$

$$= a^2 \sum_{all\ x} p_x[x - E(X)]^2 = a^2\sigma_X^2$$

A clear parallel exists between the sample variance where $S_{aX+c}^2 = a^2 S_X^2$ (Chapter 1) and the population variance where $\sigma_{aX+c}^2 = a^2\sigma_X^2$. This property of the sample and population variances is unexpectedly important in developing a number of statistical relationships in this chapter and beyond.

Examples of $E(X)$ and σ_X^2

EXAMPLE

Toss a fair coin once. Suppose $X = 0$ represents the occurrence of tails making $p_0 = P(X = 0) = 1/2$ and $X = 1$ represents the occurrence of heads making $p_1 = P(X = 1) = 1/2$, yielding perhaps the simplest possible probability distribution. The expected value of the distribution of the random variable X is

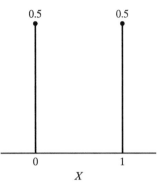

$$E(X) = \sum_{\text{all } x} p_x x = (1/2)(0) + (1/2)(1) = 1/2$$

and the variance of this binary random variable is

$$\sigma_X^2 = \sum_{\text{all } x} p_x [x - E(X)]^2 = (1/2)(0 - 1/2)^2 + (1/2)(1 - 1/2)^2 = 1/4.$$

Notice that the expected value and the variance depend only on the coin being fair $[P(heads) = P(tails) = 1/2]$ and does not involve sampled observations. ∎

In general, for any binary variable X where $P(X = 0) = 1 - p$ and $P(X = 1) = p$, then the expected value is

$$E(X) = (1 - p)(0) + (p)(1) = p$$

and the variance is

$$\sigma_X^2 = (1 - p)(0 - p)^2 + p(1 - p)^2 = [p^2 + p(1 - p)](1 - p) = p(1 - p).$$

EXAMPLE

Toss a fair die once. Define the random variable X as the number on the up-face of the die, then, as before, $x = 1, 2, 3, 4, 5,$ or 6 and $p_x = P(X = x) = 1/6$

for each value of x. The mean value of this probability distribution is

$$E(X) = \sum_{all\ x} p_x x = (1/6)(1) + (1/6)(2) + (1/6)(3) + (1/6)(4)$$

$$+ (1/6)(5) + (1/6)(6)$$

$$= 21/6 = 3.5$$

with a variance of

$$\sigma_X^2 = \sum_{all\ x} p_x [x - E(X)]^2 = (1/6)(1 - 3.5)^2 + (1/6)(2 - 3.5)^2$$

$$+ (1/6)(3 - 3.5)^2 + (1/6)(4 - 3.5)^2 + (1/6)(5 - 3.5)^2$$

$$+ (1/6)(6 - 3.5)^2 = 35/12.$$

Probability distribution for one toss of a die.

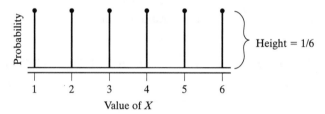

Height = 1/6

Value of X

EXAMPLE

Genetic cross of two heterozygous individuals (Aa × Aa) gives the probability distribution where

$Y = 0$ represents no A-genes inherited by an offspring (aa) and $p_0 = 1/4$

$Y = 1$ represents one A-gene inherited by an offspring (Aa) and $p_1 = 1/2$

$Y = 2$ represents two A-genes inherited by an offspring (AA) and $p_2 = 1/4$

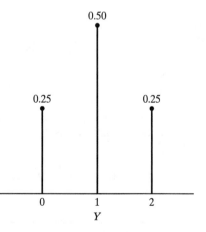

then, the expected number of A-genes inherited by an offspring is

$$E(Y) = \sum_{all\ y} p_y y = (1/4)(0) + (1/2)(1) + (1/4)(2) = 1.0$$

and the variance is

$$\sigma_Y^2 = \sum_{all\ y} p_y[y - E(Y)]^2 = (1/4)(0-1)^2 + (1/2)(1-1)^2 + (1/4)(2-1)^2 = 1/2.$$

∎

EXAMPLE

A simplified slot machine has four outcomes:

{*   *   *} is the event no bars; the casino pays 0 and $p_0 = 87/100$,
{bar   *   *} is the event one bar; the casino pays \$1.00 and $p_1 = 1/10$,
{bar   bar   *} is the event two bars; the casino pays \$5.00 and
                   $p_2 = 1/50$, and
{bar   bar   bar} is the event three bars; the casino pays \$10.00 and
                   $p_3 = 1/100$.

Suppose the random variable X represents the amount paid by the casino (won by a player), then

$$P(X = 0) = p_0 = \frac{87}{100}$$

$$P(X = \$1.00) = p_1 = \frac{1}{10}$$

$$P(X = \$5.00) = p_2 = \frac{1}{50}$$

$$P(X = \$10.00) = p_3 = \frac{1}{100}$$

is the probability distribution associated with the casino payoffs from this slot machine. What is the expected payoff? (Statistically: What is the mean of the probability distribution that describes the random variable X?) Answer:

$$E(X) = \sum_{all\ x} p_x x = \left(\frac{87}{100}\right)\$0 + \left(\frac{1}{10}\right)\$1 + \left(\frac{1}{50}\right)\$5 + \left(\frac{1}{100}\right)\$10 = \$0.30.$$

An expected payoff of $0.30 requires the casino to pay, in the "long-run," a mean of thirty cents each time the machine is played. No single payoff is thirty cents but the expected value is thirty cents. Thus, thirty cents is the theoretical cost to the casino over a large (actually infinite) number of times the machine is played. In statistical terms, it is the mean of the probability distribution describing the payoffs of the slot machine. In nonstatistical terms, when the casino charges $0.50 to play, it makes the considerable profit of $0.20, again in the "long-run."

The variance associated with the probability distribution of the random variable X is

$$\sigma_X^2 = \frac{87}{100}(0-0.30)^2 + \frac{1}{10}(1-0.30)^2 + \frac{1}{50}(5-0.30)^2 + \frac{1}{100}(10-0.30)^2 = 1.51.$$

The utility of variances, such as the value 1.51, will be taken up in Chapter 4. ■

EXAMPLE

A species of turtle (*Selvinis fictionus*) always lays exactly four eggs. This turtle has two strategies for nest building:

>Strategy A: build one nest for all four eggs, or
>Strategy B: build four separate nests, one for each of the four eggs.

Suppose a predator has a probability p of finding a single nest and destroying all the eggs in that nest. Define the random variable S as the number of surviving eggs. Which of the two strategies yields the highest expected number of surviving eggs, the highest $E(S)$?

Assuming that finding nests are independent events, then the expected values are:

>Strategy A: the values of S are $s = 0$ or 4 where $p_0 = P(S = 0) = p$ and $p_1 = P(S = 4) = 1 - p$ giving

$$E(S) = \sum_{all\ s} p_s s = (p)0 + (1 - p)4 = 4(1 - p).$$

>Strategy B: the values of S are $s = 0, 1, 2, 3,$ or 4 giving

$$E(S) = \sum_{all\ s} p_s s = [p^4]0 + [4p^3(1 - p)]1 + [6p^2(1 - p)^2]2$$
$$+ [4p(1 - p)^3]3 + [(1 - p)^4]4$$
$$= 4(1 - p).$$

The expected number of surviving eggs is the same for the one-nest (A) and four-nest (B) strategies. For example, if $p = 0.25$, then the expected number of surviving eggs is $E(S) = 4(0.75) = 3.0$ for both strategies.

The variances associated with these two strategies are:

Strategy A:

$$\sigma_S^2 = \sum_{\text{all } s} p_s[s - E(S)]^2 = p[0 - 4(1-p)]^2 + (1-p)[4 - 4(1-p)]^2$$

$$= 16p(1-p)$$

Strategy B:

$$\sigma_S^2 = \sum_{\text{all } s} p_s[s - E(S)]^2 = p^4[0 - 4(1-p)]^2 + 4p^3(1-p)[1 - 4(1-p)]^2$$

$$+ 6p^2(1-p)^2[2 - 4(1-p)]^2 + 4p(1-p)^3[3 - 4(1-p)]^2$$

$$+ (1-p)^4[4 - 4(1-p)]^2 = 4p(1-p).$$

Again, for $p = 0.25$, the variance for strategy A is $\sigma_S^2 = 3.0$ and for strategy B is $\sigma_S^2 = 0.75$.

Both strategies yield the same expected number of surviving eggs, namely $4(1-p)$. But, strategy A incurs four times the variability of strategy B, regardless of the value of p. In other words, the extremes (all eggs survive and all eggs are destroyed) are far more likely for strategy A than for strategy B. So when people say "don't put all your eggs in one basket," somewhat surprisingly, they are giving advice based on the variance and not the expected value. For $p = 0.25$, the two probability distributions are

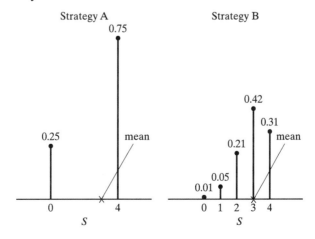

Summary of the notation:

Sample	Probability distribution
sample size $= n$	sample size not relevant
relative frequency $= f_i/n = \hat{p}_i$	probability $= p_x$
sample mean $= \bar{x}$	population mean $= E(X)$
sample variance $= S_X^2$	population variance $= \sigma_X^2$
sample standard deviation $= S_X$	population standard deviation $= \sigma_X$

Joint probability distribution

The probability that the composite event A and B occurs is denoted as $P(AB)$, which is a more compact version of $P(A$ and $B)$, as before (Chapter 2). The events A and B can represent two random variables X and Y simultaneously taking on two specific numeric values. For example, X can represent the value on the first roll of a die and Y can represent the value on the second roll of a die. The variable X takes on the values $x = 1, 2, 3, 4, 5$, or 6 and, identically, the variable Y takes on the values $y = 1, 2, 3, 4, 5$, or 6. A joint probability has the form

$$P(X = a\ specific\ value\ \text{and}\ Y = a\ specific\ value) = P(X = x_i\ \text{and}\ Y = y_j).$$

The probability of this special kind of composite event is denoted p_{ij}.

EXAMPLE

Suppose a die is tossed twice (or two dice are tossed once) where X represents {*number on first toss*} and Y represents {*number on second toss*}, then all possible $6 \times 6 = 36$ joint outcomes of X and Y are:

		Second toss $= Y$					
		$Y = 1$	$Y = 2$	$Y = 3$	$Y = 4$	$Y = 5$	$Y = 6$
	$X = 1$	(1 and 1)	(1 and 2)	(1 and 3)	(1 and 4)	(1 and 5)	(1 and 6)
	$X = 2$	(2 and 1)	(2 and 2)	(2 and 3)	(2 and 4)	(2 and 5)	(2 and 6)
first	$X = 3$	(3 and 1)	(3 and 2)	(3 and 3)	(3 and 4)	(3 and 5)	(3 and 6)
toss $= X$	$X = 4$	(4 and 1)	(4 and 2)	(4 and 3)	(4 and 4)	(4 and 5)	(4 and 6)
	$X = 5$	(5 and 1)	(5 and 2)	(5 and 3)	(5 and 4)	(5 and 5)	(5 and 6)
	$X = 6$	(6 and 1)	(6 and 2)	(6 and 3)	(6 and 4)	(6 and 5)	(6 and 6)

For each roll of the two dice, every pair of up-faces is mutually exclusive and equally likely. The 36 joint probabilities are, therefore, 1/36 for every possible pair of outcomes [$p_{ij} = P(X = i\ \text{and}\ Y = j) = 1/36$]. For example, the probability of a four on the first die and a three on the second die is $p_{43} = P(X = 4 \text{ and } Y = 3) = 1/36$. The collection of all possible probabilities p_{ij} is called the *joint probability distribution* of the random variables X and Y. ■

An important case arises when the two random variables under consideration are independent.

EXAMPLE

Suppose X represents selecting a value at random from the probability distribution given by

$$p_1 = P(X = 1) = 0.1 \qquad p_3 = P(X = 3) = 0.3$$
$$p_2 = P(X = 2) = 0.2 \qquad p_4 = P(X = 4) = 0.4.$$

The probabilities p_x denote the probability that $x = 0, 1, 2, 3,$ or 4 is selected. Suppose Y represents a second value independently and randomly selected from the same probability distribution. The symbols $q_1, q_2, q_3,$ and q_4 denote the probabilities that $y = 1, 2, 3,$ or 4 on the second selection. Since the variables X and Y are independent, the $4 \times 4 = 16$ joint probabilities are $p_{ij} = P(X = i$ and $Y = j) = P(X = i)P(Y = j) = p_i q_j$ (Chapter 2). The complete joint probability distribution is

	$P(Y = 1)$	$P(Y = 2)$	$P(Y = 3)$	$P(Y = 4)$	Marginal probabilities
$P(X = 1)$	$p_{11} = 0.01$	$p_{12} = 0.02$	$p_{13} = 0.03$	$p_{14} = 0.04$	$p_1 = 0.1$
$X = $ first $P(X = 2)$	$p_{21} = 0.02$	$p_{22} = 0.04$	$p_{23} = 0.06$	$p_{24} = 0.08$	$p_2 = 0.2$
selection $P(X = 3)$	$p_{31} = 0.03$	$p_{32} = 0.06$	$p_{33} = 0.09$	$p_{34} = 0.12$	$p_3 = 0.3$
$P(X = 4)$	$p_{41} = 0.04$	$p_{42} = 0.08$	$p_{43} = 0.12$	$p_{44} = 0.16$	$p_4 = 0.4$
marginal probabilities	$q_1 = 0.1$	$q_2 = 0.2$	$q_3 = 0.3$	$q_4 = 0.4$	1.0

$Y = $ second selection

The joint probability p_{ij} is found in the ith-row and the jth-column. For example, $p_{23} = P(X = 2 \text{ and } Y = 3) = P(X = 2)P(Y = 3) = p_2 \times q_3 = (0.2)(0.3) = 0.06.$ ■

The *marginal probabilities* (sums of the rows and sums of the columns*) are the probability distributions of X (rows) and Y (columns), respectively. In

NOTE: The subscripts, i and j, indicate the probability in the ith-row and j^{th}-column, respectively. The value represented by p_{12}, for example, is found in the first row and second column ($p_{12} = 0.02$). Rules for the summation of values with two subscripts are given in Appendix B.1.

symbols, the marginal probabilities are, for example,

$$p_{11} + p_{12} + p_{13} + p_{14} = p_1 = 0.1, \text{ and}$$
$$p_{21} + p_{22} + p_{23} + p_{24} = p_2 = 0.2$$

also

$$p_{11} + p_{21} + p_{31} + p_{41} = q_1 = 0.1, \text{ and}$$
$$p_{12} + p_{22} + p_{32} + p_{42} = q_2 = 0.2.$$

As before, $p_1 + p_2 + p_3 + p_4 = q_1 + q_2 + q_3 + q_4 = 0.1 + 0.2 + 0.3 + 0.4 = 1.0$.

When two random variables are independent, the joint probability distribution (probabilities p_{ij}) can be calculated from the individual probability distributions $p_1, p_2, p_3, \cdots$ and $q_1, q_2, q_3, \cdots$. Each joint probability is

$$p_{ij} = P(X = x_i \text{ and } Y = y_j) = P(X = x_i)P(Y = y_j) = p_i \times q_j.$$

The special case of independence is the focus of the following discussion of the joint probability distribution and is the basis for several central properties of the sample mean value. When the random variables X and Y are not independent, the probabilities p_{ij} cannot be determined from the marginal probabilities p_i and q_j (discussed in Chapters 7 and 8). Incidentally, when two dice are tossed independently, the joint distribution (first example) can also be created from the marginal probabilities.

Expectation of a sum of random variables

It should come as no surprise that the sum of a series of random variables (denoted S) is itself a random variable and has its own probability distribution. For example, if X and Y again represent random variables each described by a probability distribution, then the sum $S = X + Y$ has a probability distribution. Again not surprisingly, the properties of the variables that make up the sum determine the properties of the probability distribution describing the sum S. The probability distribution of the sum is the primary topic of the rest of this chapter and the next. To start, it is important to consider the mean (expected value) and the variance of the probability distribution that results from adding two or more independent random variables.

The simplest sum consists of two random variables, $S = X + Y$, and the sum S has its own probability distribution. The mean of this probability distribution is $E(S) = E(X + Y)$ and $E(S) = E(X + Y) = E(X) + E(Y)$ (Box 3.5). Remarkably, the expected value of a sum is simply equal to the sum of the individual expected values that make up the sum.

Box 3.5. Expectation of a Sum

To show: $E(X + Y) = E(X) + E(Y)$

$$E(X + Y) = \sum_i \sum_j p_{ij}(x_i + y_j) = \sum_i \sum_j p_{ij} x_i + \sum_i \sum_j p_{ij} y_j$$

$$= \sum_i \left(\sum_j p_{ij} \right) x_i + \sum_j \left(\sum_i p_{ij} \right) y_j$$

$$= \sum_i p_i x_i + \sum_j q_j y_j = E(X) + E(Y)$$

Note: $\sum_j p_{ij} = p_i$ and $\sum_i p_{ij} = q_j$ are the marginal probabilities.

In general, if $X_1, X_2, \cdots , X_n$ are n random variables, then the sum is a random variable represented by

$$S = X_1 + X_2 + \cdots + X_n.$$

Since values of X_i vary from sample to sample, the values of S also vary from sample to sample. To repeat, the variation of S is described by its own probability distribution. The probability distribution of S, like all probability distributions, has a mean value [expected value, denoted $E(S)$] and a variance (denoted σ_S^2). The mean value of the probability distribution of the sum S is

$$E(S) = E(X_1 + X_2 + \cdots + X_n) = E(X_1) + E(X_2) + \cdots + E(X_n).$$

Notice the important property that the expectation of a sum of a series of random variables can be calculated directly without specific knowledge of the probability distribution of the sum of the random variables. The expectation of a sum of random variables is the sum of the individual expectations of each component of the sum, the values $E(X_i)$. If the expectation of X_1 is 7 and the expectation of X_2 is 3 [$E(X_1) = 7$ and $E(X_2) = 3$], then the expectation of the random variable $S = X_1 + X_2$ is 10 [$E(S) = E(X_1 + X_2) = E(X_1) + E(X_2) = 7 + 3 = 10$], regardless of the joint distribution of X_1 and X_2.

More generally, if $a_1 X_1, a_2 X_2, \cdots , a_n X_n$ are n random variables, each multiplied by a constant value a_i, then the mean of the probability distribution of the sum of these random variables ($S = a_1 x_1 + a_2 x_2 + \cdots + a_n x_n = \sum a_i x_i$) is

$$E(S) = E(a_1 X_1 + a_2 X_2 + \cdots + a_n X_n) = a_1 E(X_1) + a_2 E(X_2) + \cdots + a_n E(X_n)$$

where, as always, $E(a_i X_i) = a_i E(X_i)$ (Box 3.2). Using the more compact summation notation,

$$E(S) = E\left(\sum a_i X_i\right) = \sum E(a_i X_i) = \sum a_i E(X_i)$$

(Box 3.2 is a special case).

Knowledge of the joint distribution is not necessary and no reference is made to the probability distribution of S to calculate the mean (expected value) of a sum.

Variance of a sum of independent random variables

If X and Y again represent two independent random variables, then the variance of the sum $S = X + Y$ (denoted σ_S^2 or σ_{X+Y}^2) is

$$\sigma_S^2 = \sigma_{X+Y}^2 = \sigma_X^2 + \sigma_Y^2.$$

A justification for this property appears later (Chapter 8—Box 8.2). Parallel to the calculation of an expected value of a sum, the variance of a sum of two independent random variables is the sum of the individual variances of the variables that make up the sum. Thus, the variance of the probability distribution describing $S = X + Y$ (denoted σ_S^2) is simply $\sigma_X^2 + \sigma_Y^2$.

In general, if $X_1, X_2, \cdots, X_n$ are n independent random variables each multiplied by a constant a_i, then the variance of the distribution describing the sum of these variables ($S = a_1 x_1 + a_2 x_2 + \cdots + a_n x_n = \sum a_i x_i$) is

$$\sigma_S^2 = \sigma_{a_1 X_1 + a_2 X_2 + \cdots + a_n X_n}^2$$
$$= \sigma_{a_1 X_1}^2 + \sigma_{a_2 X_2}^2 + \cdots + \sigma_{a_n X_n}^2$$
$$= a_1^2 \sigma_{X_1}^2 + a_2^2 \sigma_{X_2}^2 + \cdots + a_n^2 \sigma_{X_n}^2$$

where, as always, $\sigma_{a_i X_i}^2 = a_i^2 \sigma_{X_i}^2$ (Box 3.4). More concisely,

$$\sigma_S^2 = \sigma_{\sum a_i X_i}^2 = \sum \sigma_{a_i X_i}^2 = \sum a_i^2 \sigma_{X_i}^2 \qquad \text{(Box 8.2).}$$

As with the expected value of a sum, the variance of a sum is the variance of the probability distribution describing the variability of the summary variable S.

The expected value of the distribution of a sum of random variables is the sum of the individual expectations whether or not the variables are independent. The variance of this probability distribution is the sum of the individual variances only when the random variables are independent. When the random variables are independent, computation of the variance of a sum, like the expected value, does not require reference to the joint probability distribution of the random variables being considered or to the probability distribution of the sum S itself.

For most samples of observations, the joint probability distribution is extremely complex making the calculation of a complete description of the probability distribution of S difficult even for a sum made up of a few sampled values and impossible for a sum containing a large number of values. The fact that the expectation and variance of a distribution of a sum of independent observations can be calculated without dealing with the complex and certainly tedious calculations of a joint probability distribution makes many statistical techniques simple and easy to apply. Without this property of a sum of sampled values, statistical analysis would be an obscure and a rather useless topic, perhaps to the delight of some.

Examples

The next two examples illustrate, in simple cases, the calculation of the expected value and variance of the distribution of a sum of two independent random variables. First, these two quantities are calculated from the probability distribution of the sum of two random variables (a task that requires a bit of effort). Second, they are calculated directly from the individual expectations and variances of the values that make up the sum (a task that requires almost no effort). For the remainder of the text, only the second approach is used because it is simple, direct, and easy. The joint probability distribution and the probability distribution of a sum, however, continue to be basic elements in understanding statistical methods. The important property, to repeat, is that their explicit descriptions are not necessary to calculate the mean value and variance of the probability distribution of a sum.

EXAMPLE

Consider again the probability distribution where $p_x = P(X = x) = x/10$ for $x = 1, 2, 3,$ or 4. Then, for the random variable X, a sampled value from this distribution, the expected value and the variance are

$$E(X) = 0.1(1) + 0.2(2) + 0.3(3) + 0.4(4) = 3.0$$

and

$$\sigma_X^2 = 0.1(1-3)^2 + 0.2(2-3)^2 + 0.3(3-3)^2 + 0.4(4-3)^2 = 1.0.$$

Consider a second independent value Y sampled from the same probability distribution. Then, necessarily $E(Y) = E(X) = 3.0$ and $\sigma_Y^2 = \sigma_X^2 = 1.0$.

The joint probability distribution of X and Y (16 p_{ij}-values) is given in an earlier example. This joint distribution allows the calculation of the probability distribution describing the random variable $S = X + Y$ or

$S = X + Y$	$S = 2$	$S = 3$	$S = 4$	$S = 5$	$S = 6$	$S = 7$	$S = 8$	Total
$P(S = s) = p_s$	0.01	0.04	0.10	0.20	0.25	0.24	0.16	1.0

For example, from the previously derived joint probability distribution, $P(S = 4) = P(X = 1)P(Y = 3) + P(X = 2)P(Y = 2) + P(X = 3)P(Y = 1) = p_{13} + p_{22} + p_{31} = 0.03 + 0.04 + 0.03 = 0.10$. The probability distribution of the random variable S is

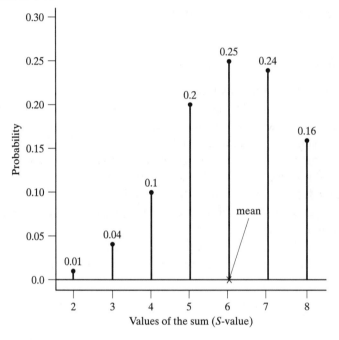

Now, the mean and variance of the probability distribution describing the random variable S, calculated in the usual way from the explicit probability distribution of S (the p_s-values), are

$$E(S) = \sum p_s = 0.01(2) + 0.04(3) + 0.10(4) + 0.20(5) + 0.25(6)$$
$$+ 0.24(7) + 0.16(8) = 6.0$$

and

$$\sigma_S^2 = \sum p_s[s - E(S)]^2 = 0.01(2 - 6)^2 + 0.04(3 - 6)^2 + 0.10(4 - 6)^2$$
$$+ 0.20(5 - 6)^2 + 0.25(6 - 6)^2 + 0.24(7 - 6)^2 + 0.16(8 - 6)^2 = 2.0.$$

These two values are also found directly and simply. The expected value is

$$E(S) = E(X + Y) = E(X) + E(Y) = 3.0 + 3.0 = 6.0.$$

Because X and Y are independent observations, the variance of S is

$$\sigma_S^2 = \sigma_{X+Y}^2 = \sigma_X^2 + \sigma_Y^2 = 1.0 + 1.0 = 2.0.$$

Both values are calculated without reference to the joint probabilities (16 joint probabilities p_{ij}) or the probability distribution of the random variable S (seven probabilities p_s). ∎

EXAMPLE

Suppose X represents the number observed on the first toss of a die and Y represents the number observed on the independent second toss of a die and, furthermore, it is the properties of the probability distribution of the sum of these two tosses that are of interest. Then, the sum $S = X + Y$ has the probability distribution shown below

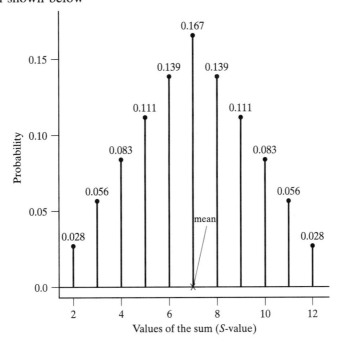

The expected value and variance of the probability distribution describing the random variable S, as before, can be calculated directly from the probability distribution of S. The explicit probability distribution of S is

$S = X + Y$	2	3	4	5	6	7	8	9	10	11	12	Total
$P(S = s) = p_s$	1/36	2/36	3/36	4/36	5/36	6/36	5/36	4/36	3/36	2/36	1/36	1.0

These probabilities result from adding the appropriate joint probabilities associated with tossing a pair of dice (a previously given example of a joint probability distribution). For example, there are four mutually exclusive ways a sum of five $(S = 5)$ can occur. The probability that the sum of five occurs is then $P(S = 5) = P(X = 1 \text{ and } Y = 4) + P(X = 2 \text{ and } Y = 3) + P(X = 3 \text{ and } Y = 2) + P(X = 4 \text{ and } Y = 1) = 1/36 + 1/36 + 1/36 + 1/36 = 4/36$.

The expected value and variance calculated directly from the probability distribution of S are

$$E(S) = \sum p_s s = (1/36)(2) + (2/36)(3) + \cdots + (1/36)(12) = 7.0$$

and

$$\sigma_S^2 = \sum p_s [s - E(S)]^2$$
$$= (1/36)(2 - 7.0)^2 + (2/36)(3 - 7.0)^2 + \cdots + (1/36)(12 - 7.0)^2 = \frac{35}{6}.$$

The expectation and the variance of the sum S are again readily calculated without reference to the joint probability distribution of X and Y or the probability distribution of S itself. Since $E(X) = E(Y) = 3.5$ and $\sigma_X^2 = \sigma_Y^2 = 35/12$ (previously calculated), then

$$E(S) = E(X + Y) = E(X) + E(Y) = 3.5 + 3.5 = 7.0$$

and

$$\sigma_S^2 = \sigma_{X+Y}^2 = \sigma_X^2 + \sigma_Y^2 = \frac{35}{12} + \frac{35}{12} = \frac{35}{6}$$

which are, as required, the same values calculated from the probability distribution of the sum (S). ■

As emphasized, calculating a joint probability distribution and the corresponding probability distribution of the sum S is certainly complex for samples of more than a few observations. When the random variables are independent, the expected value and variance of the distribution of a sum, however, are computed directly from the expected values and variances of each variable that make up the sum and, as illustrated, it is unnecessary to calculate either the joint probability distribution of the components or derive the probability distribution of the sum.

EXAMPLE

When three dice are tossed at once (a gambling game called chuck-a-luck popular during the gold rush years in California), the joint distribution is made up of $6 \times 6 \times 6 = 216$ joint probabilities. The calculation of the distribution of the sum of the three values observed on a single toss involves different combinations of these 216 probabilities. Nevertheless, the mean of the probability distribution describing possible sums of three dice is

$$E(S) = E(X_1 + X_2 + X_3) = E(X_1) + E(X_2) + E(X_3) = 3(3.5) = 10.5$$

and the variance of this probability distribution is

$$\sigma_S^2 = \sigma_{X_1+X_2+X_3}^2 = \sigma_{X_1}^2 + \sigma_{X_2}^2 + \sigma_{X_3}^2 = 3\left(\frac{35}{12}\right) = 8.75.$$

The probability distribution for the chuck-a-luck game is shown below

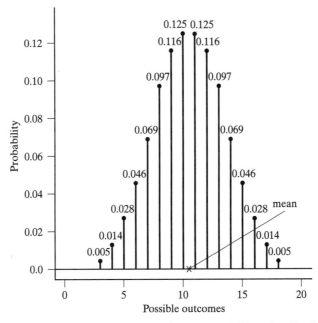

In fact, the mean and the variance of the probability distribution describing the sum (S) observed from tossing any number of independent dice are $E(S) = n(3.5)$ and $\sigma_S^2 = n(35/12)$ for n dice. ∎

Independent and identically distributed random variables

The phrase *independent and identically distributed random variables* describes a special and common kind of sampled observation. Observations are, in general, independent and identically distributed when each value is selected independently from the same probability distribution. That is, each observation sampled is unrelated to any other sampled observation and the sampled population is unchanged by the sampling process. Naturally, the expectation and variance of each sample value also remains unchanged. All observations then yield exactly the same information concerning the population sampled.

EXAMPLE

Suppose X represents a toss of a fair coin. A sample of three independent tosses each with the probability of heads equal to 1/2 constitutes a sample of three independent and identically distributed observations. Because the tosses (denoted X_1, X_2, and X_3) are sampled from the same unchanging population, it follows that $E(X_1) = E(X_2) = E(X_3) = E(X) = 1/2$ and $\sigma_{X_1}^2 = \sigma_{X_2}^2 = \sigma_{X_3}^3 = \sigma_X^2 = 1/4$, as previously calculated. ∎

More generally, for n independent and identically distributed random variables, represented by $X_1, X_2, X_3, \cdots, X_n$, the expected value and variance of each sampled value is the same or

$$E(X_1) = E(X_2) = \cdots = E(X_n) = E(X) = \text{ population mean}$$

and

$$\sigma_{X_1}^2 = \sigma_{X_2}^2 = \cdots = \sigma_{X_n}^2 = \sigma_X^2 = \text{ population variance.}$$

The expressions for the mean and variance of the probability distribution of a sum of n independent and identically distributed random variables become

$$
\begin{aligned}
E(S) &= E(a_1 X_1 + a_2 X_2 + \cdots + a_n X_n) \\
&= a_1 E(X_1) + a_2 E(X_2) + \cdots + a_n E(X_n) \\
&= a_1 E(X) + a_2 E(X) + \cdots + a_n E(X) \\
&= (a_1 + a_2 + \cdots + a_n) E(X) \\
&= \left(\sum a_i \right) E(X)
\end{aligned}
$$

and

$$
\begin{aligned}
\sigma_S^2 &= \sigma_{a_1 X_1}^2 + \sigma_{a_2 X_2}^2 + \cdots + \sigma_{a_x X_n}^2 = a_1^2 \sigma_{X_1}^2 + a_2^2 \sigma_{X_2}^2 + \cdots + a_n^2 \sigma_{X_n}^2 \\
&= a_1^2 \sigma_X^2 + a_2^2 \sigma_X^2 + \cdots + a_n^2 \sigma_X^2 \\
&= (a_1^2 + a_1^2 + \cdots + a_n^2) \sigma_X^2 \\
&= \left(\sum a_i^2 \right) \sigma_X^2
\end{aligned}
$$

where a_i represents a constant value (not a random variable). Therefore, for a specified set of a_i-values, the expected value and the variance of a sum ($S = \sum a_i x_i$) are succinctly

$$E(S) = \left(\sum a_i \right) E(X) \qquad \text{and} \qquad \sigma_S^2 = \left(\sum a_i^2 \right) \sigma_X^2.$$

EXAMPLE

Suppose a fair coin is tossed 10 independent times where again $P(heads) = P(X_i = 1) = 1/2$ and $P(tails) = P(X_i = 0) = 1/2$ for each toss. Because each toss produces an independent and identically distributed observation,

$$E(X_1) = E(X_2) = E(X_3) = \cdots = E(X_{10}) = E(X) = 1/2$$

and

$$\sigma_{X_1}^2 = \sigma_{X_2}^2 = \sigma_{X_3}^2 = \cdots = \sigma_{X_{10}}^2 = \sigma_X^2 = 1/4$$

where $E(X) = 1/2$ and $\sigma_X^2 = 1/4$ are the mean and the variance of the population sampled (as previously calculated). The sum of these 10 independent and identically distributed binary variables is $S = X_1 + X_2 + X_3 + \cdots + X_{10}$ and is the number of heads in 10 tosses. The sum S itself is a random variable described by its own probability distribution (explicitly discussed in Chapter 4). The mean of this probability distribution is

$$E(S) = E(X_1) + E(X_2) + E(X_3) + \cdots + E(X_{10})$$
$$= 1/2 + 1/2 + 1/2 + \cdots + 1/2 = 10(1/2) = 5$$

and its variance is

$$\sigma_S^2 = \sigma_{X_1}^2 + \sigma_{X_2}^2 + \sigma_{X_3}^2 + \cdots + \sigma_{X_{10}}^2 = 1/4 + 1/4 + 1/4 + \cdots + 1/4 = 10(1/4) = 2.5.$$

Or, more succinctly, since $a_1 = a_2 = \cdots = a_{10} = 1$, making $\sum a_i = \sum a_i^2 = 10$, then

$$E(S) = \left(\sum a_i\right) E(X) = (10)(1/2) = 5 \quad \text{and}$$
$$\sigma_S^2 = \left(\sum a_i^2\right) \sigma_X^2 = (10)(1/4) = 2.5.$$

The probability distribution describing the number of heads in 10 independent tosses of a fair coin (the probability distribution of the sum S) is symmetric with a minimum of 0 and a maximum of 10 is displayed on the next page.

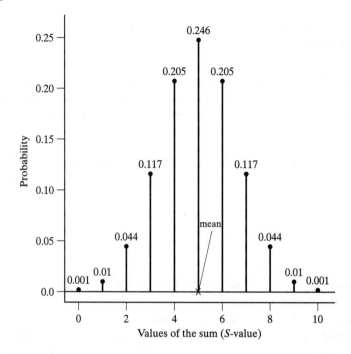

The expected value and variance are directly calculated from the population values $E(X) = 1/2$ and $\sigma_X^2 = 1/4$. Otherwise, the calculation of these two quantities involves a joint probability distribution with 2^{10} probabilities and the probability distribution of S itself.   ■

EXAMPLE

An illustration of the sum of non-independent and non-identically distributed random variables:

age	24 years
height	6 feet
weight	140 pounds
address	111 North Street

---

sum	$S = 24 + 6 + 140 + 111 = 281$

■

Expectation and variance of the sample mean

Like all sums of random variables, the sample mean has a probability distribution that, like all probability distributions, has its own mean and variance.

The observations $x_1, x_2, \cdots, x_n$ that make up a sample mean are frequently selected from the same and unchanging population. If the process of sampling these observations assures that the n selected values are independent, then the sample consists of n independent and identically distributed random variables.

Necessarily each sampled value then has the same expected value $E(X)$ and the same variance σ_X^2.

The sample mean value (weighted average, Chapter 1) is

$$\bar{x} = \frac{\sum a_i x_i}{\sum a_i} = \frac{1}{n}x_1 + \frac{1}{n}x_2 + \cdots + \frac{1}{n}x_n = \frac{1}{n}\sum x_i$$

where the weights are $a_1 = a_2 = \cdots = a_n = 1/n \left(\sum a_i = 1\right)$ and is a special case of the previous expression for the expected value and the variance of a sum of a series of independent and identically distributed random variables. Therefore, the expectation of the sample mean, denoted $E(\overline{X})$, is

$$E(\overline{X}) = \left(\sum a_i\right)E(X) = \left(\sum \frac{1}{n}\right)E(X) = n\left(\frac{1}{n}\right)E(X) = E(X)$$

$$\left[\sum a_i = \sum \frac{1}{n} = n\frac{1}{n} = 1\right].$$

The mean (the expected value) of the probability distribution describing the possible values of the sample mean and the mean of the population sampled are the same, $E(\overline{X}) = E(X)$.

The variance of the probability distribution describing the sample mean (denoted $\sigma_{\overline{X}}^2$) is (again, the weights are $a_1 = a_2 = \cdots = a_n = 1/n$)

$$\sigma_{\overline{X}}^2 = \left(\sum a_i^2\right)\sigma_X^2 = \sum \left(\frac{1}{n}\right)^2 \sigma_X^2 = n\left(\frac{1}{n}\right)^2 \sigma_X^2 = \left(\frac{1}{n}\right)\sigma_X^2$$

$$\left[\sum a_i^2 = \sum \left(\frac{1}{n}\right)^2 = n\frac{1}{n^2} = \frac{1}{n}\right].$$

The variance of the probability distribution of a sample mean is less than the variance of the distribution of the population sampled by a factor of n. In symbols, $\sigma_{\overline{X}}^2 = \sigma_X^2/n$. Miraculously, the expected value and the variance of the probability distribution describing the possible values of the sample mean is simply and directly calculated from the expected value and the variance of the population sampled.

The square root of the variance of the sample mean (denoted $\sigma_{\overline{X}}$) is the standard deviation of the probability distribution of the mean, which is sometimes called the *standard error of the mean*, and is

$$\sigma_{\overline{X}} = \sqrt{\sigma_{\overline{X}}^2} = \sqrt{\frac{\sigma_X^2}{n}} = \frac{\sigma_X}{\sqrt{n}}.$$

The variability of the sample mean decreases as the sample size increases because the averaging process typically balances observations greater than the mean with observations less than the mean producing a summary value likely closer to the population mean $E(X)$ than any single value. From another point of view, the averaging process decreases the likelihood of extreme values and increases the likelihood of "typical" values, which is just another way of saying that the variability associated with a sample mean value is reduced relative to the variance of the population sampled.

To clarify the properties of the distribution of the sample mean, envision the rather artificial situation where samples of size n are taken repeatedly from the same population and each of these samples consists of n independent and identically distributed observations. For each sample, a sample mean value $(\bar{x})$ is calculated. These estimated mean values will generally differ, since the observations making up each sample differ (sampling variation). The probability distribution describing this sampling variability, however, has the same mean as the mean of the population from which the sample was selected or $E(\overline{X}) = E(X)$. In addition, the variance of the probability distribution describing these mean values is the variance of the sampled population divided by the sample size n or $\sigma_{\overline{X}}^2 = \sigma_X^2/n$. In applied situations, a single mean is calculated but, nevertheless, the distribution that describes the properties of this mean value has a mean of $E(X)$ and a variance of σ_X^2/n.

EXAMPLE

If a die is independently tossed four times or four dice are tossed once and interest is focused on the mean of the four outcomes, then the sample mean is represented by $\bar{x} = (x_1 + x_2 + x_3 + x_4)/4$. The values on the up-face of each die constitute a sample of four independent and identically distributed observations, therefore,

$$E(X_1) = E(X_2) = E(X_3) = E(X_4) = E(X) = 3.5$$

and

$$\sigma_{X_1}^2 = \sigma_{X_2}^2 = \sigma_{X_3}^2 = \sigma_{X_4}^2 = \sigma_X^2 = 35/12.$$

The probability distribution of $\bar{x}$ (where $\bar{x}$ is based on four observations) has a specific mean value (expected value), namely

$$E(\overline{X}) = E(X) = 3.5$$

and a specific variance, namely

$$\sigma_{\overline{X}}^2 = \frac{\sigma_X^2}{n} = \frac{35/12}{4} = \frac{35}{48} = 0.729$$

and standard deviation

$$\sigma_{\overline{x}} = \sqrt{0.729} = 0.854.$$

Once again, these values are calculated directly without reference to the joint probability distribution of four dice, which is somewhat tedious to calculate because it involves $6^4 = 1296$ joint probabilities (the complete probability distribution is given in Chapter 4). The probability distribution of the mean $(\overline{x})$ generated by tossing four dice is (see following figure)

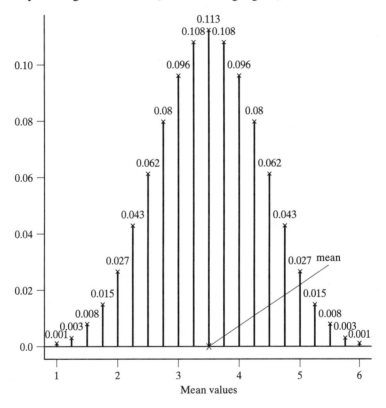

Mean values

If interest is focused on tossing 10 dice, describing the joint probability distribution requires considerable tedious calculation (6^{10} probabilities). However, the probability distribution of the mean $\overline{x}$ describing all possible observed mean values that could occur has the mean value $E(\overline{X}) = E(X) = 3.5$ and variance $\sigma_{\overline{X}}^2 = \sigma_X^2/n = (35/12)/10 = 0.291$, based entirely on the mean value ($E(X) = 3.5$) and the variance ($\sigma_X^2 = 35/12$) of the population sampled.   ■

EXAMPLE

Again let X represent a value sampled from the probability distribution $p_1 = P(X = 1) = 0.1$, $p_2 = P(X = 2) = 0.2$, $p_3 = P(X = 3) = 0.3$ and $p_4 = P(X = 4) = 0.4$. Previous calculations show that the mean value of this probability distribution $E(X)$ is 3.0 and the variance σ_X^2 is 1.0. Suppose two independent samples ($n = 2$) are selected from this probability distribution (denoted X_1 and X_2). The mean value of these two independent and identically distributed values is $\bar{x} = (x_1 + x_2)/2$ and has the following probability distribution:

$\overline{X} = (X_1 + X_2)/2$	$\overline{X}=1$	$\overline{X}=1.5$	$\overline{X}=2$	$\overline{X}=2.5$	$\overline{X}=3$	$\overline{X}=3.5$	$\overline{X}=4$	Total
$P(\overline{X}=\bar{x})=p_{\bar{x}}$	0.01	0.04	0.10	0.20	0.25	0.24	0.16	1.0

These are the same probabilities associated with the sum S (previous example) because dividing the sum S by 2 ($\overline{X} = S/2$) does not change the probabilities associated with the joint occurrences of X_1 and X_2. For example, the probability that $S = X_1 + X_2 = 4$ is the same as the probability that $\overline{X} = S/2 = (X_1 + X_2)/2 = 2$, both equal 0.10.

The mean value of this distribution of the sample mean ($n = 2$) calculated directly from its probability distribution is

$$E(\overline{X}) = \sum p_{\bar{x}}\bar{x} = 0.01(1) + 0.04(1.5) + 0.10(2) + 0.20(2.5) + 0.25(3)$$
$$+ 0.24(3.5) + 0.16(4) = 3.0,$$

verifying that $E(X) = E(\overline{X}) = 3$. The variance of the sample mean again calculated from its probability distribution is

$$\sigma_{\overline{X}}^2 = \sum p_{\bar{x}}[\bar{x} - E(\overline{X})]^2 = 0.01(1 - 3)^2 + 0.04(1.5 - 3)^2 + 0.10(2 - 3)^2$$
$$+ 0.20(2.5 - 3)^2 + 0.25(3 - 3)^2 + 0.24(3.5 - 3)^2 + 0.16(4 - 3)^2 = 0.5,$$

verifying that $\sigma_{\overline{X}}^2 = \sigma_X^2/n = \sigma_X^2/2 = 1.0/2 = 0.5$.   ∎

Summary

The essence of the preceding sections is the relationship between the mean value $E(X)$ and variance σ_X^2 of the population distribution sampled and the parallel values associated with the distribution of a sample mean, $E(\overline{X})$ and $\sigma_{\bar{x}}^2$. It is important to keep in mind that two distinct distributions are involved, the distribution from which the observations are sampled (the distribution of X) and the distribution of the sample mean calculated from the sampled observations (the distribution of $\overline{X}$). These two distributions have the same mean value $[E(X) = E(\overline{X})]$ but otherwise differ in significant ways. For example, they have different variances (as long as $n > 1$). The variance of the mean consistently deceases as the sample size increases while the variance of the sampled population (sometimes called the *parent population*) remains unchanged. Although these two probability distributions are certainly related, they play entirely different roles in the analysis of sampled data (further discussed in Chapter 4).

Two fundamental characteristics of the probability distribution of the sample mean have been identified and described, its mean and variance. A third property remains. While the mean value and variance are essential parts of the description of any probability distribution, they give only a slight hint of the shape of the probability distribution of the mean. Once the entire distribution is defined, it becomes a fundamental part of statistical analysis because it then becomes possible to completely describe the statistical properties of a sample mean. For example, it is relatively easy to calculate the probability of the occurrence of any specific sample mean value based on the mean value and variance of the population sampled. The next chapter is a discussion of several specific probability distributions, leading to completing the description of the probability distribution of the sample mean.

**There are three kinds
of statisticians:
Those who can count,
and those who can't**

PROBLEM SET 3

You and two friends buy the same brand of laptop computer. Each of the three computers is possibly defective. Suppose $P(defective) = 0.2$ and that the condition of each computer is independent of the others. Let $X =$ the number of defective computers.

1. What values can the random variable represented by X take on?
2. What are the corresponding probabilities?
3. Find the expected value of X, $E(X)$.
4. Find the variance of X, $variance(X) = \sigma_X^2$.
5. Find the standard deviation of X, σ_X.

The mean gestation period for Golden Retrievers is 63 days (expected value) with an associated variance of 1.0 $(days)^2$.

6. What is $E(X) =$ length of pregnancy in terms of weeks?
7. What is σ_X^2 in terms of weeks?
8. What is σ_X in terms of weeks?

There are four possible treatments available to patients with a specific disease. Three treatments, A, B, and C, are drugs with increasing severity of side effects and the last resort is surgery, S. The treatment pattern is to give drug A for two weeks; if that fails, drug B for two weeks. If B fails, drug C is given for two weeks. If C is ineffective, surgery is performed. For all four treatments, symptoms will diminish by the end of the two-week treatment period if the treatment is effective.

The corresponding probabilities of recovery are:

$$P(recover\ after\ treatment\ A) = 0.4$$
$$P(recovery\ after\ treatments\ AB) = 0.3$$
$$P(recovery\ after\ treatments\ ABC) = 0.2$$
$$P(recovery\ after\ treatments\ ABCS) = 0.1$$

9. What is the expected number of treatments? What is the variance of the distribution?
10. What is the expected number of weeks of treatment? What is the variance of the distribution?
11. What is the expected number of days of treatment? What is the variance of the distribution?
12. How are the three expected values related?
13. What is the standard deviation for treatments A, B, and C? How are they related?
14. If this treatment regime must be delayed for 7 days from diagnosis, what is the expected number of days under a physician's care and the corresponding variance?
15. Find the expected number of treatments a clinic would give to two patients (i.e., X_1 is patient one and X_2 is patient 2, then $E(X_1 + X_2) =$?). Assuming independence, calculate the expectation $E(X_1 + X_2)$ and the variance of this sum $[Variance(X_1 + X_2)]$ using the joint probability distribution.

Make the same two calculations without reference to the joint probability distribution.

16. What is the expected number of treatments given to 10 patients? The variance? (Don't calculate the joint probability distribution unless you have a lot of time.)

Suppose a fair coin is tossed six times and the number of heads is recorded (represented by X).

Part I. If the probability of heads is 0.5 [$P(heads) = 0.5$] and the tosses are independent, then

17. What are the possible outcomes for the variable X?
18. What is the probability of each outcome?
19. What is the mean of this probability distribution?
20. What is the variance of this probability distribution?

Part II. Consider tossing the same fair coin once (represented by X_i), then

21. What are the possible outcomes for the variable X_i?
22. What is the probability of each outcome?
23. What is the mean of this probability distribution?
24. What is the variance of this probability distribution?

Part III. Suppose S represents the sum of six of the binary variables from Part II or $S = X_1 + X_2 + X_3 + X_4 + X_5 + X_6$.

25. What are the possible outcomes for the variable S?
26. What is the mean of this probability distribution (calculate this value using Part I and then using Part II)?
27. What is the variance of this probability distribution (calculate this value using Part I and then using Part II)?

CHAPTER 4

Probability Distributions

As previously emphasized, probability distributions play a central role in statistical analysis and the important ones have specific names. The probability distributions discussed in this chapter are:

DISCRETE DISTRIBUTIONS	CONTINUOUS DISTRIBUTIONS
Uniform (discrete)	Uniform (continuous)
Binomial	Normal
Poisson	

DISCRETE DISTRIBUTIONS

Uniform probability distribution (discrete case)

A random variable X has a *uniform probability distribution* (discrete case) when it takes on a series of positive, consecutive integer values each with the same probability. The probability associated with each outcome is

$$p_x = P(X = x) = \frac{1}{k} \qquad \text{for } x = 1, 2, \cdots, k$$

where k represents the total number of possible outcomes. As with all discrete probability distributions, the sum of all possible p_x-values is 1.0. Specifically, for the uniform probability distribution

$$\sum_{all\ x} p_x = \sum_{i=1}^{k} \frac{1}{k} = k \left(\frac{1}{k} \right) = 1.0$$

because the k outcomes are mutually exclusive and exhaustive.

The probability that a random variable takes on a value less than or equal to a specified constant (denoted c) is called a *cumulative probability*. In symbols this probability is represented by $P(X \leq c)$ or, more succinctly, denoted $F(c)$. For a uniform probability distribution as well as other discrete probability distributions, the cumulative probability is defined as

$$F(c) = P(X \leq c) = p_1 + p_2 + \cdots + p_c = \sum_{all\ x \leq c} p_x.$$

A cumulative probability is the population or probability distribution equivalent of the sample relative cumulative frequency (Chapter 1). For a discrete uniform distribution, the cumulative probabilities are

$$F(c) = P(X \le c) = \sum_{x \le c} p_x = \sum_{i=1}^{c} \frac{1}{k} = \frac{1}{k} + \frac{1}{k} + \cdots + \frac{1}{k} = \frac{c}{k}.$$

The expectation of a random variable X when it has a uniform probability distribution (discrete) is

$$E(X) = \frac{k+1}{2}, \qquad \text{see Box 4.1.}$$

where k again represents the total number of outcomes.

Box 4.1. Expectation of a Discrete Uniform Random Variable

The sum of k consecutive integers can be expressed as

$$1 \; + \; 2 \; + \; 3 \; + \cdots + \; k \; = \; \sum_{i=1}^{k} i \; = \; S$$

$$k \; + (k-1) + (k-2) + \cdots + \; 1 \; = \; \sum_{i=1}^{k} i \; = \; S$$

$$(k+1) + (k+1) + (k+1) + \cdots + (k+1) = 2 \sum_{i=1}^{k} i = 2S$$

then, $S = k(k+1)/2$. So the expected value of a random variable X with a discrete uniform distribution is

$$E(X) = \sum_{all\ x} p_x x = \sum_{i=1}^{k} \frac{1}{k} i = \frac{1}{k} \sum_{i=1}^{k} i = \frac{1}{k} S = \frac{k+1}{2}.$$

The variance of a uniformly distributed variable X is

$$\sigma_X^2 = \frac{k^2 - 1}{12}. \qquad \text{Box 4.2.}$$

Box 4.2. Variance of a Discrete Uniform Random Variable

Note: $\displaystyle\sum_{i=1}^{k} i^2 = \frac{k(k+1)(2k+1)}{6}$ (a result from algebra).

So the variance is

$$\sigma_X^2 = \sum_{all\ x} p_x[x - E(X)]^2 = \sum \frac{1}{k}\left(i - \frac{k+1}{2}\right)^2$$

$$= \frac{1}{k}\sum\left[i^2 - 2i\frac{(k+1)}{2} + \frac{(k+1)^2}{4}\right]$$

$$= \frac{1}{k}\left[\sum i^2\right] - \frac{1}{k}(k+1)\sum i + \left(\frac{k+1}{2}\right)^2$$

$$= \frac{(k+1)(2k+1)}{6} - \frac{(k+1)^2}{2} + \frac{(k+1)^2}{4}$$

$$= \frac{(k+1)}{12}[2(2k+1) - 3(k+1)]$$

$$= \frac{(k+1)(k-1)}{12} = \frac{k^2-1}{12}.$$

The value k completely defines the uniform probability distribution (discrete case) and is called a *parameter*. Once the parameter or parameters of a probability distribution are known, the probabilities of all possible outcomes follow directly. These probabilities, in turn, determine the expected value and the variance. In other words, the properties of a probability distribution are completely defined by its parameters. For the uniform probability distribution, when the parameter equals k, the probabilities are $p_x = 1/k$ making $F(c) = c/k$, $E(X) = (k+1)/2$ and $\sigma_X^2 = (k^2 - 1)/12$.

EXAMPLE

Suppose a computer program produces the numbers 1, 2, 3, 4, 5, 6, 7, 8, 9, or 10 ($k = 10$) at random. The random variable X is the number produced and, if the computer program works, the random value X has a discrete uniform probability distribution with parameter $k = 10$ making $p_x = 1/10$ for all 10 possible outcomes. A cumulative probability, for example, when $c = 5$ is

$$F(5) = P(X \le 5) = \sum_{x=1}^{5} p_x = \frac{1}{10} + \frac{1}{10} + \frac{1}{10} + \frac{1}{10} + \frac{1}{10} = 5\left(\frac{1}{10}\right) = \frac{5}{10} = \frac{1}{2}.$$

In general, the cumulative probabilities are $F(c) = P(X \leq c) = c/10$. The mean value, variance and standard deviation of the distribution of X are

$$E(X) = \frac{10+1}{2} = 5.5, \quad \sigma_X^2 = \frac{10^2 - 1}{12} = \frac{99}{12} = 8.250 \text{ and}$$

$$\sigma_X = \sqrt{8.250} = 2.872.$$

These values are determined entirely by the parameter $k = 10$. ∎

EXAMPLE

Tossing a die once produces a uniform (discrete) random variable (Chapter 3). When X represents the number on the up-face of a die, the defining parameter $k = 6$ yields

$$P(X = x) = p_x = \frac{1}{6} \quad \text{for} \quad x = 1, 2, 3, 4, 5, \text{ or } 6,$$

giving the earlier results (Chapter 3) that the expected value and variance are

$$E(X) = \frac{7}{2} = 3.5 \quad \text{and} \quad \sigma_X^2 = \frac{6^2 - 1}{12} = \frac{35}{12}. \quad ∎$$

Two probability distributions

One introductory textbook refers to elementary statistical theory as the "tale of two distributions."[8] These two probability distributions are the binomial and the normal distributions and indeed they are at the heart of many statistical analyses. The binomial probability distribution provides a statistical structure for the analysis of counts of binary events making it fundamental to the interpretation of data collected to study a large variety of phenomena. The normal probability distribution is critically important to statistical methods because sample mean values frequently have normal or approximate normal distributions. These two probability distributions are occasionally used to describe sampled populations but their primary role in statistical analysis is the description of quantities calculated from sample data, such as counts and means.

Binomial probability distribution

The *binomial probability distribution* defines probabilities associated with a count of independent binary events. A binary event can be just about anything—on/off, dead/alive, male/female, little/big, ill/well, up/down or, generally, {event A}/{event not A}. The two alternatives are coded as a zero or a one. The sum of these zeros and ones is the number of times the event coded as a one occurs. Such a process is just a mathematically formal way of counting.

Two famous binary variables are: "to be or not to be" (Hamlet) and "give me liberty or give me death" (Patrick Henry). The binomial distribution was celebrated in a Gilbert and Sullivan production by the two lines:

> About the binomial theorem I'm teeming with a lot' news,
> With many cheerful facts about the square of the hypotenuse.

The fact that the binomial theorem has little to do with the hypotenuse shows that rhyming is more important than mathematics in light opera.

Formal definition of a binomial distribution

A binomial random variable arises from a sum of n independent observations where each observation has two outcomes. Specifically, for each observation x_i,

1. $x_i = 0$ or $x_i = 1$ $\quad i = 1, 2, \cdots, n$,
2. $P(X_i = 0) = 1 - p$ and $P(X_i = 1) = p$ where the probability p is constant for all n binary observations and
3. the binomial random variable (denoted X) is the sum of these n independent binary values or $X = X_1 + X_2 + \cdots + X_n$.

The binomial variable X is simply the count of the number of times X_i equals 1 out of the n observations. There are $n+1$ possible values of X with a minimum of 0 and a maximum of n. The values p and n define completely all binomial probabilities (denoted p_x) making p and n the parameters of the binomial probability distribution.

EXAMPLE

Envision n independent binary observations where an event occurs (coded $X_i = 1$) or does not occur (coded $X_i = 0$). The probability that X values of 1 occur ($X = \sum X_i$) and necessarily $n - X$ values of 0 occur is the product of probabilities p and $1 - p$. If $X = 3$ and $n = 9$, then $x_1 = 1$, $x_2 = 0$, $x_3 = 1$, $x_4 = 0$, $x_5 = 0$, $x_6 = 0$, $x_7 = 1$, $x_8 = 0$, and $x_9 = 0$ is one possible outcome. The probability of this specific outcome is $p(1-p)p(1-p)(1-p)(1-p)p(1-p)(1-p) = p^3(1-p)^6$. Other possibilities (arrangements) exist where $X = 3$ also occurs (for example, 0 1 0 0 1 0 1 0 0, 1 1 0 0 0 0 0 0 1, 0 0 0 1 0 0 0 1 1, etc.). There are $\binom{9}{3} = 84$ different (mutually exclusive) arrangements of 3 ones and 6 zeroes (Chapter 2). For each of these 84 mutually exclusive outcomes, the sum X equals 3 regardless of the arrangement and each has the same probability of occurring, namely $p^3(1-p)^6$. The probability of observing exactly $X = 3$ is then

$$P(X = 3) = \underbrace{p^3(1-p)^6 + \cdots + p^3(1-p)^6}_{84 \text{ identical terms}}$$

$$= \binom{9}{3}p^3(1-p)^6 = 84p^3(1-p)^6.$$

If $p = 1/4$ and $n = 9$, for example, then $P(X = 3) = 84(1/4)^3(3/4)^6 = 0.234$. ∎

In general, if X has a binomial probability distribution with parameters p and n, then

$$p_x = P(X = x) = \binom{n}{x}p^x(1-p)^{n-x}$$

and the cumulative probability is

$$F(c) = P(X \le c) = p_0 + p_1 + p_2 + \cdots + p_c = \sum_{x=0}^{c} \binom{n}{x}p^x(1-p)^{n-x}.$$

The mean value of the distribution of a binomial random variable X is

$$E(X) = \sum p_x x = np. \qquad \text{See Box 4.3.}$$

Box 4.3. Expectation of a Binomial Random Variable

Noting that $E(X) = E(X_1 + \cdots + X_n) = E(X_1) + \cdots + E(X_n)$ (Chapter 3).

The expected value of a single binary value X_i is

$$E(X_i) = \sum_{\text{all } x} p_x x = (1-p)(0) + (p)(1) = p,$$

which is true for all n binary observations when p is constant. Then, the expected value is

$$E(X) = E(X_1 + \cdots + X_n) = \underbrace{p + p + \cdots + p}_{n\text{-values}} = np.$$

The variance of X in the binomial case is

$$\sigma_X^2 = np(1-p). \qquad \text{See Box 4.4.}$$

Box 4.4. Variance of a Binomial Random Variable

Noting that $\sigma_X^2 = \sigma_{X_1+\cdots+X_n}^2 = \sigma_{X_1}^2 + \sigma_{X_2}^2 + \cdots + \sigma_{X_n}^2$ (Chapter 3)

because the n binary observations X_i are required to be independent. The variance of a single binary value X_i is

$$\sigma_{X_i}^2 = \sum_{all\ x} p_x[x - E(X)]^2 = (1-p)(0-p)^2 + p(1-p)^2 = p(1-p)$$

which is true for all binary n observations when p is constant. Then, the variance is

$$\sigma_X^2 = \sigma_{X_1+\cdots+X_n}^2 = \underbrace{p(1-p) + \cdots + p(1-p)}_{n\text{-}values} = np(1-p).$$

The mean value and variance of a binomially distributed random variable can also be calculated directly from the general definitions of expectation and variance. Some tricky algebra yields

$$E(X) = \sum_{all\ x} p_x x = \sum \underbrace{\left[\binom{n}{x} p^x (1-p)^{n-x}\right]}_{p_x} x = np$$

and

$$\sigma_X^2 = \sum_{all\ x} p_x[x - E(X)]^2 = \sum \underbrace{\left[\binom{n}{x} p^x (1-p)^{n-x}\right]}_{p_x} (x - np)^2 = np(1-p).$$

EXAMPLE

Suppose X represents the number of males in a family of four children. Assume the birth of each child is an independent event and the probability of a male birth is $p = 1/2$ (constant for each birth order). For a family of size four ($n = 4$), the following probabilities are associated with the occurrence of the five possible family compositions when modeled by the binomial probability distribution (binomial distribution parameters: $p = 1/2$ and $n = 4$):

$$P(no\ males) = P(X = 0) = p_0 = \binom{4}{0} p^0 (1-p)^4$$

$$= 1(1/2)^0(1/2)^4 = 1/16 = 0.0625$$

$$P(one\ male) = P(X = 1) = p_1 = \binom{4}{1}p^1(1-p)^3$$

$$= 4(1/2)^1(1/2)^3 = 4/16 = 0.250$$

$$P(two\ males) = P(X = 2) = p_2 = \binom{4}{2}p^2(1-p)^2$$

$$= 6(1/2)^2(1/2)^2 = 6/16 = 0.375$$

$$P(three\ males) = P(X = 3) = p_3 = \binom{4}{3}p^3(1-p)^1$$

$$= 4(1/2)^3(1/2)^1 = 4/16 = 0.250$$

$$P(four\ males) = P(X = 4) = p_4 = \binom{4}{4}p^4(1-p)^0$$

$$= 1(1/2)^4(1/2)^0 = 1/16 = 0.0625.$$

As always, $a^0 = 1$ for any $a > 0$ and $0! = 1$.

The cumulative probability that an observation is less than or equal to 2 ($c = 2$), for example, is $F(2) = P(X \le 2) = p_0 + p_1 + p_2 = 0.0625 + 0.250 + 0.375 = 0.688$. Thus, about 69% of the families of size four will contain two or fewer males. The entire cumulative probability distribution $F(x)$ is

$X = c$	$c = 0$	$c = 1$	$c = 2$	$c = 3$	$c = 4$
$F(c)$	$F(0)=0.0625$	$F(1)=0.3125$	$F(2)=0.6875$	$F(3)=0.9375$	$F(4)=1.000$

Also $p_0 + p_1 + p_2 + p_3 + p_4 = 0.0625 + 0.250 + 0.375 + 0.250 + 0.0625 = 1.0$ because the five possible outcomes are mutually exclusive and exhaustive.

The mean (expected value) of this binomial distribution is

$$E(X) = np = 4\left(\frac{1}{2}\right) = 2.0$$

and the variance is

$$\sigma_X^2 = np(1-p) = 4\left(\frac{1}{2}\right)\left(\frac{1}{2}\right) = 1.0.$$

These two quantities calculated directly from the binomial probability distribution are identical. Specifically, they are:

$$E(X) = 0.0625(0) + 0.250(1) + 0.375(2) + 0.250(3) + 0.0625(4) = 2.0$$

and

$$\sigma_X^2 = 0.0625(0-2)^2 + 0.250(1-2)^2 + 0.375(2-2)^2 + 0.250(3-2)^2$$
$$+ 0.0625(4-2)^2 = 1.0.$$ ∎

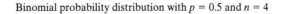

Binomial probability distribution with $p = 0.5$ and $n = 4$

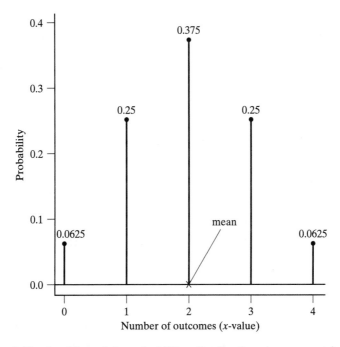

When $p = 1/2$, the binomial probability distribution is symmetric but when $p \neq 1/2$ the distribution is skewed to the right ($p < 1/2$) or to the left ($p > 1/2$) (Figure 4.1).

Three binomial probability distributions (Figure 4.1) are:

	$p = 0.2$	$p = 0.5$	$p = 0.8$
$P(X = 0) = (1 - p)^5$	0.328	0.031	0.0003
$P(X = 1) = 5p(1 - p)^4$	0.410	0.156	0.006
$P(X = 2) = 10p^2(1 - p)^3$	0.205	0.312	0.051
$P(X = 3) = 10p^3(1 - p)^2$	0.051	0.312	0.205
$P(X = 4) = 5p^4(1 - p)$	0.006	0.156	0.410
$P(X = 5) = p^5$	0.0003	0.031	0.328
Expectation of X: $E(X)$	1.0	2.5	4.0
variance of X: σ_X^2	0.80	1.25	0.80

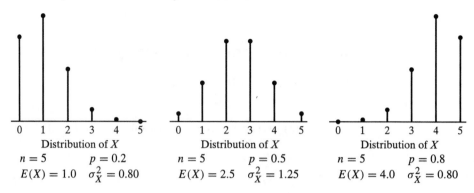

FIGURE 4.1: Three examples of the binomial probability distribution.

Estimation of the binomial parameter p

When a binomial distribution is used to describe count data, the parameter n is usually obvious but the parameter p is frequently not known. An estimate of the parameter p then comes from the fact that $E(X) = np$. The distribution of $\bar{x}$ has the mean value $E(X)$ and, therefore, it is likely that a sample value of $\bar{x}$ will be close to the population value $E(X)$, particularly for samples containing large numbers of observations (Chapter 3). This reasoning equally applies to a mean value made up of binary observations and allows an estimate of p (symbolized as $\hat{p}$) in the binomial case. In symbols,

$$\bar{x} = n\hat{p} \qquad \text{or} \qquad \hat{p} = \bar{x}/n$$

because $E(\overline{X}) = E(X) = np$. That is, the fixed and unknown population mean value $E(\overline{X})$ is estimated by its corresponding sample value $\bar{x}$. To repeat, a value with a circumflex indicates a quantity estimated from sample data, which is subject to sampling variation. The value of $\bar{x}$ is the usual mean value consisting of the sum of k observed values of the binomial variable X, where each value of X is made up of a sum of n binary components. The k values of X vary from 0 to n with most values likely in the neighborhood of np.

EXAMPLE

Suppose a sample of 15 ($k = 15$) families of size four ($n = 4$) is collected and the number of males per family (denoted X) are recorded. Specifically, the 15 families (M = male and F = female) are:

FFFF	($X = 0$)	FFMM	($X = 2$)	MMMM	($X = 4$)
FMMM	($X = 3$)	MMMM	($X = 4$)	FMFM	($X = 2$)
FFMF	($X = 1$)	FMMM	($X = 3$)	FFFF	($X = 0$)

FFFM $(X = 1)$ MMMF $(X = 3)$
MMMM $(X = 4)$ MMMM $(X = 4)$
MFMM $(X = 3)$ MMFF $(X = 2)$

producing $k = 15$ values of the binomial variable X, namely the counts of males (sums of the four binary values) in each family $\{0, 3, 1, 2, 4, 3, 4, 2, 0, 1, 4, 3, 3,$ 4, and 2\}.

Since 36 males (Table 4.1) are among the $k = 15$ families sampled, then $\bar{x}$ (the mean number of males per family) is

$$\bar{x} = \frac{0 + 3 + 1 + \cdots + 2}{15} = \frac{36}{15} = 2.4 = n\hat{p},$$

and

$$\hat{p} = \frac{\bar{x}}{n} = \frac{36/15}{4} = \frac{2.4}{4} = 0.6.$$

Binomial count data are displayed frequently in a table such as Table 4.1, grouped by the number of occurrences of the variable X.

Therefore, since $n = 4$, $k = 15$ and the total number of males observed remains 36, the estimate of p is unchanged and is

$$n\hat{p} = \bar{x} \quad \text{or} \quad \hat{p} = \frac{\bar{x}}{n} = \frac{[(0)(2) + (1)(2) + (2)(3) + (3)(4) + (4)(4)]/15}{4}$$

$$= \frac{36/15}{4} = \frac{2.4}{4} = 0.6.$$

In general,

$$\hat{p} = \frac{\bar{x}}{n} = \frac{\sum x_i / k}{n} = \frac{\sum x_i}{nk} = \frac{\sum x_i}{N}$$

$$= \frac{total\ outcomes\ counted}{total\ number\ of\ all\ possible\ binary\ outcomes}$$

where $N = nk$ represents the total number of binary observations sampled.

TABLE 4.1: Grouped binomial data: again, the 15 families.

Frequency of males per family of four	$X = 0$	$X = 1$	$X = 2$	$X = 3$	$X = 4$	Total
Number of families with X males	2	2	3	4	4	15

By directly counting binary outcomes without regard to family composition, the estimate of the proportion of males is again

$$\hat{p} = \frac{\sum x_i}{N} = \frac{36}{60} = 0.6 \qquad i = 1, 2, 3, \cdots, N = 60$$

where x_i is the original binary variable describing each person sampled where $x_i = 1$ (male) and $x_i = 0$ (female). The estimate $\hat{p} = 0.6$ is the proportion of the males among all $N = nk = (4)(15) = 60$ sampled individuals. ∎

In the binomial case, an estimate of a population parameter p is obtained by using the sample mean $\bar{x}$ to estimate the population or probability distribution mean value $E(X)$. The sample mean $\bar{x}$ is always an estimate of the mean value for any probability distribution as seen in the last chapter. This approach, therefore, applies to other probability distributions yielding other useful estimates (for example, the next section).

Poisson distribution

A *Poisson distributed* random variable summarizes a series of values that take on one of two distinct outcomes much like a binomial variable. Again, the random variable X represents a count of binary observations. In the Poisson case, $p = P(X_i = 1)$ is usually small and the number of possible occurrences of outcomes (x_i) is large (theoretically infinite). As with the binomial distribution, the probability p is the same for all binary observations x_i ($p =$ constant). In fact, when p is small and the number of possible binary events is large, little difference exists between the probabilities generated by the Poisson and binomial distributions. The Poisson probability distribution, however, depends on only a single parameter (denoted λ; the Greek letter lambda). Unlike the binomial distribution, it is not necessary to know or estimate the two parameter values, p and n. A single parameter value λ defines a Poisson probability distribution.

When a random variable X has a Poisson distribution, the probabilities p_x are given by the expression

$$P(X = x) = p_x = \frac{e^{-\lambda}\lambda^x}{x!}, \qquad x = 0, 1, 2, \cdots.$$

A complete justification of these Poisson probabilities is left to more advanced texts[9] but a brief explanation is given in the appendix (B.3). The symbol e represents the mathematical constant 2.71828 and values of $e^{-\lambda}$ can be found with most scientific calculators.

The expected value of a Poisson random variable X is λ or

$$E(X) = \sum p_x x = \lambda. \qquad \text{See Box 4.5.}$$

The value represented by λ is not only the parameter that defines the Poisson distribution, it is also the expected number of occurrences of the binary variable being observed. As with all expected values, it is the mean of the Poisson probability distribution.

Box 4.5. Expected Value of the Poisson Distribution (Population Mean)

$$E(X) = \sum_{all\ x} p_x x = \sum_{x=0}^{\infty} \left[\frac{e^{-\lambda}\lambda^x}{x!} \right] x = e^{-\lambda}\lambda \sum_{x=1}^{\infty} \frac{\lambda^{x-1}}{(x-1)!}$$

$$= e^{-\lambda}\lambda \left(1 + \lambda + \frac{\lambda^2}{2} + \cdots \right) = e^{-\lambda}\lambda e^{\lambda} = \lambda$$

The reason $e^{\lambda} = 1 + \lambda + \cdots$ is found in most elementary calculus textbooks.

The variance of a random variable with a Poisson probability distribution is

$$\sigma_X^2 = \sum p_x (x - \lambda)^2 = \lambda.$$

The Poisson probability distribution is characterized by the property that its mean and variance are identical.

A Poisson probability distribution is an asymmetric and discrete probability distribution with an infinite number of possible outcomes. A typical Poisson distribution defined by the parameter $\lambda = 2$, making the mean and variance of the probability distribution also equal to 2, is

k	$P(X = k)$	Expression	Probability	Cumulative probability
0	$P(X = 0)$	$\lambda^0 e^{-\lambda}/0!$	$e^{-2.0} = 0.135$	0.135
1	$P(X = 1)$	$\lambda^1 e^{-\lambda}/1!$	$(2.0)e^{-2.0} = 0.271$	0.406
2	$P(X = 2)$	$\lambda^2 e^{-\lambda}/2!$	$(2.0)^2 e^{-2.0}/2 = 0.271$	0.677
3	$P(X = 3)$	$\lambda^3 e^{-\lambda}/3!$	$(2.0)^3 e^{-2.0}/3! = 0.180$	0.857
4	$P(X = 4)$	$\lambda^4 e^{-\lambda}/4!$	$(2.0)^4 e^{-2.0}/4! = 0.090$	0.947
5	$P(X = 5)$	$\lambda^5 e^{-\lambda}/5!$	$(2.0)^5 e^{-2.0}/5! = 0.036$	0.983
6	$P(X = 6)$	$\lambda^6 e^{-\lambda}/6!$	$(2.0)^6 e^{-2.0}/6! = 0.012$	0.995
7	$P(X = 7)$	$\lambda^7 e^{-\lambda}/7!$	$(2.0)^7 e^{-2.0}/7! = 0.003$	0.999
—	—	—	—	—
—	—	—	—	—
—	—	—	—	—

The mean and variance calculated directly from this probability distribution are

$$E(X) = 0.135(0) + 0.271(1) + 0.271(2) + 0.180(3) + \cdots = 2.0$$

and

$$\sigma_X^2 = 0.135(0-2)^2 + 0.271(1-2)^2 + 0.271(2-2)^2 + 0.180(3-2)^2 + \cdots = 2.0.$$

The plot of this typical Poisson probability distribution is given below

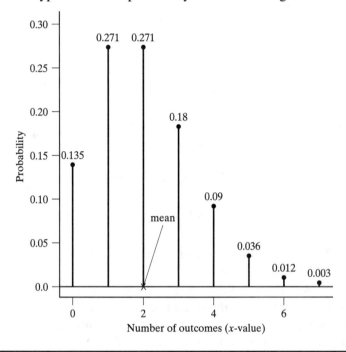

EXAMPLE

During World War II the German military attacked London using "pilotless flying-bombs." It was critical for the British military to determine if these bombs had an effective guidance system or whether they fell on London at random. To investigate the pattern of flying-bomb strikes, a map of London was divided into 576 small squares each with the same area (0.25 square kilometers). If the flying-bombs had an effective guidance system, then strategic areas would have a high frequency of hits per square and less strategic areas would experience a lower frequency. If the German weapon, however, did not possess an effective guidance system, each of these 576 squares would have the same small probability (denoted p) of being hit, regardless of its location. A constant value of p for all 576 areas is a formal way of saying that the flying-bombs fell on London at random. That is, all areas are equally likely to be hit. In this instance, the Poisson distribution would then describe the frequency of hits per square. In other words, the probability a specific bomb falls within one of the large number of squares is small and constant ($p = 1/576$) making the Poisson distribution an accurate description of the number of hits per square. Specifically, these Poisson probabilities are

$$p_x = P(\text{exactly } x \text{ hits in a specific square}) = \frac{\lambda^x e^{-\lambda}}{x!}.$$

When the expected number of hits per square is hypothetically 0.9 ($E(X) = \lambda = 0.9$), the Poisson distribution describing the distribution of flying-bomb strikes would be

Hits per square	p_x	Expression	Probability	Value
0	p_0	$\lambda^0 e^{-\lambda}/0!$	$e^{-0.9}$	0.407
1	p_1	$\lambda^1 e^{-\lambda}/1!$	$(0.9)e^{-0.9}$	0.366
2	p_2	$\lambda^2 e^{-\lambda}/2!$	$(0.9)^2 e^{-0.9}/2!$	0.165
3	p_3	$\lambda^3 e^{-\lambda}/3!$	$(0.9)^3 e^{-0.9}/3!$	0.049
4	p_4	$\lambda^4 e^{-\lambda}/4!$	$(0.9)^4 e^{-0.9}/4!$	0.011
5	p_5	$\lambda^5 e^{-\lambda}/5!$	$(0.9)^5 e^{-0.9}/5!$	0.002

and the probability of more than five hits in a single square is 0.0003. These theoretical frequencies can be compared to the observed values (Chapter 7) to assess the conjecture that all 576 areas (squares) in London have the same probability of a hit. For example, the theoretical distribution of hits (if random) predicts a bit more than 40% of the 576 square areas should have no hits and the rest should have one of more hits. If the data correspond poorly to the theoretical Poisson distribution, then it is likely that the German weapons have a guidance system that produces clusters (p is not constant). Conversely, if the data conform to a Poisson distribution, then no evidence emerges that the bombs have an effective guidance system (p is constant).

The World War II data and the Poisson estimated values are:

Flying-bomb hits (x)	0	1	2	3	4	≥ 5
observed	229	211	93	35	7	1
theoretical	226.7	211.4	98.5	30.6	7.1	1.6

The analysis of these flying-bomb data has been published a number of times[10] because the observed values closely correspond to the theoretical values derived from the Poisson probability distribution (discussed further in Chapter 7).   ■

A partial list of phenomena described accurately by a Poisson distributions is: cases of leukemia per county, numbers of radioactive decaying particles per minute, arrivals of patients at a doctor's waiting room per hour, typographical errors per page, numbers of individuals over 100 years old per Swiss canton, Supreme Court appointments per U.S. president, occurrences of suicide per week, and telephone calls arriving at a switchboard per second. The versatility of the Poisson distribution produced the comment:

> On rats arriving in random profusion
> "I know nothing of math,
> Probability or stats,
> But I handle'em with the Poisson distribution."

EXAMPLE

The California lottery provides another example of an application of the Poisson distribution. The probability of winning the "super" payoff is 1 in 41 million (p). When 41 million lottery tickets are sold (n), the expected number of winners is one [$\lambda = np = $ (41 million)(1/41 million) $= 1$]. However, there is not always a single winner. Sometimes no one wins and other times two or even more individuals win. Based on the Poisson distribution (p is small and constant while the number of possible outcomes is large), the probabilities of a specific number of winners for a single lottery drawing are

$$P(x \; number \; of \; winners) = P(X = x) = p_x = \frac{e^{-\lambda}\lambda^x}{x!}$$

and, specifically, for $\lambda = 1$

no winners:	$P(X = 0) = e^{-1}/0! = 0.368$
one winner:	$P(X = 1) = e^{-1}/1! = 0.368$
two winners:	$P(X = 2) = e^{-1}/2! = 0.184$
three winners:	$P(X = 3) = e^{-1}/3! = 0.061$
four winners:	$P(X = 4) = e^{-1}/4! = 0.015$
five winners:	$P(X = 5) = e^{-1}/5! = 0.003$

If there is no winner for a specific drawing, the payoff is carried over to the next drawing ("rolled over") and the probability of this occurring is 0.368.   ■

CONTINUOUS DISTRIBUTIONS

Introduction

A continuous probability distribution can be viewed as the ultimate result of plotting a histogram based on larger and larger amounts of data. As

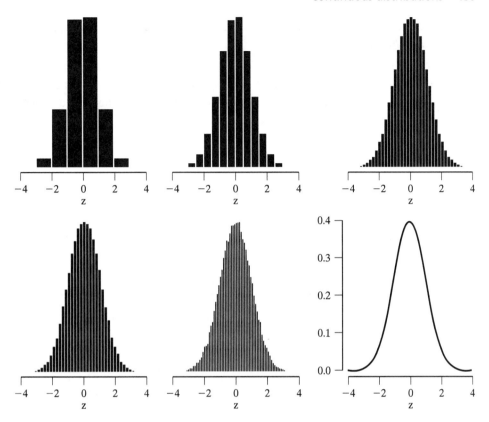

FIGURE 4.2: The progression of a histogram to a continuous distribution as the sample size increases.

more observations are available, larger numbers of histogram rectangles can be constructed with smaller widths. As the widths become smaller, the histogram becomes a smoother representation of the underlying continuous distribution. Figure 4.2 displays this progression, starting with few observations (upper left) and ending in a smooth continuous probability distribution (lower right).

Uniform probability distribution (continuous case)

The *uniform probability distribution* (continuous case) is similar to the discrete uniform probability distribution but differs in one critical respect, the number of possible outcomes is infinite. Therefore, unlike the discrete uniform distribution, the probability that a uniform random variable X (continuous case) takes on a specific predetermined value x is zero. In symbols, $P(X = x) = 0$. Cumulative probabilities, nevertheless, can be calculated and used to describe the properties of a variable with a continuous uniform distribution.

EXAMPLE

Suppose an infant can be born at any time during a 24-hour period and the continuous random variable X represents the time (hours + fractions of hours) of birth. The uniform probability distribution of X defined for a 24-hour period ($0 \leq X \leq 24$) displayed graphically is

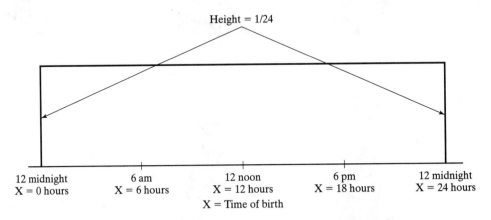

Height = 1/24

12 midnight	6 am	12 noon	6 pm	12 midnight
X = 0 hours	X = 6 hours	X = 12 hours	X = 18 hours	X = 24 hours

X = Time of birth

Five notable properties of this probability distribution are:

1. the random variable X represents a continuous random variable (results from measuring),
2. the probability distribution has height = 1/24 for all outcomes x, making
3. the total area = 1.0 (total probability = 1.0) and, of most importance,
4. area corresponds to cumulative probability: $F(x) = P(X \leq x) =$ total area to the left of x,
5. with special cases $F(0) = 0$ and $F(24) = 1$.

The area to the left of an arbitrary time x equals the probability that an infant is born before that specific time; that is, a cumulative probability. Some examples are:

$$P(X \leq 12 \ noon) = (height)(width) = area = \frac{1}{24}(12) = 0.5$$

or

$$P(X \leq 6 \ am) = \frac{1}{24}(6) = 0.25$$

and

$$P(X \leq 6 \ pm) = P(X \leq 18) = \frac{1}{24}(18) = 0.75.$$

∎

In general, the probability distribution describing the variability of a uniform continuous random variable X defined between a and b ($a \leq X \leq b$) displayed graphically is below

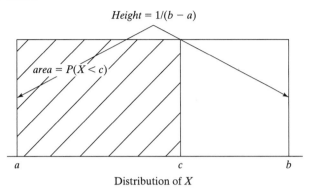

Distribution of X

where

$$height = 1/(b-a) \text{ for all } x$$

and

$$F(x) = P(X \leq x) = area = (height)(width) = \frac{1}{b-a}(x-a)$$

is the cumulative probability for a specific value of x (shaded area). Two parameters a and b define the uniform probability distribution (continuous case). The cumulative probabilities, like all probabilities, range from $F(a) = 0$ to $F(b) = 1$. An essential property is that the area associated with a continuous uniform probability distribution is geometrically equivalent to cumulative probability. A similar relationship exists between cumulative relative frequency and area from histogram and polygon plots (Chapter 1).

A commonly used uniform probability distribution has parameters $a = 0$ and $b = 1$, then

$$F(1) = P(X \leq 1) = 1,$$

$$F(0) = P(X \leq 0) = 0,$$

$$F(0.25) = P(X \leq 0.25) = 0.25,$$

$$F(0.50) = P(X \leq 0.50) = 0.50$$

and, in general, $P(X \leq x) = x$.

The total area enclosed by a uniform probability distribution, to repeat, is 1.0 allowing a variety of probabilities to be calculated from cumulative probabilities. For example,

$$P(X \leq 0.6) + P(X \geq 0.6) = 1,$$

$$\text{then } P(X \geq 0.6) = 1 - P(X \leq 0.6) = 1 - 0.6 = 0.4$$

and

$$P(X \leq 0.4) + P(0.4 \leq X \leq 0.6) + P(X \geq 0.6) = 1, \text{ then}$$

$$P(0.4 \leq X \leq 0.6) = 1 - P(X \leq 0.4) - P(X \geq 0.6)$$

$$= 1 - P(X \leq 0.4) - [1 - P(X \leq 0.6)]$$

$$= P(X \leq 0.6) - P(X \leq 0.4) = 0.6 - 0.4 = 0.2.$$

The mean value of a uniform (continuous) distribution X is

$$E(X) = (a + b)/2$$

with variance

$$\sigma_X^2 = (b - a)^2/12.$$

Again, the cumulative probabilities, the mean and variance are completely determined by the parameters a and b.

For the example concerning the time of birth of an infant ($a = 0$ and $b = 24$), the expected value and variance are:

$$E(X) = (0 + 24)/2 = 12$$

and

$$\sigma_X^2 = (24 - 0)^2/12 = 48.$$

If $a = 0$ and $b = 1$, then similarly $E(X) = 1/2$ and $\sigma_X^2 = 1/12$.

A continuous uniform distributed variable illustrates two basic features common to all continuous random variables, namely, for a specific value x,

$$P(X = x) = 0$$

and the cumulative probability associated with a specific value x is

$$F(x) = P(X \leq x) = \text{area to the left of } x.$$

The mean of two values sampled independently from a rectangular shaped uniform probability distribution (Figure 4.3 with $a = 0$ and $b = 1$—left) has a triangular shaped probability distribution (Figure 4.3—right). As anticipated, the expected value of the distribution of mean values is 0.5, which is the mean of the parent population sampled ($E(\overline{X}) = E(X) = 0.5$; Chapter 3). Otherwise, the probability distribution describing the values of the mean does not resemble the probability distribution of the population sampled (Figure 4.3). Equally anticipated, the variance associated with the distribution of the sample mean is reduced. This reduction occurs because a triangular shaped distribution dictates

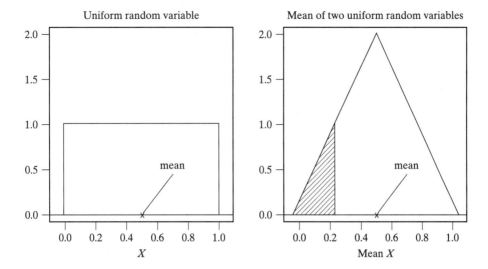

FIGURE 4.3: The rectangular distribution of a random uniform variable X between 0 and 1 (left) and the triangular distribution of the mean of two such random uniform variables (right).

that extreme values in the neighborhood of 0 and 1 are considerably less likely than values near 0.5 (mean value). This change in shape is the reason that the variance decreases from $\sigma_X^2 = 1/12 = 0.083$ to $\sigma_{\overline{X}}^2 = \sigma_X^2/2 = (1/12)/2 = 0.042$, because $\sigma_{\overline{X}}^2 = \sigma_X^2/n$ even when the sample size n is only two (Chapter 3).

The cumulative probability associated with a mean value is again the area to the left of a specified value. For example, the probability that the mean of two independently selected uniform variables is less than 0.25 equals 0.125 (the area of the shaded triangle in Figure 4.3). In symbols, the cumulative probability is

$$F(0.25) = P([X_1 + X_2]/2 \le 0.25) = P(\overline{X} \le 0.25) = 0.125.$$

Using usual geometry (area of a triangle $= \frac{1}{2} \times base \times altitude$), then $P(\overline{X} \le 0.25) = [\frac{1}{2}(0.25)(1.0)] = 0.125$, which is the area to the left of 0.25.

Normal probability distribution

The importance of the *normal probability distribution* in the analysis of sampled data cannot be overstated. This fundamental probability distribution is sometimes called an "error" curve, a Gaussian distribution, or a "bell-shaped" curve. Its special properties place it at the center of statistical estimation and inference for both discrete and continuous data.

A normal probability distribution is defined by two parameters, its mean value (denoted μ) and its variance (denoted σ^2). When a random variable has a normal distribution, the probability distribution looks like Figure 4.4.

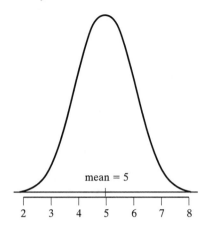

FIGURE 4.4: A typical normal probability distribution ($\mu = 5, \sigma^2 = 1$).

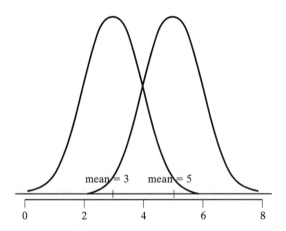

FIGURE 4.5: Two normal distributions with different mean values and the same variance ($\mu_1 = 3, \mu_2 = 5$ and $\sigma^2 = 1$).

The expected value, denoted previously by $E(X)$, gets a special symbol μ because of the importance of the normal probability distribution but it differs only in notation and not in principle. As with any expected value, the expected value μ is the mean value (location) of the normal probability distribution (Figure 4.5).

The variance σ^2 indicates the dispersion or spread associated with a normally distributed random variable. Figure 4.6 shows two normal probability distributions with different variances and the same mean value.

Four notable properties of the normal probability distribution are:

1. parameters: the normal distribution is completely defined by its mean and variance, μ and σ^2,

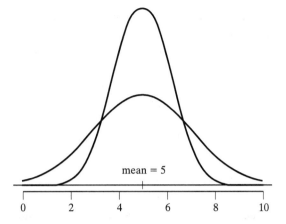

FIGURE 4.6: Two normal distributions with different variances and the same mean value ($\sigma_1^2 = 4$, $\sigma_2^2 = 1$ and $\mu = 5$).

2. symmetry: mean = median = mode,
3. range: a normally distributed value can be large (theoretically infinite) in both positive and negative directions, and
4. continuous: the probability of any specific value is zero, as before, $P(X = x) = 0$.

As with all continuous probability distributions, the total area enclosed by the normal distribution curve is 1.0 and the cumulative probabilities are given by $F(x) = P(X \leq x)$. Geometrically, the cumulative probability $F(x)$ is again the area to the left of the value x enclosed by the normal curve. For example, if $z = 1.5$, $\mu = 0$ and $\sigma^2 = 1$, then $F(1.5) = P(Z \leq 1.5) = 0.933$ or

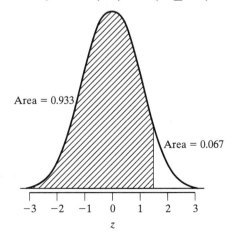

The shaded area enclosed by the normal curve equals 93.3% of the total area. Thus, a randomly selected value from this normal distribution has a probability of 0.933 of being less than 1.5.

Calculating cumulative probabilities from the normal distribution (area under normal curve) is a numeric problem; no easy formula exists. Computer programs are used typically to compute these probabilities. Table A.1 contains selected values for $F(z) = P(Z \le z)$ when Z represents a normally distributed random variable (mean $= \mu = 0$ and variance $= \sigma_Z^2 = 1$), called the *standard normal distribution*. The letter Z will be used to refer exclusively to a value randomly selected from this normal distribution. The value z correspondingly represents any specified value. The standard deviation of this specific normal distribution is also 1 since $\sqrt{\sigma_Z^2} = \sigma_Z = 1$. The standard normal distribution is an essential statistical tool used extensively in this chapter and the following chapters, as well as statistics in general.

The values in Table A.1 are a population version of a relative cumulative frequency polygon (Chapter 1). They relate specified values (denoted z) from the standard normal distribution (mean $= \mu = 0$ and variance $= \sigma_Z^2 = 1$) to their corresponding cumulative probabilities. The cumulative probabilities $F(z)$ listed in the table refer to the likelihood that a randomly selected value Z is equal to or less than a given value z, or $F(z) = P(Z \le z)$. Figure 4.7 displays the values found in Table A.1. A value z leads to a probability $F(z)$. For example, if $z = 1$, then $F(1) = P(Z \le 1) = 0.841$ and similarly, if $z = -1$, then $F(-1) = P(Z \le -1) = 0.159$ (shown in Figure 4.7). The plot (table) can also be read "backwards." A probability $F(z)$ leads to a value of z. For example, if $F(z) = 0.95$, then $z = 1.645$ and similarly, if $F(z) = 0.05$, then $z = -1.645$ (Figure 4.7 again displays the values found in Table A.1.)

Some additional examples of the relationship between selected values of z and the cumulative normal probabilities $F(z) = P(Z \le z)$ from Table A.1 are:

$$z = 0 : F(0) = P(Z \le 0) = 0.500$$

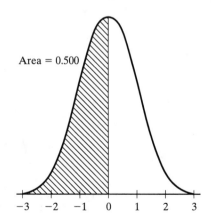

Area = 0.500

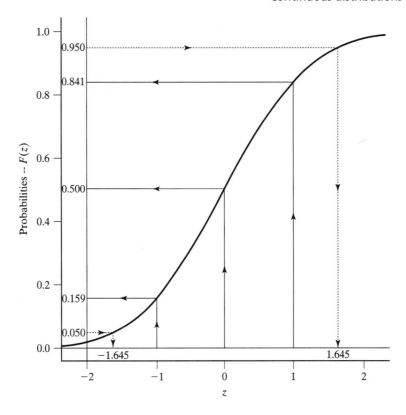

FIGURE 4.7: Graphic representation of the standard normal probability distribution (Table A.1).

$$z = 1 : F(1) = P(Z \leq 1) = 0.841$$

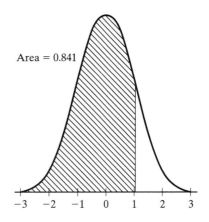

$z = -1 : F(-1) = P(Z \le -1) = 0.159$

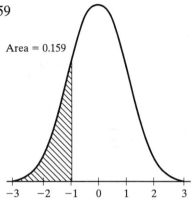

Area = 0.159

$z = 2 : F(2) = P(Z \le 2) = 0.997$

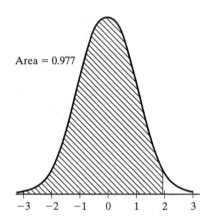

Area = 0.977

Since the total area enclosed by the normal probability distribution equals one, it follows that $P(X \le x) + P(X \ge x) = 1$, then

$$P(X \ge x) = 1 - P(X \le x) = 1 - F(x)$$

for any value x. Again, for example, consider the special case of a standard normal variable Z and $z = 2$, then

$$P(Z \ge 2) = 1 - P(Z \le 2) = 1 - F(2) = 1 - 0.977 = 0.023.$$

The value of $F(2) = 0.977$ comes from Table A.1.

The probability that a normally distributed random variable takes on a value between two specified limits (denoted x_1 and x_2) is

$$P(x_1 \le X \le x_2) = P(X \le x_2) - P(X \le x_1). \qquad \text{See Box 4.6.}$$

Box 4.6. $P(x_1 \leq X \leq x_2) = ?$

Noting that $P(X \leq x_1) + P(x_1 \leq X \leq x_2) + P(X \geq x_2) = 1.0$, then

$$P(x_1 \leq X \leq x_2) = 1 - P(X \leq x_1) - P(X \geq x_2)$$
$$= 1 - P(X \leq x_1) - [1 - P(X \leq x_2)]$$
$$= P(X \leq x_2) - P(X \leq x_1).$$

Note: $P(X < x_1) + P(X = x_1) = P(X \leq x_1)$ and because $P(X = x_1) = 0$, $P(X < x_1) = P(X \leq x_1)$, which is a property of all continuous probability distribution.

For example, consider again a random variable symbolized by Z with a standard normal distribution, then

$$P(-1.5 \leq Z \leq 1.5) = P(Z \leq 1.5) - P(Z \leq -1.5)$$
$$= F(1.5) - F(-1.5)$$
$$= 0.933 - 0.067 = 0.866$$

from Table A.1.

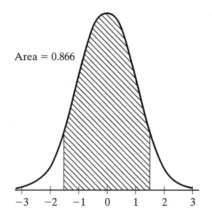

The shaded area corresponds to $P(z_1 \leq Z \leq z_2)$ where $z_1 = -1.5$ and $z_2 = 1.5$ and area = probability = $P(-1.5 \leq Z \leq 1.5)$ is 0.866.

For a normal distribution with mean = μ, for any value b,

$$P(X \leq \mu - b) = P(X \geq \mu + b),$$

which is a formal statement of the fact that all normal distributions are symmetric. For the standard normal distribution, the mean is zero ($\mu = 0$) making

$P(Z \le -b) = P(Z \ge b)$. For example, if $b = 1.5$, then $P(Z \le -1.5) = 0.067$ (Table A.1) and $P(Z \ge 1.5) = 0.067$.

Table A.1 is also used to find the percentiles associated with a standard normal distribution. Instead of associating a probability (area) with a specified value, a percentile is the value that corresponds to a specified probability (area). Instead of values of z leading to probabilities $F(z)$, probabilities $F(z)$ lead to values of z. In general, when $z_{1-\alpha}$ represents the value such that $(1-\alpha)\%$ of the distribution is below $z_{1-\alpha}$ and $\alpha\%$ is above $z_{1-\alpha}$, the value $z_{1-\alpha}$ is the $(1-\alpha)^{\text{th}}$-percentile of the standard normal distribution because $P(Z \le z_{1-\alpha}) = 1 - \alpha$. The 50th percentile is the median, mode, and mean of all normal distributions and is represented by μ. For the standard normal distribution, then $\mu = z_{0.5} = 0$ and $P(Z \le \mu) = P(Z \le z_{0.5}) = P(Z \le 0) = 0.5$. Calculations of percentiles from a standard normal distribution are displayed in Figure 4.7 (dotted lines).

The last two columns in Table A.1 are designed specifically to find selected values of $z_{1-\alpha}$ (percentiles) associated with specified probabilities (areas) of the standard normal distribution.

EXAMPLE

For the 90th percentile, $P(Z \le z_{0.90}) = 0.90$, then $z_{0.90} = 1.282$ is the 90th percentile because $P(Z \le 1.282) = 0.90$ and $P(Z \ge 1.282) = 0.10$ (from the last two columns of Table A.1). ∎

EXAMPLE

For the 75th, $P(Z \le z_{0.75}) = 0.75$, then $z_{0.75} = 0.674$ is the 75th percentile because $P(Z \le 0.674) = 0.75$ and $P(Z \ge 0.674) = 0.25$. The 25th percentile $z_{0.25}$ is similarly equal to -0.674 because $P(Z \le -0.674) = 0.25$ making the interquartile range 1.348 (IQR $= z_{0.75} - z_{0.25} = 0.674 - (-0.674) = 1.348$). ∎

The percentiles $z_{1-\alpha}$ from the standard normal distribution are used in a large number of contexts in the following chapters. Two frequently occurring percentiles are:

for $1 - \alpha = 0.95$, the 95th percentile is $z_{0.95} = 1.645$ because

$P(Z \le 1.645) = 0.95$

and

for $1 - \alpha = 0.975$, the 97.5th percentile is $z_{0.975} = 1.960$ because

$P(Z \leq 1.960) = 0.975$.

The 97.5th percentile is important because $P(-1.960 \leq Z \leq 1.960) = P(Z \leq 1.960) - P(Z \leq -1.960) = 0.975 - 0.025 = 0.95$. That is, 95% of random values from a standard normal distribution are between -1.960 and 1.960.

Standardization of a normally distributed variable

The probabilities associated with any normally distributed random variable (any parameters μ and σ^2) are determined by redefining the variable in terms of the distance from its mean, measuring distance in units of standard deviation ($\sqrt{variance} = \sigma$). The probability that a normally distributed value is a specific number of standard deviations above or below its mean value μ is the same for all normal distributions. Therefore, the probabilities associated with any normal distribution (mean = μ and variance = σ^2) can be calculated from the standard normal distribution using units of standard deviations σ relative to the mean μ (Table A.1).

More formally, when X has a normal distribution with mean μ and variance σ_X^2, the quantity $Z = (X - \mu)/\sigma_X$ has a normal distribution with mean $= \mu = E(Z) = 0$ and variance $= \sigma_Z^2 = \sigma_Z = 1$ (Box 4.7). The value of Z is the number of standard deviations above or below the mean associated with the value of X. Therefore, the associated cumulative probability is

$$F(x) = P(X \leq x) = P\left(Z \leq \frac{x - \mu}{\sigma_X}\right) = P(Z \leq z)$$

and $P(Z \leq z)$ is found in Table A.1. Thus, for a normally distributed variable, subtracting the mean and dividing by its standard deviation (calculating z) does not change the cumulative probability associated with X. The only difference between variables X and Z, in terms of probability, is that the probability associated with Z can be found in a table (for example, A.1). When a variable X measured in natural units is standardized, the standardized variable Z becomes the distance, measured in standard deviations, above or below the mean and, to repeat, the associated cumulative probability is the same for both normal distributions of X and Z.

EXAMPLE

Suppose $x = 9$ weeks with $\mu = 6$ weeks and $\sigma_X = 3$ weeks, then 9 weeks corresponds to $z = (9 - 6)/3 = 1.0$ standard deviation above the mean and when X has a normal distribution, $F(x) = F(9) = P(X \leq 9) = P(Z \leq 1.0) = 0.841$ (Table A.1). A value of nine weeks is one standard deviation above the mean and, for any normal distribution, the probability is that a randomly selected value is less than one standard deviation above the mean is 0.841, making the probability that a random observation X is less than 9 weeks equal to 0.841. ∎

Box 4.7. Standardization of the Normal Variable X

Noting that $E(aX + c) = aE(X) + c$ and $\sigma^2_{aX+c} = a^2\sigma^2_X$ for any variable X, then

$$E(Z) = E\left(\frac{X - \mu}{\sigma_X}\right) = \frac{1}{\sigma_X}E(X - \mu) = \frac{1}{\sigma_X}(E(X) - \mu) = \frac{1}{\sigma_X}(\mu - \mu) = 0$$

and

$$\sigma^2_Z = variance\ (Z) = variance\left(\frac{X - \mu}{\sigma_X}\right) = \frac{1}{\sigma^2_X}\ variance\ (X - \mu)$$

$$= \frac{1}{\sigma^2_X}\ variance\ (X) = \frac{\sigma^2_X}{\sigma^2_X} = 1.$$

Regardless of the units of measurement (inches, feet, miles, etc., or standard deviations) the standard normal distribution (Table A.1) provides probabilities from any normal distribution. For example, the probability that a randomly selected newborn infant weighs less that 5.5 pounds or 88 ounces or 2500 grams or 2.5 kilograms is 0.055 when the weights of newborn infants are normally distributed with mean = 7.5 lbs and standard deviation = 1.25 lbs. The four birth weights are all 1.6 standard deviations below the mean and for all normal distributions $P(Z \leq -1.6) = 0.055$ (Table A.1).

EXAMPLE

As already noted, the cumulative probability for any normally distributed random variable is found using the standardized value $Z = (X - \mu)/\sigma_X$. One deals simply in terms of units of standard deviation above or below the mean. Suppose a sample of heights of army recruits is known to come from a normal distribution with mean = $\mu = 6$ feet and standard deviation = $\sigma_X = 2$ inches; then

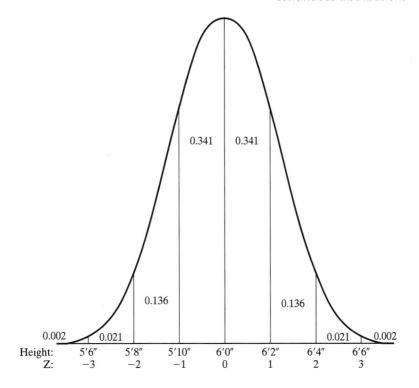

The numbers (0.021, 0.136, and 0.341) below the curve represent the areas (probabilities) between the vertical lines and come from Table A.1 using the corresponding units of standard deviation. For example, an army recruit whose height is 5′ 10″ is 2 inches below the mean of 6 feet. Since one standard deviation equals 2 inches, then 5′ 10″ lies one standard deviation below the mean. Thus, $P(X \leq$ 5′ 10″) corresponds to $P(less\ than\ one\ standard\ deviation\ below\ the\ mean) = P(Z \leq -1)$. From Table A.1, then $F(5′\ 10″) = P(X \leq 5′\ 10″) = P(Z \leq -1) = 0.159$.

Three additional examples are:

$$P(X \leq 6′\ 2″) = P(less\ than\ one\ standard\ deviation\ above\ the\ mean)$$
$$= P(Z \leq 1) = 0.841,$$
$$P(X \geq 6′\ 4″) = P(more\ than\ two\ standard\ deviations\ above\ the\ mean)$$
$$= P(Z \geq 2) = 1 - P(Z \leq 2) = 1 - 0.977 = 0.023$$

and the probability that a randomly selected recruit is between 6′ 2″ and 6′ 4″ is

$$P(6′\ 2″ \leq X \leq 6′\ 4″) = P(1 \leq Z \leq 2)$$
$$= P(Z \leq 2) - P(Z \leq 1)$$
$$= 0.977 - 0.841 = 0.136. \qquad \blacksquare$$

ANOTHER EXAMPLE

Suppose X represents the weight of a five-year-old male child sampled from a normal distribution ($\mu = 43$ lbs and $\sigma_X = 5$ lbs), then

$$P(X \le 35.5 \text{ lbs}) = P\left(\frac{X - \mu}{\sigma_X} \le \frac{35.5 - 43}{5}\right)$$

$$= P\left(Z \le \frac{35.5 - 43}{5}\right) = P\left(Z \le \frac{-7.5}{5}\right) = P(Z \le -1.5)$$

$$= 0.067.$$

Less technically, the weight 35.5 lbs is 1.5 standard deviations below the mean implying that 6.7% of these five-year-old males weigh less than 35.5 lbs. Also,

$$P(34 \text{ lbs} \le X \le 52 \text{ lbs}) = P(X \le 52) - P(X \le 34)$$

$$= P\left(Z \le \frac{52 - 43}{5}\right) - P\left(Z \le \frac{34 - 43}{5}\right)$$

$$= P(Z \le 1.8) - P(Z \le -1.8)$$

$$= 0.964 - 0.036 = 0.928$$

showing that 92.8% of these five-year-old males weigh between 34 and 52 lbs. Or equally, 92.8% of five-year-old children have weights within -1.8 and $+1.8$ standard deviations of the mean of 43 lbs ($\mu = 43$ lbs). Lastly,

$$P(X \ge 56 \text{ lbs}) = 1 - P(X \le 56) = 1 - P\left(Z \le \frac{56 - 43}{5}\right)$$

$$= 1 - P(Z \le 2.6) = 1 - 0.995 = 0.005$$

indicates that only rarely (0.5%) do these five-year-old children weigh more than 56 lbs. From another prospective, a randomly selected five-year-old male child is not likely to weigh more than 56 lbs (probability $= 0.005$). ■

What is the 75th percentile weight for five-year-old male children? or what weight x yields $P(X \le x_{0.75}) = 0.75$? That is, what weight divides the distribution of five-year-olds so the 75% are below and 25% are above the selected value. From Table A.1, $P(Z \le 0.674) = 0.75$. For a standard normal distribution, the 75th percentile is 0.674 standard deviation above the mean. The 75th percentile for weights of five-year-old males is then 3.372 lbs above the mean, because one standard deviation equals five lbs ($\sigma_X = 5$) making $(0.674)\sigma_X = (0.674)5 = 3.372$ lbs. Therefore, $x_{0.75} = \mu + z_{0.75}\sigma_X = 43 + 3.372 = 46.372$ lbs and is the 75th percentile. Thus, $P(Z \le 0.674) = P(X \le 46.372) = 0.75$.

Similarly, the 95th percentile is 51.224 lbs because $P(Z \leq 1.645) = 0.95$ making $(1.645)\sigma_X = (1.645)5 = 8.224$ lbs, which is the distance above the mean in natural units (lbs). The 95th percentile is then $43 + 8.224 = 51.224$ and $P(Z \leq 1.645) = P(X \leq 51.224) = 0.95$. The fact that 51.224 lbs is the 95th percentile is directly verified because $z = (51.224 - 43)/5 = 1.645$ and $P(Z \leq 1.645) = 0.95$.

Mechanically, when the random variable X has a normal distribution with mean $= \mu$ and variance $= \sigma_X^2$, the value

$$Z = \frac{X - \mu}{\sigma_X}$$

has a normal distribution with $\mu = 0$ and $\sigma_Z = 1$ and relates any value x to a probability or $F(x) = P(X \leq x) = P(Z \leq z)$. Conversely,

$$x_{1-\alpha} = z_{1-\alpha}\sigma_X + \mu$$

and is, for any normally distributed value X, the $[(1 - \alpha) \times 100]^{\text{th}}$-percentile because $P(X \leq x_{1-\alpha}) = 1 - \alpha$ and $P(X \geq x_{1-\alpha}) = \alpha$. In both cases (probability or percentile), the desired values are derived from the standard normal distribution (Table A.1). As mentioned, the exact probabilities are also readily available from computer programs and some scientific calculators.

Central limit theorem

The essence of the *central limit theorem* is that a sample mean value frequently has an approximate normal distribution. Formally, the central limit theorem states:

if $X_1, X_2, \cdots, X_n$ are n independent and identically distributed random variables selected from a population with mean $= \mu$ and variance $= \sigma_X^2$, then the sample mean $\bar{x}$ has an approximate normal distribution, for large values of n. Furthermore,

$$Z = \frac{\bar{X} - E(\bar{X})}{\sigma_{\bar{X}}} = \frac{\bar{X} - \mu}{\sqrt{\sigma_X^2/n}} = \frac{\sqrt{n}(\bar{X} - \mu)}{\sigma_X}$$

has an approximate standard normal distribution (mean $= E(Z) = 0$ and variance $= \sigma_Z^2 = 1$).

What is not stated in the central limit theorem leads to its importance. Its remarkable feature is that the observed values used to calculate a mean value $\bar{x}$ can be sampled from any probability distribution (any parent distribution) and the sample mean value will have at least an approximate normal distribution.

If the n sample values $x_1, x_2, \cdots, x_n$ are themselves normally distributed, then the mean value $\bar{x}$ has an exact normal distribution. Thus, a sample mean value $\bar{x}$ calculated from normally distributed data is always (1) normally distributed with (2) mean value $= E(\overline{X}) = E(X)$ and (3) variance $= \sigma_{\overline{X}}^2 = \sigma_X^2/n$. Otherwise, the sample mean has an approximate normal distribution, again with mean value $= E(\overline{X}) = E(X)$ and variance $\sigma_{\overline{X}}^2 = \sigma_X^2/n$. The central limit theorem makes it possible to use the normal distribution to calculate probabilities or at least approximate probabilities that indicate the likelihood of the occurrence of a mean value made up of observations sampled from most any parent probability distribution as long as the number of sampled values is large.

EXAMPLE

The properties of the central limit theorem are illustrated by considering four tosses ($n = 4$) of a fair die (denoted x_1, x_2, x_3, and x_4) and computing the mean value from the four observed values where the mean value is, as usual, $\bar{x} = (x_1+x_2+x_3+x_4)/4$. The outcome of each toss (each observation) has a discrete uniform probability distribution, which is the parent distribution. Each toss of the die then comes from a uniform distribution with a mean value of $E(X) = 3.5$ and a variance of $\sigma_X^2 = 35/12$ (Chapter 3). The probability distribution describing the possible values of the mean $\bar{x}$ (calculated from four observed tosses of a die), therefore, has mean value

$$E(\overline{X}) = E(X) = 3.5$$

and variance

$$\sigma_{\overline{X}}^2 = \frac{\sigma_X^2}{n} = \frac{35/12}{4} = \frac{35}{48} = 0.729.$$

In addition, the central limit theorem states that $\bar{x}$ is a single observation from an approximate normal probability distribution. Furthermore, the value

$$Z = \frac{\bar{x} - 3.5}{\sqrt{\dfrac{35/12}{4}}} = \frac{\bar{x} - 3.5}{\sqrt{0.729}}$$

has an approximate standard normal distribution.

There are $6 \cdot 6 \cdot 6 \cdot 6 = 1296$ possible outcomes of four independent tosses of a die. Table 4.2 and Figure 4.8 show the exact probability distribution of $\bar{x}$ based on 1296 joint probabilities of these outcomes. The distribution was derived by enumerating (with a computer) all possible combinations of four dice and calculating all 1296 possible mean values. The frequencies of the 21 different mean values are given in Table 4.2 (first row). ∎

TABLE 4.2: Cumulative probability distributions of the sample mean $\bar{x}$ based on a sample of $n = 4$ observations, exact (G), and approximate (F).

Mean ($\bar{x}$)	1.0	1.25	1.5	1.75	2.0	2.25	2.5	2.75	3.0	3.25	3.5	Total
frequency	1	4	10	20	35	56	80	104	125	140	146	
cumulative	1	5	15	35	70	126	206	310	435	575	721	
$G(\bar{x})$	0.001	0.004	0.012	0.027	0.054	0.097	0.159	0.239	0.336	0.444	0.556	
Z	−2.928	−2.635	−2.342	−2.049	−1.757	−1.464	−1.171	−0.878	−0.586	−0.293	0.000	
$F(\bar{x})^*$	0.003	0.006	0.014	0.029	0.054	0.094	0.153	0.232	0.330	0.442	0.558	

mean ($\bar{x}$)	3.75	4.0	4.25	4.5	4.75	5.0	5.25	5.5	5.75	6.0	Total
frequency	140	125	104	80	56	35	20	10	4	1	1296
cumulative	861	986	1090	1170	1226	1261	1281	1291	1295	1296	—
$G(\bar{x})$	0.664	0.761	0.841	0.903	0.946	0.973	0.988	0.996	0.999	1.000	—
Z	0.293	0.586	0.878	1.171	1.464	1.757	2.049	2.342	2.635	2.928	—
$F(\bar{x})^*$	0.670	0.768	0.847	0.906	0.946	0.971	0.986	0.994	0.997	0.999	—

*normal distribution based approximation $= P(\bar{X} \leq \bar{x}+0.125)$ where $\bar{x} = 1.125, 1.375, 1.625, \ldots, 5.625, 5.875, 6.125$.

This enumerated distribution of mean values illustrates the underlying reason that a mean value has at least an approximately symmetric probability distribution that is often accurately described by a normal probability distribution (central limit theorem). Extreme mean values (for example: 1, 1.25, 1.5, or 5.5, 5.75, 6) rarely occur because only a few combinations of the four outcomes (15/1296 about 1.2%) produce these small or large mean values. At the most extreme, only one set of four values produces a mean value of 1.0 and only one set produces a mean value of 6.0, each with probability less than 0.001 (1/1296). Conversely, values in the neighborhood of the expected value (3.5) occur with a much higher frequency. For example, a relatively large number of ways exist for a more typical mean value of 3.0 (125 ways) or mean value of 4.0 (125 ways) to occur, making up about 20% of all possible combinations of outcomes (250/1296 = 0.193). Each of the 1296 sets of four outcomes are equally likely (1/1296). It is the mean (sum) of these four values, however, that defines the probability distribution and the 21 possible mean values are far from equally likely. The central limit theorem is a formal statement of the simple fact that extreme sample mean values are unlikely because only a few combinations produce extreme values and "typical" sample mean values occur frequently because they are produced in a large number of ways. This pattern yields a distribution that becomes normal-like as the number of sampled observations increases regardless of the distribution of the population sampled.

The exact cumulative probabilities arising from the mean of four dice are directly calculated from the enumerated frequencies in Table 4.2. That is, the cumulative probability $G(\bar{x}) = P(\bar{X} \leq \bar{x})$ is the cumulative frequency of the values less than or equal to $\bar{x}$ divided by 1296 (the second and third rows of Table 4.2). For example, when $\bar{x} = 4$, $G(4) = P(\bar{X} \leq 4) = 986/1296 = 0.761$.

The distribution of the up-face numbers on a die has a discrete uniform distribution; nevertheless, the sample mean has an approximate normal distribution (central limit theorem—Figure 4.8). Using a normal distribution (mean $= \mu = 3.5$ and variance $= \sigma^2 = 0.729$), even for this small sample of four values, yields an accurate approximate, cumulative probabilities associated with any mean $\bar{x}$. A sample mean $\bar{x}$ translates into a specific value of Z with an approximate standard normal distribution. The value of Z then determines an approximate, cumulative probability (Table A.1). For example, the approximate probability of observing a sample mean value less than or equal to 3, found by employing the central limit theorem approximation, is

$$F(3) = P(\bar{X} \leq 3) = P\left(Z \leq \frac{3 - 3.5}{\sqrt{0.729}}\right) = P\left(Z \leq \frac{-0.5}{0.854}\right)$$
$$= P(Z \leq -0.586) = 0.279.$$

The selected sample mean value $\bar{x} = 3$ is 0.586 standard deviations below the expected value 3.5 and the associated cumulative probability is $F(3) =$

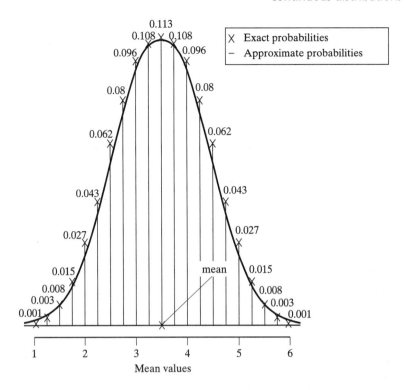

FIGURE 4.8: The distribution of the mean value of four tosses of a fair die, exact (G), and normal distribution approximation (F).

$P(\overline{X} \le 3) = P(Z \le -0.586) = 0.279$ using the standard normal probability distribution to calculate an approximate probability. The exact probability based on enumerating all 1296 outcomes shows $1 + 4 + 10 + \cdots + 104 + 125 = 435$ sample mean values are in fact less than or equal to 3 or $G(3) = 435/1296 = 0.336$. The approximate value calculated from the normal distribution is not very different from the exact value, especially since the sample size is small, only $n = 4$ observations.

Note that the distribution $G(\overline{x})$ is discrete and each possible value of $\overline{x}$ is separated by 0.25. The normal distribution approximation is substantially improved by adding 1/2 of this interval width $= (1/2)(0.25) = 0.125$ to 3 and finding $F(3.125) = P(\overline{X} \le 3.125) = P(Z \le -0.439) = 0.330$ (an explanation for this correction factor follows). The approximate (0.330) and the exact (0.336) probabilities are now the same for all practical purposes.

The calculation of an exact probability requires a complete enumeration of the probability distribution of $\overline{x}$, which depends on the joint probability distribution of X_1, X_2, X_3, and X_4; a process that is tedious in this case and not possible in most applied situations, as mentioned. Application of the central limit theorem requires only knowledge of the expected value $[E(X) = 3.5]$ and the variance ($\sigma_X^2 = 35/12$) of the sampled distribution (parent population) to find approximate probabilities associated with the occurrence of any possible mean value of $\overline{x}$. All exact and approximate cumulative probabilities are contained in the Table 4.2 [$F(x)$ and $G(x)$]. The largest difference is 0.007. A difference of this magnitude is typically unimportant.

Samples are frequently collected because little is known about the sampled population. The central limit theorem, nevertheless, usually allows a rigorous evaluation of the sample mean in terms of, at least approximate, probabilities. These probabilities become the foundation underlying a number of statistical techniques, such as confidence intervals and statistical tests (topics of the next two chapters).

A question remains: How large a sample assures an accurate approximation? Many investigators feel "safe" when the sample size exceeds 20 or 30 observations. This rule of "20 or 30" is probably a good guideline but does not guarantee any specific degree of accuracy. Critical to the accuracy of the central limit theorem approximation is the degree of symmetry of the parent distribution. Symmetric parent distributions yield sample mean values with distributions that are accurately approximated using a normal distribution, even for small sample sizes. If the parent distribution is close to symmetric, a sample size in the neighborhood of $n = 10$ yields a mean value with a nearly normal distribution. A sample size of $n = 4$ works well for the dice example (symmetric parent = uniform probability distribution). As the parent distribution becomes less symmetric, a larger sample size is necessary to obtain accurate probabilities using a normal distribution as an approximation.

Figure 4.9 illustrates three parent distributions (left-most column); a normal distribution, a continuous uniform distribution and an asymmetric distribution (skewed to the right). The corresponding rows display the distribution of the sample mean value resulting from $n = 3, 10$, and 30 observations sampled from each distribution. The illustration confirms that the distribution of the sampled mean value (1) has at least an approximate normal distribution, (2) has a mean value equal to the mean value of the sampled distribution [as always, $E(\overline{X}) = E(X)$], and (3) has a variance that decreases as the sample size increases ($\sigma_{\overline{X}}^2 = \sigma_X^2/n$). As mentioned, if the parent probability distribution is normally distributed, then a mean value based on sampled observations is itself normally distributed (top row, Figure 4.9). The central limit theorem is not relevant since the distribution of the sample mean has an exact normal distribution regardless of sample size.

Once again, it is critical to keep in mind that the central limit theorem links two distributions—the distribution of sampled observations and the distribution of the sample mean constructed from the sampled observations. These two distribution are certainly related but equally important is the fact that they are often completely different distributions and always play entirely different roles in evaluating an observed mean value.

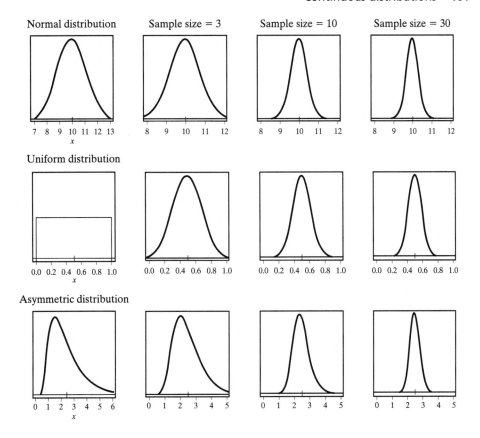

FIGURE 4.9: Three sampled distributions (parent distributions) and the distribution of the sample mean $\bar{x}$ for samples of size $n = 3$, 10, and 30.

A section in Gail Howard's book *State Lotteries: How to get in $\cdots$ and how to win it!* describes a lottery strategy she calls the "well-balanced game." She suggests that

> in a lotto game where you select six numbers out of a range of 1 to 40, the ideal total of those numbers would be 120. (In 6/40 Lotto the midnumber is 20. You play six numbers, $6 \times 20 = 120$) $\cdots$ and the greatest percentage of possible six-number combinations in the 6/40 game add up to 120. There is only one six-number combination that adds to 21 $(1+2+3+4+5+6 = 21)$ and only one six-number combination that adds to 225 and that is $35 + 36 + 37 + 38 + 39 + 40 = 225$. These two combinations are at the tails of the bell curve [normal distribution], making it virtually impossible for these numbers to be drawn as a winning combination.

Ms. Howard's statement of the central limit theorem is correct. The mean of six selected lottery numbers will more likely be in the neighborhood of 20 (sum = 120) than in the tails of an approximate normal distribution because the central limit theorem accurately applies to the mean of six numbers sampled from the symmetric discrete distribution. Unfortunately, a lottery payoff is determined by each value selected and not the mean value making the central limit theorem irrelevant to the probability of winning. The individual selected lottery values remain entirely unpredictable and no reason exists for any specific selected number to be particularly close to the expected value 20.5. All values, 1 through 40, are equally likely on each drawing. It is the mean that has an approximate normal distribution, and it is the mean that is likely be in the neighborhood of 20.5, not each individual lottery number. Therefore, picking a balanced set of lottery numbers has absolutely no positive or negative impact on the probability of winning. A sampled value and a sample mean value have different probability distributions and, as emphasized, the properties of the sampled values (x_i) that make up the mean value are different from the properties of a mean value $(\bar{x})$. Ms. Howard has confused the distribution sampled with the distribution of the sample mean (approximately normal with $\mu = 20.5$).

AN ADDITIONAL EXAMPLE

The following example illustrates a theorem called *the law of large numbers*. This law loosely translates into what every school child knows: There is safety in large numbers.

Each of $n = 64$ Western Tiger Swallowtail butterflies (*Papilio rutulus*) was collected independently from a population in Baja, California. It is known that the distribution of wing lengths (X) has a mean value of $E(X) = 4$ cm and a variance of $\sigma_X^2 = 25$ cm^2. What is the probability that a sample mean value calculated from the 64 sampled butterflies will fall between the values 3.5 cm and 4.5 cm? In symbols, $P(3.5 \text{ cm} \leq \bar{X} \leq 4.5 \text{ cm}) = ?$

The central limit theorem states that mean values have at least approximate normal distributions; therefore, standardizing the values 3.5 and 4.5 and using Table A.1 gives a good approximate answer, or

$$P(3.5 \text{ cm} \leq \bar{X} \leq 4.5 \text{ cm}) = P(\bar{X} \leq 4.5) - P(\bar{X} \leq 3.5)$$

$$= P\left(Z \leq \frac{4.5 - 4}{\sqrt{25/64}}\right) - P\left(Z \leq \frac{3.5 - 4}{\sqrt{25/64}}\right)$$

$$= P(Z \leq 0.8) - P(Z \leq -0.8)$$

$$= 0.788 - 0.212 = 0.576.$$

About 57.6% of mean wing lengths, based on a sample of $n = 64$ observations, fall between 3.5 cm and 4.5 cm.

When the sample size is increased to $n = 225$, the same calculation gives

$$P(3.5 \text{ cm} \leq \bar{X} \leq 4.5 \text{ cm}) = P(Z \leq 1.5) - P(Z \leq -1.5)$$

$$= 0.933 - 0.067 = 0.866.$$

The probability that the sample mean is contained in the same interval increases as the sample size increases (from 0.576 to 0.866). If $n = 625$, then

$$P(3.5 \text{ cm} \leq \overline{X} \leq 4.5 \text{ cm}) = P(Z \leq -2.5) - P(Z \leq 2.5) = 0.988. \quad \blacksquare$$

The fact that the estimated mean $(\overline{x})$ is increasingly likely to be close to the population mean as the sample size n increases is certainly not surprising, since the variance of a mean $(\sigma_{\overline{X}}^2 / n)$ decreases as the sample size increases. Small variances make extreme values less likely and "typical" values more likely. This calculation illustrates the law of large numbers, which simply states that if the sample size is large enough, the mean value $\overline{x}$ will hardly differ from its expected value $E(X)$.

In general, a mean value based on many independent observations becomes stable and predictable regardless of the sampled population (parent population). Many activities depend on such stability. Insurance companies earn a specific profit based on an expected number of deaths; stores stock specific quantities of goods based in expected sales; government budgets depend on expected amounts of tax revenues; concerts expect specific size audiences; and numerous other examples show that a sample made up of a large number of observations allows precise predictions to be made.

Robert M. Coates writes[11] about the situation where the law of large numbers is repealed. He envisions the New York City bridge personnel overcome by nearly everyone trying to cross the Triborough Bridge between the hours of seven and nine o'clock, the theaters on Eighth Avenue practically empty; two hundred and seventy-four successive customers asking for a spool of pink thread; and the Twentieth Century Limited leaving New York with three passengers. If the law of large numbers were not already a statistical phenomenon, it is likely that Congress would certainly mandate such a law to maintain "the averageness of the American way of life."

Normal approximation for the binomial distribution

As before, an estimated value of the binomial parameter p, denoted $\hat{p}$, is

$$\hat{p} = \frac{x_1 + x_2 + \cdots + x_n}{n} = \frac{\sum x_i}{n} = \overline{x}$$

where x_i takes on values of 0 or 1 making the value $\hat{p}$ the mean number of occurrences of the value 1 among a total of n binary observations. The estimate $\hat{p}$ is usually called a *proportion* but is no more than a special kind of mean value. For a proportion (a mean), therefore,

$$E(\overline{X}) = E(\hat{p}) = E(X_i) = p \qquad \text{Chapter } 3 - E(X_i) = p$$

and, furthermore, the variance is

$$\sigma_{\overline{X}}^2 = \sigma_{\hat{p}}^2 = \frac{\sigma_{X_i}^2}{n} = \frac{p(1-p)}{n} \qquad \text{Chapter 3} - \sigma_{X_i}^2 = p(1-p).$$

When the binary values $x_1, x_2, \cdots, x_n$ are sampled independently from the same distribution ($p = $ constant), the central limit theorem applies to a proportion for large values of n (the meaning of "large" will be discussed), even though each observation takes on only the values 0 or 1. The parent distribution is not normally distributed; in fact, it is not even continuous. It is a simple discrete probability distribution made up of two alternatives (Chapter 3). The central limit theorem, nevertheless, applies and the quantity

$$Z = \frac{\overline{x} - E(\overline{X})}{\sigma_{\overline{X}}} = \frac{\hat{p} - p}{\sqrt{p(1-p)/n}}$$

is a special case and has an approximate standard normal distribution for large n. Thus, a normal distribution with a mean value of p and variance of $p(1-p)/n$ approximately describes the sampling variation of the sample estimate $\hat{p}$.

The assessment of an estimated proportion, like all estimates, requires an estimate of the associated variability. As noted, this variance is

$$variance(\hat{p}) = \frac{p(1-p)}{n} \qquad \text{see Box 4.8.}$$

where n represents the number of independent and identically distributed binary observations used to estimate $\hat{p}$ ($\hat{p} = \sum x_i/n$—Chapter 3).

Box 4.8. The Variance of an Estimated Proportion

Noting that $\sigma_{aX}^2 = a^2 \sigma_X^2$ for any random variable X, then

$$variance(\hat{p}) = variance\left(\frac{X}{n}\right) = \left[\frac{1}{n}\right]^2 \sigma_X^2$$

Therefore,

$$\sigma_{\hat{p}}^2 = \left[\frac{1}{n}\right]^2 \sigma_X^2 = \left[\frac{1}{n}\right]^2 np(1-p) = \frac{p(1-p)}{n}$$

where the count X represents a random variable with a binomial probability distribution with parameters p and n (Chapter 3).

EXAMPLE

If $n = 50$ and $p = 0.5$, then

$$E(\hat{p}) = p = 0.5, \quad \sigma_{\hat{p}}^2 = \frac{\sigma_{X_i}^2}{n} = \frac{p(1-p)}{n} = \frac{(0.5)(0.5)}{50} = 0.005 \quad \text{and}$$

$$Z = \frac{\hat{p} - 0.5}{\sqrt{0.005}}$$

has an approximate standard normal distribution. Now suppose one wishes to calculate the probability of observing a sample proportion $\hat{p}$, based on 50 observations, between 0.44 and 0.56, then

$$P(0.44 \leq \hat{p} \leq 0.56) = P(\hat{p} \leq 0.56) - P(\hat{p} \leq 0.44)$$

$$= P\left(Z \leq \frac{0.56 - 0.5}{\sqrt{0.005}}\right) - P\left(Z \leq \frac{0.44 - 0.5}{\sqrt{0.005}}\right)$$

$$= P(Z \leq 0.849) - P(Z \leq -0.849) = 0.802 - 0.198 \quad \text{Table A.1}$$

$$= 0.604.$$

Again, the use of a correction factor improves this approximation producing the approximate probability $P(0.42 + 0.01 \leq \hat{p} \leq 0.56 + 0.01) = 0.678$ ($0.5 \times$ interval width $= 0.5 \times 1/50 = 0.01$).

The exact probability calculated directly but tediously from the binomial probability distribution is

$$P(0.44 \leq \hat{p} \leq 0.56) = P(22 \leq X \leq 28) = \sum_{k=22}^{28} \binom{50}{k}(0.5)^k(0.5)^{50-k} = 0.678$$

where $50(0.44) = 22$ and $50(0.56) = 28$. ∎

The use of the continuous normal distribution as an approximation for the more complicated discrete binomial distribution by way of the central limit theorem produces accurate probabilities when p is near 0.5 and the sample size is moderately large (about 30—Table 4.3) but requires larger sample sizes when p differs from 0.5. Binomial distributions with a parameter p not equal to 0.5 ($p \neq 0.5$) are not symmetric (Chapter 3). As the sample size increases, however, the distribution of a proportion (sample mean) becomes increasingly symmetric producing a distribution that is more accurately approximated by the symmetric normal distribution. Table 4.3[12] gives values for p and n that allow accurate use of the normal approximation (central limit theorem).

TABLE 4.3: Sample size n for accurate use of the normal distribution as an approximation for the binomial distribution.

p	0.5	0.4	0.3	0.2	0.1	0.05
n	30	50	80	200	600	1400

When a sample size is not large enough to use the normal distribution to produce an approximate probability, computer routines or tables exist to find exact binomial probabilities.

Continuity correction factor

A specific and correctable error occurs when a continuous distribution such as the normal distribution is used to approximate probabilities from a discrete probability distribution such as the binomial or uniform distributions. The source of error is best seen by an example.

If a random variable X has a binomial distribution with parameters $p = 1/2$ and $n = 4$ $[E(X) = np = 2]$, then

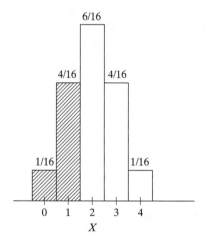

and, exactly,

$$G(1) = P(X \le 1) = 1/16 + 4/16 = 5/16 = 0.3125.$$

An approximation using the normal distribution looks like:

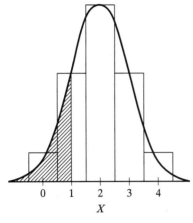

$$E(X) = np = 4(1/2) = 2$$
$$\sigma_X^2 = np(1 - p) = 4(1/2)(1/2) = 1$$
$$\sigma_X = 1$$

The approximate probability based on the normal distribution is

$$F(1) = P(X \leq 1) = P(Z \leq -1) = 0.159.$$

Most of the difference between the exact probability $[G(1) = 0.3125]$ and the approximate probability $[F(1) = 0.159]$ occurs because the area between 1 and 1.5 is part of the binomial probability distribution but is not included in the area under the normal curve. The accuracy of the approximation is improved by simply including the missing area, which means using the normal distribution approximation starting 1/2 unit to the right. For the example,

$$F(1 + 0.5) = P(X \leq 1 + 0.5) = P(X \leq 1.5) = P(Z \leq -0.5) = 0.309$$

(approximate + correction factor).

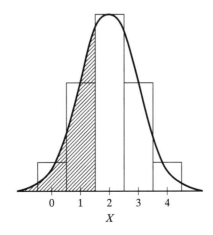

In general, the normal approximation is improved by adding 0.5 times the width of the interval between discrete values to the value x when the cumulative probability $P(X \leq x)$ is approximated. In symbols,

$$P(X \leq x) = P\left[Z \leq \frac{x + [0.5 \times (\textit{interval width})] - E(X)}{\sigma_X}\right]$$

where X is a value from a discrete probability distribution and Z is the corresponding value from the continuous standard normal distribution. The quantity $[0.5 \times (\textit{interval width})]$ added to a specified point (x) increases the accuracy of using a continuous normal distribution to approximate cumulative probabilities from a discrete distribution and is called the *continuity correction factor*. As the sample size increases, the interval width decreases and the importance of the correction factor becomes less of an issue.

Review: The expected value and variance of the distribution of a weighted average of independently sampled observations is determined by the expected values and variances of each of its components. The sum $\sum a_i x_i$ is a special kind of a weighted average where the sum of the weights is one ($\sum a_i = 1$). For any sample of n observations $x_1, x_2, \cdots, x_n$, then the expected value of this sum (the mean of its probability distribution) is

$$E\left(\sum a_i X_i\right) = \sum a_i E(X_i)$$

and if the x_i-values are independent, then the variance is

$$\sigma^2_{\sum a_i X_i} = \sum a_i^2 \sigma^2_{X_i}.$$

Furthermore, if these sampled values have the same expectations and variances (identically distributed), which is frequently the case, then

$$E\left(\sum a_i X_i\right) = \left(\sum a_i\right) E(X)$$

and

$$\sigma^2_{\sum a_i X_i} = \left(\sum a_i^2\right) \sigma^2_X$$

where $E(X)$ and σ^2_X are the mean value and variance of the population sampled (parent population).

When the x_i-values are independently and identically distributed values with a normal distribution, then a weighted average $\sum a_i x_i$ has normal distribution with mean $= (\sum a_i) E(X)$ and variance $= (\sum a_i^2) \sigma^2_X$. In addition, when the data are not sampled from a normal distribution, the weighted average $\sum a_i x_i$ has an approximate normal distribution with the same mean and variance when the sample size n is large (central limit theorem).

Because a sample mean ($\bar{x}$) is a weighted average (all weights $= a_i = 1/n$) frequently calculated from a sample of independent and identically distributed values, three fundamental properties apply:

1. **expectation:** The expected value (mean) of the distribution describing the possible values of the sample mean is the mean of the probability distribution that produced the sampled observations or $E(\overline{X}) = E(X)$, since $\sum a_i = 1$,

2. **variance:** The variance of the distribution describing the sample mean is the variance of the probability distribution that produced the sampled observations divided by the sample size or $\sigma^2_{\overline{X}} = \sigma^2_X/n$, since $\sum a_i^2 = 1/n$, and

3. **distribution:** The distribution of the sample mean value is, in most cases, at least an approximate normal distribution for moderately large sample sizes regardless of the probability distribution that produced the sampled observations.

These three properties of the sample mean make it possible to calculate probabilities associated with a specific observed mean value based on the normal distribution. The application of many statistical techniques, in this text and throughout statistics, capitalize on these three fundamental properties because they involve special kinds of weighted averages (for example, a sample mean or a sample proportion).

A review of five specific statistical distributions described in Chapter 4 is:

Distributions	Parameters	Mean values	Variances
uniform (discrete)	k	$(k+1)/2$	$(k^2 - 1)/12$
binomial	n, p	np	$np(1-p)$
Poisson	λ	λ	λ
uniform (continuous)	b, a	$(a+b)/2$	$(b-a)^2/12$
normal	μ, σ^2_X	μ	σ^2_X

the
normal
law of errors
stands out in the
endeavors of mankind
as one of the broadest
generalizations of natural
philosophy. It serves as the
guiding instrument for research
in the physical and social sciences
and in medicine, agriculture and in the
biological world in general. It is a tool
important for the analyses and interpretations
of the basic information obtained by observation and by
experimental design to produce fundamental statistical inferences.

W. J. Youden

PROBLEM SET 4

Using data from the 1926 epidemic of measles in St. Pancras (England) a study was made of the occurrence of secondary cases. Out of 250 families of four children, each family had a case of measles and three additional susceptible children under the age of 10, the following data were recorded:

Number ill out of three susceptibles (number of secondary cases) x_i	Number of families f_i
0	95
1	80
2	50
3	25
Total	250

The hypothesis that measles is not contagious implies that there is a constant probability p of contracting the disease within each family, which means that the chance of getting measles is not related to within family exposure.

Assume each susceptible has the same chance p of getting measles regardless of other factors.

1. Estimate the probability of measles $\hat{p}$ from the St. Pancras data.
2. Based on this estimate, estimate the number of families with 0, 1, 2, and 3 secondary cases which you would expect to find under the hypothesis p is constant.
3. Does this hypothesis seem reasonable in light of the data? Why or why not? (No further calculations are necessary.)

The following data were collected to study a genetic trait (a kind of blue eyes) and focuses on families of size four ($k = 143$ families and $n = 4$ persons per family involving a total of $N = 4(143) = 572$ persons).

Cases	0	1	2	3	4	Total
Families	45	71	20	6	1	143

Suppose $p =$ the probability of inheriting this genetic trait (a specific individual has blue eyes).

4. Compute the number of families with 0, 1, 2, 3, and 4 blue-eyed children using a family size of 4 and probability $p = 0.25$.
5. Estimate the same probability of the blue-eyed child ($\hat{p}$) from the data.
6. Estimate the number of families with 0, 1, 2, 3, and 4 blue-eyed children using the estimate $\hat{p}$.
7. Which set of estimated values best corresponds to the data ("fits")? Speculate why or why not?

For two hundred years, the northern Japanese have recorded the number of severe typhoons that strike their islands each year. For one island, the data are given below:

Number of typhoons each year (x_i)	0	1	2	3	4	5	Total
Frequency of years with x_i typhoons (f_i)	149	24	15	5	4	3	200

8. Estimate the mean number of typhoons per year.

9. Assuming the number of typhoons per year is described accurately by a Poisson distribution, find the probabilities for years with 0, 1, 2, 3, 4, 5, and 6 or more storms.

10. Do you think the distribution of these typhoons is described by a Poisson distribution? Speculate why or why not? (No further calculations are necessary.)

Suppose Z represents a normal random variable with a mean of zero and a variance of one ($\mu = 0$ and $\sigma^2 = 1$). Find:

11. $P(0 \leq Z \leq 1)$

12. $P(-1.960 \leq Z \leq 1.960)$

13. $P(Z \geq 1.645)$

Suppose Z represents a normal random variable with a mean of zero and a variance of one. Find, in each case, the percentile z such that

14. $P(Z \geq z) = 0.50$

15. $P(Z \geq z) = 0.05$

16. $P(Z \leq -z \text{ or } Z \geq z) = 0.10$

Given a normal distribution with mean $\mu = 50$ and variance $\sigma^2 = 25$, find:

17. The probability that a single random observation is larger than 50.

18. What is the probability that a single random observation falls between 40 and 60?

19. Find 10th-percentile, the 30th-percentile, the 50th-percentile, and the 95th-percentile.

Suppose the heights of male graduate students are normally distributed with a mean of $\mu = 70$ inches with a standard deviation of $\sigma = 2$ inches.

20. What is the probability that a male graduate student chosen at random will be over 74 inches tall?

21. What is the probability that a male graduate student chosen at random is less than 68 inches but more than 66 inches tall?

22. In a group of 1000 male graduate students, how many would you expect to find over 73 inches tall?

23. Suppose that a dormitory orders beds for these students. The beds should be of such a size that it is expected that only one man in one hundred will be too tall for his bed. What should the length of the beds be?

The birth weight of white female infants is normally distributed with a mean of $\mu = 7.6$ lbs with a standard deviation of $\sigma = 1.1$ lbs.

24. What is the probability that a white female infant will weigh less than 4 lbs?

25. What is the probability that a sample mean ($n = 121$) is 7.85 lbs or more?

26. In view of your answer in (b), do you think that a mean of $\bar{x} = 7.85$ based on $n = 121$ birth weights is a typical sample of all white female births? Speculate why or why not?

Assume the wing lengths of wild adult female mosquitoes, *Culex tarsalis*, are normally distributed with a mean $\mu = 4.4$ mm and a variance $\sigma^2 = 0.09$ mm^2.

27. What is the probability that the sample mean $\bar{x}$, based on $n = 25$ observations, will be more than 0.15 mm from the population mean μ?

28. If the mean of a sample of size $n = 9$ is computed, what is the probability that this sample mean will be within 0.1 mm of the population mean μ?

29. If the mean of a sample of size $n = 36$ is computed, what is the probability that this sample mean will be within 0.1 mm of the population mean μ?

30. If the sample size is huge, what is an approximate value of $\bar{x}$?

PART TWO
STATISTICS: PROPERTIES OF SAMPLED POPULATIONS

CHAPTER 5

Statistical Inference I

Typically a statistical inference results from comparing a summary value calculated from sampled data to a nonrandom value derived primarily from theory. When observed and theoretical values are similar, confidence in the theory is increased. Conversely, when the two values differ substantially, the theory becomes suspect. A statistical inference is a formal and usually a quantitative statement about this comparison. Since sampling variation influences a statistical summary, these comparisons always incur a degree of uncertainty. Values can appear to agree when they actually differ and values can appear to differ when they actually agree. The agreement between theory and observations, therefore, is measured in terms of a probability reflecting the plausibility that the observed difference or differences arose strictly by chance. The statistical concepts and tools developed in the first four chapters provide the basis for calculating this probability.

Point estimation

A *point estimate* is a single value (a point in the geometrical sense) used to estimate a population parameter from a sample of observations. Point estimates, like all estimates, are subject to sampling variation. The following three examples of point estimates along with expressions for estimating their associated variability have already been encountered:

Probability distribution	Population parameter	Point estimate	Measure of sampling variation
normal	μ	$\hat{\mu} = \bar{x}$	$S_{\bar{x}}^2 = S_X^2/n$
Poisson	λ	$\hat{\lambda} = \bar{x}$	$S_{\hat{\lambda}}^2 = \hat{\lambda}/n = \bar{x}/n$
binomial	p	$\hat{p} = \bar{x}/n$	$S_{\hat{p}}^2 = \hat{p}(1 - \hat{p})/N$

These point estimates originate from the same principle. The expected value of the distribution of the mean $\bar{x}$ is $E(X)$ suggesting that the unknown population mean value $E(X)$ can be estimated by the sampled value $\bar{x}$. Specifically, the estimated mean for a normal distribution is $\hat{\mu} = \bar{x}$ since $E(\bar{X}) = E(X) = \mu$. The parameter of the Poisson distribution (mean of the Poisson distribution) is estimated in a similar manner. Because $E(\bar{X}) = E(X) = \lambda$, the parameter λ

is estimated by $\bar{x}$ or $\hat{\lambda} = \bar{x}$. The mean value of the binomial distribution is $E(\bar{X}) = E(X) = np$ and the parameter p is again estimated by the sample mean $\bar{x}$ where $\hat{p} = \bar{x}/n$ (Chapter 4). All three population parameters are directly estimated by using the sample mean. In addition, the variance of each estimate (measure of precision) is a function of sample size and decreases as the number of observations increases. In other words, the estimate becomes increasingly more precise as the sample size becomes larger.

Description of a confidence interval

An alternative to a point estimate of a parameter is an interval that, with high probability, contains the unknown parameter of interest (for example, parameters μ, λ, or p). The location of the interval identifies a range of likely values of the parameter and the width indicates the confidence that can be placed in this sample generated estimate; thus, the name *confidence interval*. If a confidence interval is wide, the sample does not give much information about a parameter. As the width of the interval decreases, knowledge about the value of the parameter becomes increasingly more precise.

In a particular state, it was noted that more than half the women in prison for murder had killed their husbands and less than a fifth of the men in prison for murder had killed their wives. Before drawing conclusions about wife/husband relationships, it is useful to know that only four women were convicted for murder and 660 men. A confidence interval based on these data would indicate immediately their vastly different precisions. The confidence interval associated with the women would be extremely wide since the number of women involved is small (4). The data convey little information about the "true" proportion of women who murder their husbands because the considerable impact of sampling variation makes the credibility of the estimate extremely low. The confidence interval associated with the men would be narrow, indicating a much more precise (reliable) estimate because it is based on a relatively large number of observations (660), which substantially reduces the impact of sampling variation.

EXAMPLE

Suppose $\bar{x} = 6.5$ lbs is the estimated mean birth weight calculated from a sample of 30 newborn female infants with Asian mothers. To identify likely values of the population mean and provide simultaneously a measure of the impact of the sampling variability, an interval is constructed so that, with a high probability, the unknown parameter μ is contained within its limits (μ = the mean birth weight of the sampled distribution). The location of the interval indicates a range of likely values of the unknown "true" birth weight μ and the width of the interval reflects the precision of the sample mean $\bar{x} = 6.5$ as an estimate of μ. Such an interval is a confidence interval for the population mean birth weight μ. ∎

confidence interval $= \bar{x} \pm 1.960\sqrt{\frac{1}{10}} = \bar{x} \pm 0.620$ (justified in the next section).

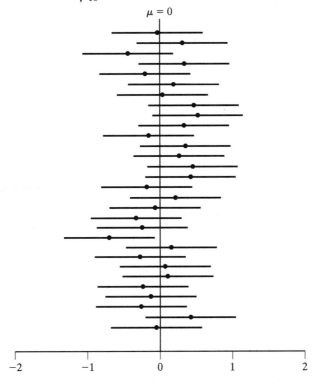

FIGURE 5.1: Confidence intervals (95%) for 30 different random samples of size $n = 10$ from a normal distribution with $\mu = 0$ and $\sigma_X^2 = 1$.

The location of the confidence interval is determined by the value of the mean $\bar{x}$ and, therefore, is itself subject to sampling variation. Its endpoints (denoted $\hat{A}$ and $\hat{B}$) vary because they are estimated from the sampled values (details are discussed in the next section). A confidence interval from $\hat{A}$ to $\hat{B}$ has the form $P(\hat{A} \leq \mu \leq \hat{B}) = 1 - \alpha$ where $1 - \alpha$ is the level of confidence. It is not correct to state that "There is a $1 - \alpha$ probability that the parameter μ is contained in the interval $\hat{A}$ to $\hat{B}$." Since μ is not a variable, it does not vary from sample to sample. It is not subject to sampling variation. The correct statement is, "There is a $1 - \alpha$ probability that the estimated confidence interval $(\hat{A}, \hat{B})$ contains the unknown population mean μ." The confidence interval varies, not μ. To repeat, the interval endpoints $\hat{A}$ and $\hat{B}$ are constructed from the sample mean and will differ from sample to sample. The distinction, at first, may seem slight but it is vital to distinguish clearly between population values (never vary) and sample values (always vary). Figure 5.1 illustrates 30 confidence intervals (95%), each constructed from 30 different samples of size $n = 10$ from a normal population with mean $= \mu = 0$ and variance $= \sigma^2 = 1$.

The confidence interval was invented by Jerzy Neyman (b. 1894) and presented in 1934. His work was immediately criticized and even called a "confidence trick." Today, however, confidence intervals appear as part of most statistical analyses regardless of the field.

Construction of a $(1 - \alpha)$-level confidence interval for a population mean (σ_X^2 known)

Consider a sample mean value $\bar{x}$, then for a moderately large sample size n,

$$Z = \frac{\overline{X} - E(\overline{X})}{\sigma_{\overline{X}}} = \frac{\overline{X} - \mu}{\sqrt{\sigma_X^2/n}} = \frac{\sqrt{n}(\overline{X} - \mu)}{\sigma_X}$$

usually has an approximate normal distribution (exact, if the values $x_1, x_2, \cdots, x_n$ are sampled from a normal distribution) with mean $= 0$ and variance $= 1$ (central limit theorem). The variance is assumed to be a known value for this chapter. The more realistic case where the variance is unknown but estimated is discussed in the next chapter.

To start, from the normal distribution

$$P(-1.960 \le Z \le 1.960) = 0.95 \qquad\qquad \textit{(from Table A.1)}$$

$$P\left(-1.960 \le \frac{\sqrt{n}(\overline{X} - \mu)}{\sigma_X} \le 1.960\right) = 0.95 \qquad \textit{(by definition of Z)}$$

$$P\left(-1.960\frac{\sigma_X}{\sqrt{n}} \le (\overline{X} - \mu) \le 1.960\frac{\sigma_X}{\sqrt{n}}\right) = 0.95 \qquad \textit{(multiplying by } \sigma_X/\sqrt{n})$$

and a 95% confidence internal is then

$$P\left(\overline{X} - 1.960\frac{\sigma_X}{\sqrt{n}} \le \mu \le \overline{X} + 1.960\frac{\sigma_X}{\sqrt{n}}\right) = 0.95.$$

$$\textit{(subtracting } \overline{X} \textit{ and multiplying by } -1)$$

The estimated lower bound of the 95% confidence interval based on a sample of $n = 30$ birth weights, the mean $\bar{x} = 6.5$ lbs, and a known variance of $\sigma_X^2 = 1$ is

$$\hat{A} = \bar{x} - 1.960\frac{\sigma_X}{\sqrt{n}} = 6.5 - 1.960\frac{1}{\sqrt{30}} = 6.5 - 0.358 = 6.142$$

and the estimated upper bound is

$$\hat{B} = \bar{x} + 1.960\frac{\sigma_X}{\sqrt{n}} = 6.5 + 1.960\frac{1}{\sqrt{30}} = 6.5 + 0.358 = 6.858$$

giving the 95% confidence interval (6.142, 6.858), length = 0.72 lbs. The interval from 6.142 lbs to 6.858 lbs has a 0.95 probability of containing the "true" but unknown mean birth weight μ of the sampled population. Or, conversely, it is not likely that the parameter μ is less than 6.142 lbs or greater than 6.858 lbs (probability = 0.05).

It is important to remember that the expression "a $(1-\alpha)$-level confidence interval" refers to one specific confidence interval among the many possible confidence intervals that could have occurred, because $\bar{x}$ is one mean value among the many possible sample means that could have occurred (see Figure 5.1). The sampling variation that influences the estimated value $\bar{x}$ equally influences the confidence interval constructed from the mean $\bar{x}$.

In general, a $(1-\alpha)$-level confidence interval based on a sample mean value is constructed from the relationship that

$$P\left(\bar{X} - z_{1-\alpha/2}\sigma_{\bar{X}} \leq \mu \leq \bar{X} + z_{1-\alpha/2}\sigma_{\bar{X}}\right) = 1 - \alpha$$

or

$$P\left(\bar{X} - z_{1-\alpha/2}\frac{\sigma_X}{\sqrt{n}} \leq \mu \leq \bar{X} + z_{1-\alpha/2}\frac{\sigma_X}{\sqrt{n}}\right) = 1 - \alpha.$$

The symbol $z_{1-\alpha/2}$ represents the $(1-\alpha/2)^{\text{th}}$-percentile of the standard normal distribution. Because the lower bound of the $(1-\alpha)\%$ confidence interval is $\hat{A} = \bar{x} - z_{1-\alpha/2}(\sigma_X/\sqrt{n})$ and the upper bound is $\hat{B} = \bar{x} + z_{1+\alpha/2}(\sigma_X/\sqrt{n})$, the length of the interval becomes $l = \hat{B} - \hat{A} = 2z_{1-\alpha/2}(\sigma_X/\sqrt{n})$. The length of a confidence interval reflects the precision of $\bar{x}$ as an estimate of μ, as already noted, and depends on the choice of the confidence level (α), the variability of the population sampled (σ_X^2), and the number of observations sampled (n).

Associated with a confidence interval is the term *margin of error*. The margin of error is defined as the length of the confidence interval divided by two [i.e., *margin of error = (upper bound − lower bound)/2*] and also directly indicates the precision of an estimate. For an estimated mean value, the margin of error is $z_{1-\alpha/2}\sigma_{\bar{X}}$. The evening television news and newspaper articles that refer to statistical estimates, such as results from election polling or results from surveys, occasionally report the relevant margin of error.

The percentile values $z_{1-\alpha/2}$ are found in tables of the standard normal distribution (Table A.1, last two columns). Three typical values are:

$1-\alpha$	α	$1-\alpha/2$	$z_{1-\alpha/2}$	Limits	Margin of error
0.90	0.10	0.95	1.645	$\bar{x} \pm 1.645\sigma_{\bar{X}}$	$1.645\sigma_{\bar{X}}$
0.95	0.05	0.975	1.960	$\bar{x} \pm 1.960\sigma_{\bar{X}}$	$1.960\sigma_{\bar{X}}$
0.99	0.01	0.995	2.576	$\bar{x} \pm 2.576\sigma_{\bar{X}}$	$2.576\sigma_{\bar{X}}$

Increasing the sample size decreases the length of a confidence interval. This property is certainly expected because the larger the sample, the more precise the estimated mean value. More mechanically, increasing the sample size n reduces the variance of the sample mean $\sigma_{\bar{X}}^2$ (σ_X^2/n), which in turn reduces the amount added to $\bar{x}$ and subtracted from $\bar{x}$ to form the endpoints of the confidence interval. For example, suppose the sample mean birth weight $\bar{x}$ remains 6.5 lbs but the sample size is increased to 120 observations. The confidence bounds are ($\sigma_X^2 = 1$)

$$\hat{A} = upper\ bound = 6.5 - 1.960\frac{1}{\sqrt{120}} = 6.5 - 0.179 = 6.321$$

and

$$\hat{B} = lower\ bound = 6.5 + 1.960\frac{1}{\sqrt{120}} = 6.5 + 0.179 = 6.679.$$

The 95% confidence interval is now (6.321, 6.679), length $= 0.36$, reduced from 0.72. Increasing the sample size by a factor of four reduces the length of the confidence interval by a factor of two.

Three notable properties of a confidence interval are:

1. when the sample size n is increased, the variance of the sample mean $\sigma_{\bar{X}}^2$ decreases and, necessarily, the confidence interval length l decreases (again, $l = 2z_{1-\alpha/2}\sigma_{\bar{X}}$),
2. when confidence level $(1 - \alpha)$ is decreased, the percentile $z_{1-\alpha/2}$ decreases and the confidence interval length l decreases, and
3. when variance σ_X^2 of the population sampled is reduced (by experimental techniques such as sampling more homogeneous observations), the sample variance $\sigma_{\bar{X}}^2$ decreases, also decreasing the confidence interval length l.

An Analogy

When a handgun is fired at a target, an assessment of the shooter's ability is not difficult. The distances from the bullet holes to the bull's-eye indicate the accuracy of the shooter. The spread among the holes reflects the precision. Assessing the accuracy and the precision of a statistical estimate is not as simple. The observations (the "bullet holes") are combined to estimate a parameter (the "bull's-eye") but, unlike target shooting, the location of the "bull's-eye" is unknown. Clearly, the results from target shooting would also be more difficult to assess if the location of the bull's-eye was unknown. For example,

Target one   Target two

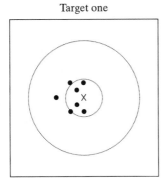
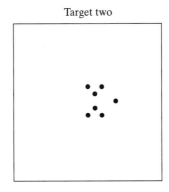

The second target with the bull's-eye removed is certainly not as useful as the first, but it is not useless. The placement of the seven bullet holes gives some indication of the location of the bull's-eye (accuracy) and the spread again reflects the skill (precision) of the shooter.

A confidence interval, like the second target, allows an assessment of an estimate without knowledge of the underlying population parameter, the "bull's-eye." This seemingly difficult task is accomplished in a simple fashion. The placement of a confidence interval suggests (with high probability) the location of the "bull's-eye," giving an indication of the accuracy of the estimated value. In addition, the width of the interval directly reflects the precision of the estimate regardless of the accuracy.

Construction of a $(1 - \alpha)$-confidence interval for a population proportion

A confidence interval also indicates the impact of sampling variation on a proportion (an estimated probability) and can be constructed using a normal distribution. The construction and interpretation of this confidence interval is the same in principle as the previously discussed confidence interval constructed from a sample mean but differs in a few technical details.

As noted earlier, a proportion is a special kind of mean value and, therefore, has an approximate normal distribution for a sample with a large number of observations n (Chapter 4—central limit theorem). Suppose again that the symbol $\hat{p}$ represents this special case of a mean value. An approximate $(1 - \alpha)$-level confidence interval for the underlying "true" proportion p is then constructed from the relationship that

$$P\left(\hat{p} - z_{1-\alpha/2}\sigma_{\hat{p}} \leq p \leq \hat{p} + z_{1-\alpha/2}\sigma_{\hat{p}}\right) \approx 1 - \alpha$$

or

$$P\left(\hat{p} - z_{1-\alpha/2}\left[\sqrt{\frac{\hat{p}(1-\hat{p})}{n}}\right] \le p \le \hat{p} + z_{1-\alpha/2}\left[\sqrt{\frac{\hat{p}(1-\hat{p})}{n}}\right]\right) \approx 1 - \alpha.$$

The calculations involved are not very different from those used to create the confidence interval for μ. The proportion $\hat{p}$ corresponds to the mean $\bar{x}$ and the expression $\sqrt{\hat{p}(1-\hat{p})/n}$; the estimated standard deviation associated with the estimate of $\hat{p}$ (Chapter 3), corresponds to $\sigma_{\bar{X}}$.

EXAMPLE

Suppose that $n = 25$ newborn infants of obese women are sampled and $x = 10$ weigh less than 2500 grams, then $\hat{p} = x/n = 10/25 = 0.4$, yielding a 95% confidence interval with an estimated lower bound of $\hat{A} = 0.4 - 1.960\sqrt{0.4(0.6)/25} = 0.208$ and an estimated upper bound of $\hat{B} = 0.4 + 1.960\sqrt{0.4(0.6)/25} = 0.592$. These bounds define an approximate 95% confidence interval (0.208, 0.592). Thus, the underlying proportion of infants weighing less than 2500 grams (p), estimated by $\hat{p} = 0.4$, is unlikely (probability = 0.05) to be less than 0.208 or greater than 0.529. The estimated upper and lower bounds indicate a range of likely values of the unknown parameter p. As before, the confidence interval has a 95% chance of containing the probability estimated by $\hat{p}$, namely p. ∎

If the sample size is small or the probability p is close to zero or one, using the normal distribution approximation (relying on the central limit theorem) can fail to give accurate confidence interval bounds (Table 4.3). Exact statistical methods, however, exist to construct a $(1 - \alpha)$-level confidence interval and the somewhat complicated calculations are usually implemented with a computer program.[13]

An application of a confidence interval: capture/recapture estimation

To estimate the size of a closed population, a preliminary sample is collected and these "captured" observations are marked. The marked observations are returned to the population, which is then resampled. The number of marked observations in the second sample ("recaptured") relates to the size of the population. When a high proportion of resampled observations are marked, the population is likely to be relatively small. When a low proportion of the second sample are marked, the population is likely to be large.

This *capture/recapture* technique has been used to estimate the size of a variety of populations such as the number of gray whales in the Pacific ocean, the number of wild dogs in the city of Baltimore, and the number of children with Down's syndrome in the state of Michigan. Once the population size is estimated, a confidence interval enriches its interpretation.

The first sample produces m marked and $N - m$ unmarked population members where N represents the unknown and to be estimated total population size. The second sample of n observations produces a count x of the marked observations and the proportion of marked observations in the resample is $\hat{p} = x/n$.

To assess the impact of sampling variation on this estimated proportion, it is treated no differently than any other proportion. An approximate $(1 - \alpha)$-level confidence interval is, again,

$$\hat{p} \pm z_{1-\alpha/2}\sigma_{\hat{p}} \qquad \text{where} \qquad \sigma_{\hat{p}}^2 = \frac{\hat{p}(1 - \hat{p})}{n}.$$

The proportion $\hat{p} = x/n$ is an estimate of p, the actual proportion of marked individuals in the population, which is $p = m/N$. The value m is known but the value N is not. An estimate of the population size is then $\hat{N} = m/\hat{p}$ since m is known and $\hat{p}$ is estimated. That is, the population size estimate answers the question: $\hat{p}$ times what population size equals m? Answer: $\hat{N}\hat{p} = m$ or $\hat{N} = m/\hat{p}$.

A confidence interval for the unknown population size N follows, because

$$P(\hat{p}_{lower} \leq p \leq \hat{p}_{upper}) = 1 - \alpha$$

where, as before, $\hat{A} = \hat{p}_{lower} = \hat{p} - z_{1-\alpha/2}\sigma_{\hat{p}}$ and $\hat{B} = \hat{p}_{upper} = \hat{p} + z_{1-\alpha/2}\sigma_{\hat{p}}$. Then,

$$P\left(\frac{1}{\hat{p}_{upper}} \leq \frac{1}{p} \leq \frac{1}{\hat{p}_{lower}}\right) = 1 - \alpha \qquad \textit{(confidence interval for the reciprocal)}$$

and

$$P\left(\frac{m}{\hat{p}_{upper}} \leq \frac{m}{p} \leq \frac{m}{\hat{p}_{lower}}\right) = 1 - \alpha \qquad \textit{(multiplying by m, a known quantity)}$$

giving

$$P(\hat{N}_{lower} \leq N \leq \hat{N}_{upper}) = 1 - \alpha \qquad \textit{(definition of N)}$$

which is an approximate $(1 - \alpha)$-level confidence interval for the population size N, constructed from the estimated population size $\hat{N}$.

EXAMPLE

To estimate the size of the population of a species of fish living in a Mexican high altitude lake, $m = 120$ fish were caught, tagged, and placed back in the lake. Now, the population proportion of marked fish is $p = 120/N$ or the population size $N = 120/p$ but N is unknown. To estimate N, all that is needed is an estimate of p. During a recapture phase, $x = 64$ tagged fish were caught in a second sample of $n = 180$ fish. An estimate of p is then $\hat{p} = 64/180 = 0.356$.

The evaluation of this estimate, as with many statistical estimates, requires the observations to be sampled independently. Explicitly, all fish, previously caught or not, have the same probability of being recaptured. The proportion of marked fish ($\hat{p} = x/n$) generates an approximate 95% confidence interval for the "true" population proportion ($p = m/N$) of marked fish in the lake where $\hat{p}_{lower} = 0.356 - 1.960(0.036) = 0.286$ and $\hat{p}_{upper} = 0.356 + 1.960(0.036) = 0.425$ or (0.286, 0.425).

The estimated size of the fish population N is a simple function of the estimate $\hat{p}$, namely $\hat{N} = m/\hat{p} = 120/0.356 = 337.5$. The estimated bounds of an approximate 95% confidence interval for the population size N, based on the estimate $\hat{N}$, are the same simple function of the previously estimated upper and lower confidence interval bounds, namely $(m/\hat{p}_{upper}, m/\hat{p}_{lower})$ or (120/0.425, 120/0.286) or (282.0, 420.1). Like all confidence intervals, this confidence interval indicates a likely range for the total number of these fish living in the lake while displaying simultaneously the precision associated with the estimated size of the fish population ($\hat{N} = 337.5$). ∎

Sample size and confidence interval length

"To that objection our Don Quixote answered: 'One swallow makes not a summer.'" This early concern with sample size might be followed by the question: How many swallows need to be observed to safely conclude summer has arrived? To calculate the sample size needed to reach a precise estimate requires a sometimes elaborate argument (Chapter 6). A simple and fundamental approach to determining the sample size necessary to produce a sample mean with a chosen level of precision is based on a confidence interval. In more specific statistical language, the question becomes: What sample size is required to estimate μ, based on the estimated mean $\bar{x}$, to attain a specific degree of precision? The length of a confidence interval provides one way to define precision and answer this question.

Suppose it is decided that sufficient data should be collected so that the sample mean $\bar{x}$ is not likely to differ from μ by more than a given amount; such a sample size can be calculated. The sample size is then the number of observations that produces a $(1 - \alpha)$-level confidence interval of length l. The length l of a $(1 - \alpha)$-level confidence interval is, as before,

$$l = \text{(upper bound)} - \text{(lower bound)} = (\bar{x} + z_{1-\alpha/2}\sigma_{\bar{X}}) - (\bar{x} - z_{1-\alpha/2}\sigma_{\bar{X}})$$

$$= 2(z_{1-\alpha/2})\sigma_{\bar{X}} = 2(z_{1-\alpha/2})\sqrt{\sigma_X^2/n}.$$

The sample size (denoted n_0) necessary to meet the requirement of length l at confidence level $1 - \alpha$ is found by rearranging this expression relating the confidence interval length to sample size. The sample size necessary to produce a $(1 - \alpha)\%$ confidence interval of length l is

$$n_0 = 4 \left[\frac{z_{1-\alpha/2}(\sigma_X)}{l} \right]^2.$$

The value n_0 is exact when the values sampled come from a normal distribution and approximate otherwise (central limit theorem).

EXAMPLE

For the infant birth weight example, suppose $l = 0.5$ lbs (within 0.25 lbs of the "true" mean or a margin of error of 0.25), a 95% confidence level is chosen ($z_{0.975} = 1.960$) and again $\sigma_X = 1$ lb, then

$$n_0 = 4 \left[\frac{1.960(1.0)}{0.5} \right]^2 = 61.463 \text{ or } 62 \text{ observations.}$$

A sample size of 62 observations produces a sample mean $\bar{x}$ with the precision desired, namely an estimated mean value likely (probability $= 0.95$) within 0.25 lbs of the population mean birth weight μ. That is,

$$length = (\bar{x} + 1.960\sigma_{\bar{X}}) - (\bar{x} - 1.960\sigma_{\bar{X}})$$

$$= (\bar{x} + 1.960\sqrt{1/62}) - (\bar{x} - 1.960\sqrt{1/62}) = 2(1.960)\sqrt{1/62} = 0.5. \quad \blacksquare$$

Statistical hypothesis testing

> There was a young man from Cascade
> who thought statistics was quite a charade.
> He hated the first weeks of class and more.
> He found means, variances, and probabilities a bore.
> But, hypothesis testing paid for all the effort and fuss he made.

In his book *The Design of Experiments*,[14] early statistician/geneticist R. A. Fisher (b. 1890) describes a lady who said she could taste whether milk was added to the tea or the other way around, the tea was added to the milk. To test her claim, eight cups of tea were prepared, four with milk added to the tea and four with the tea added to the milk. Upon tasting each of the eight cups of tea, the tea-drinking lady identified all eight correctly.[15] One now faces two explanations: She guessed and was lucky or she is rather sensitive to the way tea is prepared. Fisher suggested it is useful to know the probability of identifying correctly all eight cups of tea by guessing. If this probability is large, identifying the eight cups of tea correctly provides no substantial evidence to separate just guessing from an ability to taste the difference. Luck is a plausible explanation. If this probability is small, guessing becomes a less likely explanation and it becomes likely that the tea-tasting lady is not guessing and can tell the difference between the two methods of preparation. Incidentally, the probability of identifying all eight cups correctly by guessing is not likely ($1/70 = 0.014$), which strongly supports the lady's claim that she can tell the method used to prepare her tea. This experiment contains the essence of hypothesis testing, which is the subject of the remainder of the chapter.

In its simplest terms, a *statistical hypothesis* is a conjecture about the probability distribution of the sampled variable. Four examples are:

1. the distribution that produced the observed values has a mean value equal to zero ($\mu = 0$),
2. the two distributions have the same mean values ($\mu_x = \mu_y$),
3. the sampled binomial distribution has a specific parameter ($p = 1/2$), or
4. the collected data come from a Poisson distribution.

A formal statistical test of hypothesis is designed to choose between two possibilities. One possibility is called the *null hypothesis* (symbolized by H_0) and the other the *alternative hypothesis* (symbolized by H_1). A statistical hypothesis test provides a process for accepting or rejecting H_0 (rejecting or accepting H_1) while knowing the error rates associated with the decision. The null hypothesis H_0 is either true or false and there are two possible decisions, reject H_0 or accept H_0, creating four possible outcomes to a statistical hypothesis test (Table 5.1). Among the four possibilities, there are two correct decisions and two ways errors can occur, called *Type I* and *Type II* errors.

TABLE 5.1: The four possible outcomes of a test of hypothesis.

Decision	H_0 is true = H_1 is false	H_0 is false = H_1 is true
accept H_0 = reject H_1	correct decision	error (Type II)
reject H_0 = accept H_1	error (Type I)	correct decision

Ideally, the probability of committing an error should be zero. When dealing with quantities subject to sampling variation, uncertainty always exists and, therefore, error rates of zero are not possible. The next best strategy is to create a decision process with known and acceptably low error rates. In the context of a hypothesis test, these error rates are expressed as conditional probabilities (Chapter 2).

The null hypothesis H_0 always states that no systematic differences (only random differences) exist between a sample summary value and its corresponding theoretical value. When H_0 is true (H_1 false), observed differences between sample and theoretical values only arise because of random variation. In other words, any difference between a value calculated from the data and a value generated from theory is due to chance alone. When the alternative hypothesis H_1 is true (H_0 false), differences between sample and theoretical values are caused by both random variation and a systematic effect. Rejecting the null hypothesis H_0 implies that the data exhibit evidence of a systematic effect in addition to the influence of random variation. It is said that the data then indicate a "real" difference between observed and theoretical values. Or, stated more simply, the theoretical value is likely incorrect.

A Type I error occurs when a true null hypothesis (H_0 is true) is rejected, or equally, when a false alternative hypothesis is accepted (Table 5.1). A Type I error means that random variation has been mistaken for a "real" difference. The *level of significance*, another term for the probability of this kind of error, is denoted as α. In symbols, this conditional probability is

$$\text{level of significance} = \alpha = P(\textit{Type I error}) = P(\textit{reject } H_0 \mid H_0 \textit{ is true}).$$

The complement of a Type I error is the conditional probability $1 - \alpha$ and is the probability of correctly declaring that a random difference is due to chance alone. In symbols,

$$1 - \alpha = 1 - P(\textit{Type I error}) = P(\textit{accept } H_0 \mid H_0 \textit{ is true}).$$

A Type II error occurs when a null hypothesis is accepted when the alternative is true (H_0 is false—Table 5.1). A Type II error means that a "real" difference between observed and theoretical values has been mistaken for random variation. The conditional probability of Type II error is denoted as β. Again, in symbols,

$$\beta = P(\textit{Type II error}) = P(\textit{accept } H_0 \mid H_0 \textit{ is false}).$$

The power of a statistical test is measured by the conditional probability that the null hypothesis H_0 is correctly rejected when it is false (complement of a Type II error), In symbols,

$$\textit{power of the test} = 1 - \beta = 1 - P(\textit{Type II error})$$
$$= P(\textit{reject } H_0 \mid H_0 \textit{ is false}).$$

A powerful test is likely to identify correctly an underlying systematic difference when it exists. These four conditional probabilities completely characterize the performance of a statistical hypothesis test in light of sampling variation.

The terms Type I and Type II error come from R. A. Fisher's statistical contributions published in the early 20th century. The concept is, however, extremely old. From the *Book of Common Prayer* (1789): "We have left undone those things which we ought to have done [Type II]; and we have done those things which we ought not to have done [Type I]." One is frequently faced with such choices—

	One kind of error	The other kind of error
monetary policy	spending money when it is not needed	not spending money when it is needed
justice	an innocent person goes to jail	a guilty person goes free
alarms	alarm sounds when there is no fire	alarm does not sound when there is a fire
cheap Rolex watch	real deal, did not buy it	fake, did buy it
snake	believe it is poisonous when it is not	believe it is not poisonous when it is
cooking	thinking the roast is done and it is not	thinking the roast is not done and it is
weather	it does not rain and you have an umbrella	it rains and you do not have an umbrella

EXAMPLE

The following example illustrates a specific hypothesis test; more realistic applications are taken up in Chapter 6. The variable under study is systolic blood pressure. Furthermore, the systolic blood pressure levels of the population sampled are normally distributed with a mean $\mu = 130$ mm Hg (slightly hypertensive population) and variance $\sigma^2 = 400$ (mm Hg)^2. The claim is made that a new drug reduces blood pressure to normal levels, to $\mu = 120$ mm Hg. The newly developed drug is tested on a random sample of $n = 16$ of these slightly hypertensive individuals. To evaluate its effectiveness the mean blood pressure level of the 16 treated individuals is calculated.

Null hypothesis

The null hypothesis postulates that the blood pressure of the treated individuals is totally unaffected by the new treatment. In symbols, $\mu = 130$ or $H_0 : \mu = 130$. Any observed difference between the sample mean $\bar{x}$ and the population mean of $\mu = 130$ is then due entirely to the variation in blood pressure levels among the 16 randomly selected individuals and not to the treatment (no treatment effect exists). The distribution of the blood pressure levels (denoted X) of the treated individuals, under the null hypothesis (H_0), is identical to the population sampled, where

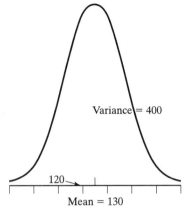

Variance = 400

120

Mean = 130

Distribution under the null hypothesis

The alternative hypothesis postulates that the blood pressure of the treated individuals is reduced to normal levels by the drug (a treatment effect exists) or the population mean associated with the 16 sampled individuals is 120. In symbols, $\mu = 120$ or $H_1 : \mu = 120$. The distribution of the blood pressure levels of the treated individuals, under the alternative hypothesis (H_1), is also identical to the population sampled but shifted 10 mm Hg to the left, where

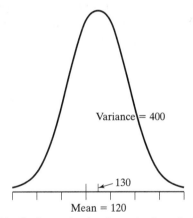

Variance = 400

130

Mean = 120

Distribution under the alternative hypothesis

A sample mean value in the neighborhood of 130 mm Hg makes it likely that the null hypothesis is true and the treatment has no effect. On the other hand, a sample mean value in the neighborhood of 120 mm Hg makes it likely that the mean level observed among the 16 treated individuals is not a chance deviation from $\mu = 130$ but rather the drug systematically lowers blood pressure. On the basis of the sample mean ($\overline{x}$), a choice is to be made between "no treatment effect exists" ($H_0 : \mu = 130$) and a "treatment effect exists" ($H_1 : \mu = 120$). In practical terms, if $\overline{x}$ is close to 130, then the null hypothesis is accepted and if $\overline{x}$ is close to 120, then the null hypothesis is rejected. It remains to define "close" and to find the error rates associated with the choice.

The first step is to decide which values of the sample mean will lead to rejecting the null hypothesis. A value (denoted c) is calculated such that the null hypothesis will be rejected in favor of the alternative hypothesis when the observed sample mean $\bar{x}$ is less than c, "close to 120." As mentioned, values of $\bar{x}$ in the neighborhood of 120 are consistent with a "real" reduction in blood pressure (consistent with a treatment effect). The value c is a preselected constant called the *critical value*. The critical value c defines the *critical region*. The critical region consists of all values of the sample mean $\bar{x}$ that lead to rejecting the null hypothesis. For the hypertension data, any observed sample mean value less than c ($\bar{x} < c$) leads to inferring that the "true" mean value, reflected by the sample mean of the 16 treated individuals, is not $\mu = 130$, but $\mu = 120$.

The critical value c follows directly from selecting an acceptably low level of a Type I error (the level of significance). This conditional probability (again, denoted α) can be set at any desired level. A typical choice is $\alpha = 0.05$ or

$$level\ of\ significance = \alpha = 0.05 = P(Type\ I\ error)$$

$$= P(reject\ H_0: \mu = 130\,|\,H_0\ true).$$

Selecting the probability α determines the critical value of c. Because the sampled blood pressures have a normal distribution, the sample mean also has a normal distribution (mean $= \mu$ with variance $= \sigma_{\bar{X}}^2$) and

$$\alpha = 0.05 = P(\bar{X} \leq c) = P\left(Z \leq \frac{c - \mu}{\sigma_{\bar{X}}}\right).$$

From Table A.1, $P(Z \leq -1.645) = 0.05$; therefore,

$$\frac{c - \mu}{\sigma_{\bar{X}}} = -1.645 \quad \text{or} \quad c = \mu - 1.645\sigma_{\bar{X}}.$$

Specifically, when $\mu = 130$ (H_0 is true) and since $\sigma_{\bar{X}} = \sqrt{400/16} = 5$, the critical point is $c = 130 - 1.645(5) = 121.8$. The critical region is all values of the sample mean less than 121.8. When the sample mean $\bar{x}$ is less the 121.8, the null hypothesis is rejected ("reject H_0") in favor of the inference that the new treatment lowers blood pressure. Otherwise, it is said that no evidence of a treatment effect exists ("accept H_0"). Because $P(\bar{X} \leq 121.8\,|\,\mu = 130) = P(Z \leq -1.645) = 0.05$, a Type I error occurs with the selected level of significance of 0.05. The value $c = 121.8$ is no more than the 5th-percentile of the normal distribution with mean $= \mu = 130$ and variance $= \sigma_{\bar{X}}^2 = 25$ (Chapter 4). The probability is 0.05 that an apparent lowering of the mean blood pressure caused by sampling variation alone will be mistaken for a treatment effect.

Data are usually collected to prove a point. For example, the blood pressure data were collected to answer the question, "Is the newly developed treatment effective?" At first, the null hypothesis appears quite the opposite because it states that any observed effects arose entirely by chance. That is, the data show nothing but random variation. A statistical test appears to address an issue that has little to do with the question being asked. This "backwards" approach, however, provides a straw man that the data are used to nullify. The statistical strategy produces a comparison between a value generated by the data and a theoretical value generated by the null hypothesis. Without a null hypothesis, no clear comparison exists. When the data produce substantial evidence that random variation is not a plausible explanation of the observed difference, the null hypothesis (the straw man) is rejected, shedding light on the issues that data were collected to investigate.

Power of the test

Once a critical region is established based on a selected Type I error probability, the next issue becomes the Type II error. The possibility always exists that the null hypothesis will be accepted when the alternative hypothesis is true, again because of the unavoidable random variation associated with sampled data. Randomly high values of $\bar{x}$ can occur when the underlying mean of the treated individuals is $\mu = 120$ mm Hg (H_1 is true), causing a Type II error to be made. An observed mean blood pressure $\bar{x}$ greater than c leads to accepting H_0 (no treatment effect) and can certainly occur when H_1 is true. Thus, a "real" treatment effect will not be identified. The probability of this kind of error (a Type II error, β) and the power ($1 - \beta$) are important and sometimes unappreciated aspects of a statistical test.

For the blood pressure example, what is the power of the test of the hypothesis H_0: $\mu = 130$ versus H_1: $\mu = 120$ based on $\bar{x}$? In symbols, the question becomes

$$power = P(reject\ H_0 \mid H_1\ is\ true) = P(reject\ H_0: \mu = 130 \mid \mu = 120) = ?$$

Power is the probability of making the correct decision when the null hypothesis is not true (H_1 is true). Or, more simply, it is the probability of detecting a systematic effect.

Specifically,

$$power = 1 - \beta = P(reject\ H_0: \mu = 130 \mid \mu = 120)$$
$$= P(\overline{X} \leq c \mid \mu = 120)$$
$$= P\left(Z \leq \frac{c - \mu}{\sigma_{\overline{X}}} \mid \mu = 120\right).$$

Because $\sigma_{\overline{X}} = \sqrt{400/16} = 5$, $c = 121.8$, and $\mu = 120$ when H_1 is true, then the associated power is

$$1 - \beta = P(\overline{X} \le 121.8 \mid \mu = 120) = P\left(Z \le \frac{121.8 - 120}{5}\right)$$

$$= P(Z \le 0.355) = 0.639 \text{ (Table A.1)}$$

and

$$P(Type\ II\ error) = \beta = P(\overline{X} \ge 121.8 \mid \mu = 120)$$

$$= P(Z \ge 0.355) = 1 - 0.639 = 0.361.$$

To summarize:

Decision	Null hypothesis is true $\mu = 130$	Null hypothesis is false $\mu = 120$
accept H_0: $\mu = 130$	$1 - \alpha = 0.95$	$\beta = 0.361$ (Type II error)
reject H_0: $\mu = 130$	$\alpha = 0.05$ (Type I error)	$1 - \beta = 0.639$

The mean value $\overline{x}$ under the hypothesis H_0 for a sample of $n = 16$ individuals has a normal distribution with variance $= \sigma_{\overline{X}}^2 = 25$ and

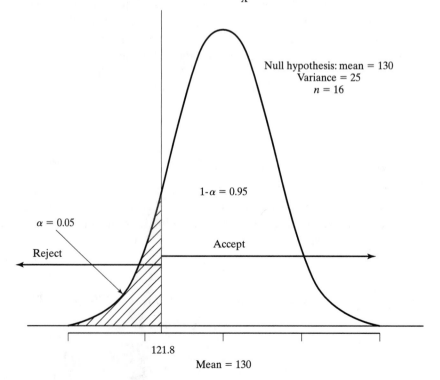

Null hypothesis: mean = 130
Variance = 25
$n = 16$

$1 - \alpha = 0.95$

$\alpha = 0.05$

Accept

Reject

121.8

Mean = 130

This normal distribution describes the behavior of the sample mean $\bar{x}$ under H_0 and is not a description of the sampled population of blood pressures.

When the number of individuals sampled (treated) is increased from 16 to 36, the effectiveness of the sample mean to discriminate between H_0 and H_1 increases (Type II error rate decreases). As with the resolution of a microscope, larger sample sizes increase the "resolution power" of the sample mean to choose correctly between the two hypotheses. For the hypertension example, an increase in statistical power produces the increased likelihood that the mean $\bar{x}$ will be close to $\mu = 130$ when H_0 is true or close to $\mu = 120$ when H_1 is true. The variability of $\bar{x}$ is reduced, which is another way of saying that the sample mean is more likely to be close to its expected value (law of large numbers).

For $n = 36$ randomly sampled and treated individuals, the critical value of c is calculated in the same manner as before, except now the standard deviation of the mean value (standard error) is reduced and $\sigma_{\bar{X}} = \sqrt{400/36} = 3.333$ (instead of 5). The level of significance, again set at 0.05, gives

$$\alpha = 0.05 = P(\bar{X} \le c \,|\, \mu = 130) = P\left(Z \le \frac{c - \mu}{\sigma_{\bar{X}}} \,\Big|\, \mu = 130\right)$$

producing a larger critical value of c (closer to $\mu = 130$) where

$$c = 130 - 1.645(3.333) = 124.5 \text{ (instead of 121.8)}.$$

The new critical region is then any $\bar{x}$ less than 124.5 and, as before, $\alpha = P(\bar{X} \le 124.5 \,|\, \mu = 130) = 0.05$.

The power of the test using $n = 36$ randomly sampled individuals (instead of 16) is

$$power = 1 - \beta = P(reject\ H_0\text{: } \mu = 130 \,|\, \mu = 120)$$
$$= P(\bar{X} \le c \,|\, \mu = 120)$$

and, specifically, the probability of identifying a treatment effect, if it exists, is

$$power = 1 - \beta = P(\bar{X} \le 124.5 \,|\, \mu = 120) = P\left(Z \le \frac{124.5 - 120}{3.333}\right)$$
$$= P(Z \le 1.355) = 0.912.$$

For a sample of 36 treated individuals, the probability of rejecting the null hypothesis when it is false (power) has substantially increased from 0.639 to 0.912. Not surprisingly, as the sample size increases, the power of the test to detect a systematic treatment effect also increases. For example, when more than 60 sampled individuals are treated for hypertension with the new drug, the power of the hypothesis test is greater than 0.99. The increased power occurs because of the reduced variability of the sample mean. In other words, a very large sample size produces a sample mean that essentially equals its population mean ($\bar{x} \approx \mu_0$ or $\bar{x} \approx \mu_1$) reducing the probability of a Type II error to close to zero making the power of the test close to one.

To summarize, the power of a statistical test depends on four quantities:

1. the size of the sample n,
2. the selected level of significance α,
3. the variance of the sampled population σ^2, and
4. the difference between μ_0 and μ_1 ($|\mu_0 - \mu_1|$), specified by the null and alternative hypotheses.

The sample size $n = 16$, $\alpha = 0.05$, $\sigma^2 = 200$, and $\mu_0 - \mu_1 = 10$ completely defines power for the hypertension example ($1 - \beta = 0.639$).

Additional example

A "modern-day astrologer" claims to be able to determine correctly the astrological sign of one out of five individuals (20%) when he knows a few facts about their personal lives. To test whether this "astrologer" has unusual powers, he reads the biographical descriptions of 100 individuals and predicts their astrological signs. The following analysis is performed:

1. null hypothesis (H_0): proportion correct $= p_0 = 1/12 = 0.083$ (the "astrologer" does no better than guessing since there are 12 close to equally likely astrological signs),
2. alternative hypothesis (H_1): proportion correct $= p_1 = 1/5 = 0.20$ (the "astrologer" can determine astrological signs with some accuracy),
3. set the level of significance at $\alpha = P(Type\ I\ error) = P(reject\ H_0 \mid p = 0.083) = 0.05$,
4. determine the critical region (c), and
5. compute the test statistic, the proportion observed correct, $\hat{p}$.

Steps 1 through 5 are no more than a formal way of using the observed proportion of correct answers to choose between the two theoretical probabilities $p_0 = 0.083$ and $p_1 = 0.20$ in such a way that the error rates associated with the choice are known.

The null hypothesis generates $p_0 = 1/12 = 0.083$ as well as a standard deviation associated with the estimated probability of a correct answer $\hat{p}$, which is

$$\sigma_{\hat{p}} = \sqrt{p_0(1 - p_0)/n} = \sqrt{0.083(1 - 0.083)/100} = 0.028 \qquad \text{(Chapter 4)}$$

based on reading $n = 100$ biographical descriptions. The test statistic $\hat{p}$ has an approximate normal distribution (central limit theorem) with mean $p_0 = 1/12 = 0.083$, and standard deviation $\sigma_{\hat{p}} = 0.028$, when H_0 is true.

Setting the level of significance α at 0.05 produces the critical point $c = p_0 + z_{1-\alpha}\sigma_{\hat{p}} = 0.083 + 1.645(0.028) = 0.129$. The critical point 0.129 is the 95th-percentile of a normal distribution ($\mu = 0.083$ and $\sigma_{\hat{p}} = 0.028$) describing the possible values of $\hat{p}$. The critical region is, therefore, $\hat{p} \geq 0.129$. If the "astrologer" correctly identifies the signs of 13 or more people out of the 100 biographies read (more than 12.9%), the inference is made that evidence exists of a special ability, as claimed. Furthermore, the Type I error rate is

$$\alpha = P(\textit{Type I error}) = P(\hat{p} \geq 0.129 \,|\, H_0 \textit{ true})$$

$$= P(\hat{p} \geq 0.129 \,|\, p = 0.083) = 0.05.$$

The power of this test of hypothesis is

$$power = 1 - \beta = P(\textit{reject } H_0 \,|\, H_0 \textit{ is false})$$

$$= P(\textit{reject } H_0\text{: } p = 0.083 \,|\, p = 0.20)$$

$$= P(\hat{p} \geq c \,|\, p = 0.20)$$

$$= P(\hat{p} \geq 0.129 \,|\, p = 0.20)$$

$$= P(Z \geq (0.129 - 0.20)/0.04)$$

$$= P(Z \geq -1.780) = 0.962$$

where the standard deviation associated with the distribution of $\hat{p}$ is $\sigma_{\hat{p}} = \sqrt{p_1(1 - p_1)/n} = \sqrt{(0.2)(0.8)/100} = 0.040$ when H_1 is true ($p_1 = 0.20$). Therefore, a probability of 0.962 (power) exists that the test of hypothesis based on 100 biographies will correctly verify the "astrologer's" claim when in fact he can determine astrological signs with a frequency of 20%.

The "astrologer" did identify correctly the signs of 12 individuals ($\hat{p} = 12/100 = 0.12$), which leads to accepting the null hypothesis (just barely). Schematically, the structure of this statistical test of hypothesis is

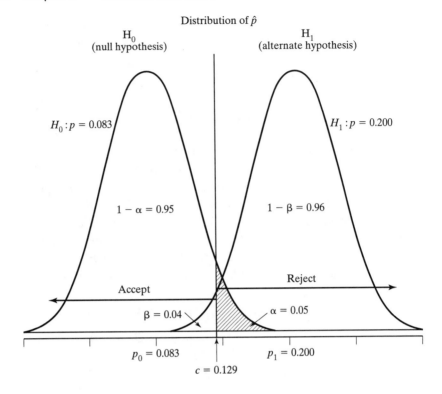

Distribution of $\hat{p}$

Computation of sample size

The fable of five blind men failing to describe an elephant after each touches a separate part of the elephant's body is a story of sample size. Touching only five parts of the elephant's body (number of observations) to get an idea of the entire animal (population) was, as the tale goes, ineffective (low power). Similarly, the number of sampled observations necessary to identify precisely specific properties of a population is frequently an issue. More specifically, it is important to have some idea of the number of observations necessary to effectively choose between two hypotheses. To decide between a null hypothesis H_0 and an alternative hypothesis H_1 with specific error rates α and β based on a sample mean, a sample size can be found (again denoted n_0).

As before, the critical point c defining the critical region is

$$c = \mu_0 + z_{1-\alpha}\sigma_{\overline{X}} \qquad \text{where } H_0\colon \mu = \mu_0 \text{ and } H_1\colon \mu = \mu_1 > \mu_0$$

and the power of the test is

$$power = 1 - \beta = P(\overline{X} \geq c \mid H_1\colon \mu = \mu_1) = P\left(Z \geq \frac{c - \mu_1}{\sigma_{\overline{X}}}\right).$$

Therefore,

$$\frac{c - \mu_1}{\sigma_{\overline{X}}} = z_\beta$$

when $\mu_1 > \mu_0$. The value z_β represents the percentile from a standard normal distribution that gives a Type II error of β; thus

$$\beta = P(Z \le z_\beta) = P\left(Z \le \frac{c - \mu_1}{\sigma_{\overline{X}}}\right).$$

Because

$$z_\beta = \frac{c - \mu_1}{\sigma_{\overline{X}}} = \frac{(\mu_0 + z_{1-\alpha}\sigma_{\overline{X}}) - \mu_1}{\sigma_{\overline{X}}} = z_{1-\alpha} + \frac{1}{\sigma_{\overline{X}}}(\mu_0 - \mu_1)$$

and $\sigma_{\overline{X}} = \dfrac{\sigma_X}{\sqrt{n_0}}$, then

$$\frac{z_\beta - z_{1-\alpha}}{\mu_0 - \mu_1} = \frac{\sqrt{n_0}}{\sigma_X}.$$

Noting that $z_\beta = -z_{1-\beta}$ and solving for n_0 gives

$$n_0 = \frac{\sigma^2(z_{1-\beta} + z_{1-\alpha})^2}{(\mu_0 - \mu_1)^2}.$$

A test of hypothesis based on n_0 observations will have the error rates α and β. When $\mu_1 < \mu_0$, the expression for the required sample size n_0 is the same.

EXAMPLE

The example concerning a blood pressure treatment where $\mu_0 = 130$, $\sigma^2 = 400$, and $\mu_1 = 120$ produces a typical sample size calculation. Setting $\alpha = 0.05$ and $\beta = 0.10$ (*power* $= 1 - \beta = 0.90$) makes $z_{0.95} = 1.645$ and $z_{0.90} = 1.282$ and gives a sample size of

$$n_0 = \frac{400(1.282 + 1.645)^2}{(130 - 120)^2} = 34.255 \quad \text{or} \quad 35.$$

Thus, a sample of 35 observations produces a test of hypothesis with a level of significance (Type I error) of 0.05 with power equal to 0.90.

For $\alpha = 0.05$ and $\beta = 0.05$ (*power* $= 1 - \beta = 0.95$), then a slightly higher sample size is required and

$$n_0 = \frac{400(1.645 + 1.645)^2}{(130 - 120)^2} = 43.289 \quad \text{or} \quad 44. \qquad \blacksquare$$

The sample size expression shows how the quantities α, β, μ_0, μ_1, and σ^2 combine to produce the required number of observations. For example, the number of required observations increases as σ^2, $1 - \alpha$, or $1 - \beta$ increase and decrease as $(\mu_1 - \mu_0)^2$ increases.

The error rates α and β are related. For example, decreasing the level of significance (decreasing α) makes it necessary to increase the sample size to maintain the same Type II error rate (β). The converse is also true. For example, increasing the level of significance from $\alpha = 0.05$ to $\alpha = 0.2$ requires a sample size of 24 rather than 44 (above example) to maintain a Type II error rate of 0.05. Specifically, for $\alpha = 0.2$ and $\beta = 0.05$, then

$$n_0 = \frac{400(0.842 + 1.645)^2}{(130 - 120)^2} = 24.730 \quad \text{or} \quad 25 \qquad \text{(reduced from 44)}.$$

From a slightly different point of view, increasing the level of significance (increasing α) associated with a test of hypothesis increases the power of the test (increases $1 - \beta$) and does not change the sample size. From the previous hypertension example, a sample size of 16 treated individuals yields a power of $1 - \beta = 0.639$ when $\alpha = 0.05$. When α is increased to 0.2, the power $1 - \beta$ substantially increases to 0.877. Previously, for α at 0.05 and $\sigma_{\overline{X}} = 5$, then the critical value was $c = 121.8$. Increasing α to 0.2 produces a larger critical value $c = 130 - 0.842(5) = 125.8$. Specifically,

$$\alpha = P(\overline{X} \leq 125.8 \mid \mu = 130) = 0.2$$

but the power of the test is now

$$power = P(\overline{X} \leq c \mid \mu = 120) = P(\overline{X} \leq 125.8 \mid \mu = 120)$$

$$= P\left(Z \leq \frac{125.8 - 120}{5}\right) = P(Z \leq 1.158) = 0.877. \quad \text{(instead of 0.639)}$$

In both cases, the sample size n is 16. Increasing the probability of a Type I error is occasionally an effective way to improve the power of a test without collecting additional observations.

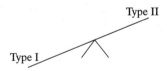

A sample size calculation to determine the precise number of observations to be sampled is rarely realistic in applied situations. First, it is not obvious what levels of Type I (α) and Type II (β) error rates should be chosen. These values depend on considerations that are usually not clear and frequently difficult to define unequivocally. Along the same lines, a meaningful alternative hypothesis is rarely available and the alternative hypothesis (μ_1) is generally no more than an "educated" guess. In addition, the variance (σ^2) is critical to a sample size calculation and an accurate value is rarely available. It is unlikely that the mean value is unknown but its associated variance is known. Sometimes pilot studies or "parallel" data sets suggest a variance σ^2, but these values are usually not satisfactory.

The expression for calculating a sample size, however, remains useful. It allows a variety of sample sizes to be explored for a number of different conditions determined by various values of α, β, μ_0, μ_1, and σ^2. For example, Figure 5.2 shows three sample size curves associated with the hypertension test of hypothesis, one for each of three selected variances ($\sigma^2 = 100$, 400, and 700).

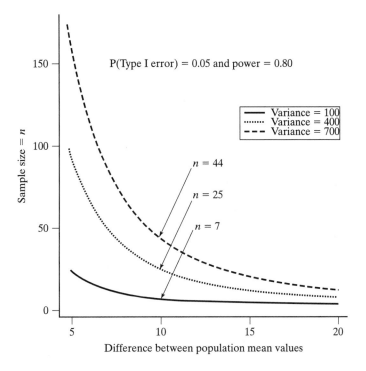

FIGURE 5.2: Sample size curves for the hypothesis test (H_0: $\mu = 130$).

Each curve indicates the sample size (vertical axis) necessary for error probabilities $\alpha = 0.05$ and $\beta = 0.2$ (*power* $= 1 - \beta = 0.8$) for a range of values generated by a series of alternative hypotheses (horizontal axis). For example, a sample size of $n = 25$ observations is necessary to detect the difference of $\mu_0 - \mu_1 = 10$ between null and alternative hypotheses with error rates of $\alpha = 0.05$ and $\beta = 0.2$ when $\sigma^2 = 400$ (Figure 5.2). For $\mu_0 - \mu_1 = 10$, sample sizes $n = 7$ and $n = 44$ are necessary to produce the same error rates when $\sigma^2 = 100$ and 700, respectively. Clearly, sample sizes can be found for other differences in mean values and other variances. These kinds of calculations do not pinpoint an unequivocal number of observations (n_0) but allow the exploration of the relationship of sample size to relevant values of the major elements of testing a specified hypothesis, namely α, β, μ_0, μ_1, and σ^2. A series of such sample size calculations produces a general picture of the number of observations that are needed to be sampled for a variety of conditions.

A sample size calculation makes it clear that a test of a hypothesis depends on five quantities (α, β, μ_0, μ_1, and σ^2) and does not depend on the number of observations in the population sampled. For example, California state law requires that ice cream have a specific butterfat content. State inspectors collect one-ounce samples for compliance testing. It is immaterial whether these samples come from a pint, a quart, a gallon, or a truckload of ice cream. Regardless, a sample of one ounce produces the desired test (power). Similarly, the precision of a presidential election poll depends on the number of individuals questioned (typically about 2000) and precisely describes (margin of error $= \pm 2\%$) the attitude of a population of 5 million voters, or 150 million voters. In more technical terms, the variance of an estimate, which primarily determines the power of a hypothesis test, depends on the sample size (n) and not the size of the population sampled as long as the sample size is small relative to size of the sampled population.

Summary

The hypothesis testing strategy is summarized by the following where the critical region is found in the right tail of the distribution generated by the null hypothesis ($\mu_1 > \mu_0$). The curves describe the distribution of the sample mean $\bar{x}$.

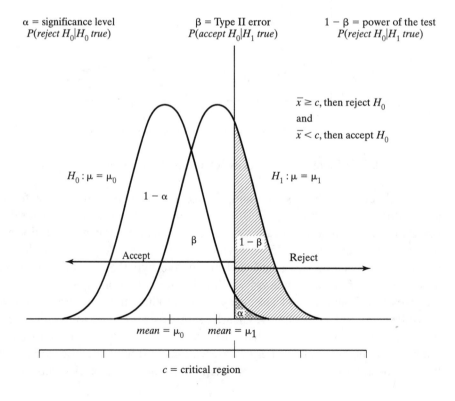

α = significance level
$P(reject\ H_0 | H_0\ true)$

β = Type II error
$P(accept\ H_0 | H_1\ true)$

$1 - \beta$ = power of the test
$P(reject\ H_0 | H_1\ true)$

$\bar{x} \geq c$, then reject H_0
and
$\bar{x} < c$, then accept H_0

$H_0 : \mu = \mu_0$

$1 - \alpha$

$H_1 : \mu = \mu_1$

β

$1 - \beta$

Accept

Reject

α

$mean = \mu_0$ $mean = \mu_1$

c = critical region

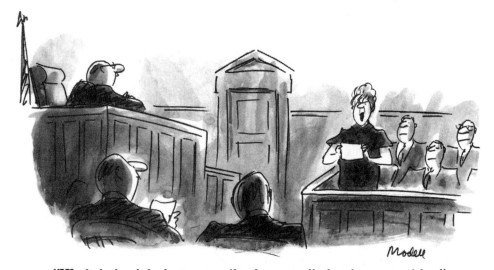

"We find the defendant not guilty but not all that innocent, either."

PROBLEM SET 5

For a normal distribution with $\sigma = 10$, H_0: $\mu = 100$, and H_1: $\mu = 107$;

1. find the critical point and power for $n = 25$ and $\alpha = 0.05$,
2. find the critical point and power for $n = 25$ and $\alpha = 0.01$,
3. find the critical point, and power for $n = 64$ and $\alpha = 0.05$, and
4. find the sample size required for $\alpha = 0.05$ and $1 - \beta = 0.9$.

In healthy males, the distribution of CD4 T-lymphocytes is normally distributed with a mean of $\mu = 1500$ cells per cubic mm. In males with HIV infection present but with no diagnosis of AIDS, the CD4 cells are normally distributed with $\mu = 600$ and $\sigma = 150$. If a drug could increase the mean cell count to 700 cells per cubic mm and maintain that level, then the drug would be of value.

5. Select H_0: $\mu = 600$ versus H_1: $\mu = 700$ with $\sigma = 150$. What sample size is needed to detect a difference of 100 cells at $\alpha = 0.05$ with $\beta = 0.10$? Complete the table below:

Type I error	$\alpha = 0.05$	$\alpha = 0.10$	$\alpha = 0.05$	$\alpha = 0.05$	$\alpha = 0.05$
Type II error	$\beta = 0.10$	$\beta = 0.10$	$\beta = 0.05$		
Critical point	_____	_____	_____	_____	_____
Sample Size	_____	_____	_____	$n = 9$	$n = 36$

6. On the basis of the completed table, what can be said about the power and the Type II error as sample size increases?

Will the sample size n, remain the same or decrease or increase under the following conditions (assume all else remains constant)?

7. increasing α, n will _____.
8. increasing $1 - \beta$, n will _____.
9. decreasing $|\mu_1 - \mu_0|$, n will _____.
10. decreasing σ, n will _____.
11. Suppose that the mean duration of hospitalization for pneumonia patients is $\mu = 4.4$ days, with a variance of $\sigma^2 = 3$ days^2. A sample of 25 patients treated with a new "wonder" drug produces a sample mean duration of $\bar{x} = 3$ days in the hospital. Test the effect of the "wonder" drug at the 5% level assuming that length of stay in the hospital is normally distributed.
12. Suppose the mean wing beats per second of the European-American honeybee is $\mu = 500$ and $\sigma = 60$. A sample of 16 African honeybees gave a sample mean of $\bar{x} = 460$ wing beats per second. Based on this information and the assumption that the data are normally distributed, assess the evidence that the wing beats per second of the African honeybees is less than that of the European-Americans bees at $\alpha = 0.01$. At $\alpha = 0.001$.

Suppose the weights of adult males are normally distributed with $\sigma = 10$ pounds. You decide to estimate the mean adult weight (μ) by taking a sample of size n and use the sample mean $\bar{x}$ to estimate μ.

13. If $n = 9$, what is the probability that your estimate $\bar{x}$ will be within 2 lbs of μ?

14. If $n = 81$, what is the probability that your estimate $\bar{x}$ will be within 2 lbs for μ?

15. If $n = 81$, within what interval around μ will $\bar{x}$ fall 95% of the time?

16. If $n = 81$, within what interval around μ will $\bar{x}$ fall 90% of the time?

17. Two methods of estimating the potency (ED_{50}) of a new antihistamine exist. Method A has a variance of $\sigma^2 = 50$ milligrams^2, while method B has a variance of $\sigma^2 = 36$ milligrams^2. Each determination costs 10 cents by method A and 12.5 cents by method B. A confidence interval for μ (the ED_{50}) can be constructed by taking a sample using either method A or method B. For a 95% confidence interval of length 3 milligrams, which method is cheaper (assuming the data are normally distributed)?

C H A P T E R 6

Statistical Inference II

The t-test procedure, which is the central topic of this chapter, was pioneered by William Sealy Gosset (b. 1879) who used the pseudonym "Student." Near the beginning of the 20th century, Gosset developed several significant biometric solutions to problems in agriculture and genetics. His most important contribution, the t-test, was contained in a 1908 paper entitled "On Probability Error of a Mean," which opened the door to the analysis of small samples of data based on a single statistical summary. The t-distribution is frequently called by the sometimes confusing name, Student's t-distribution. W. S. Gosset was not only a statistician but a master brewer. He worked for the famous Guinness brewing company and ultimately became the chief brewer for the London branch. In fact, Gosset used the pseudonym Student because the Guinness brewing company had a rule against employees participating in scientific publications. Gosset was part of a select group of scientists who, during the first part of the 20th century, laid the foundation to modern statistical analysis. Some of the others in this group were Karl Pearson, Ronald A. Fisher, E. J. G. Pitman, J. B. S. Haldane, Jerzy Neyman, and E. S. Pearson (Karl Pearson's son).

> There was a young man named Gosset
> who one day emerged from the closet.
> So around nineteen hundred and three
> he invented a distribution called the "t."
> And, statistics flowed like water from a faucet.

An unknown mean of a sampled population can be hypothesized (null hypothesis) or estimated ($\overline{x}$). As might be imagined, a realistic value for the population variance (σ_X^2) is also almost always unknown. When a value for σ_X^2 is needed, like the mean, it is typically hypothesized or estimated. The estimate, as before (Chapter 1), is $S_X^2 = \sum(x_i - \overline{x})^2/(n-1)$. The basic principles of statistical hypothesis testing and confidence interval construction using an estimated variance are the same as those discussed previously (Chapter 5). A number of details, however, need to be considered.

Student's *t*-distribution

The following theorem describes the probability distribution called *Student's t-distribution*:

> *if $X_1, X_2, \cdots, X_n$ are n independent normally distributed random variables with mean $= \mu$ $[E(X) = \mu]$ and variance σ_X^2, then*
>
> $$T = \frac{\overline{x} - E(\overline{X})}{S_{\overline{X}}} = \frac{\sqrt{n}(\overline{x} - \mu)}{S_X}$$
>
> *has a t-distribution with n − 1 degrees of freedom.*

A *t*-distribution is a symmetric probability distribution with a mean of zero similar in shape to the standard normal distribution but with greater probability in the tails (Figure 6.1). Unlike the normal distribution, no single standard *t*-distribution exists. Instead, different *t*-distributions are used to assess mean values calculated from samples, each depending on the number of sampled observations. A single parameter defines each of these *t*-distributions called the *degrees of freedom*, which are determined primarily by the sample size. For the case of assessing a single sample mean value, the degrees of freedom are

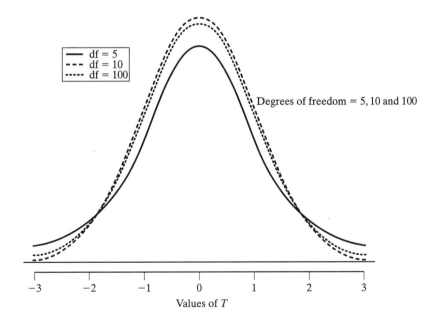

FIGURE 6.1: Three examples of Student's *t*-distributions.

$n - 1$ (n = sample size). More extensive applications of the t-distribution require different degrees of freedom (to be discussed).

Probabilities for selected t-distributions are given in Table A.2. A few percentiles from a t-distribution are:

95th-percentile

degrees of freedom = 5 $t_{0.95} = 2.015$ degrees of freedom = 10 $t_{0.95} = 1.812$

5th-percentile

degrees of freedom = 5 $t_{0.05} = -2.015$ degrees of freedom = 10 $t_{0.05} = -1.812$

80th- and 90th-percentile

degrees of freedom = 20 $t_{0.80} = 0.860$ degrees of freedom = 20 $t_{0.90} = 1.325$

95th- and 99th-percentile

degrees of freedom = 20 $t_{0.95} = 1.725$ degrees of freedom = 20 $t_{0.99} = 2.528$.

As the degrees of freedom (the sample size n) become moderately large, the probabilities associated with the t-distribution (Table A.2) differ very little from those of the standard normal distribution (Table A.1). For example, if the degrees of freedom are 30, then the 95th-percentile of the corresponding t-distribution is $t_{0.95} = 1.697$ (Table A.2) and the 95th-percentile of a standard normal distribution is $z_{0.95} = 1.645$ (Table A.1) or $P(T \leq 1.697) = P(Z \leq 1.645) = 0.95$.

The t-distribution theorem is similar in purpose to the central limit theorem (Chapter 4). Both theorems describe probability distributions used to assess a sample mean value. The application of the t-distribution, however, differs from employing the central limit theorem in three important respects:

1. The unknown population variance (σ_X^2) is replaced by an estimated variance (S_X^2) calculated from the sampled observations. Instead of $\sigma_{\overline{X}}^2 = \sigma_X^2/n$, the estimate $S_{\overline{X}}^2 = S_X^2/n$ is used. The central limit theorem requires that the population variance to be a known or a theoretical value (nonrandom).

2. The t-distribution depends directly on the number of observations collected. Different sample sizes produce different t-distributions, each identified by its degrees of freedom. Unlike central limit theorem, the t-distribution applies to any sample size, even $n = 2$.

3. For the application of a t-distribution, the data are required to be sampled from a normal distribution (parent population). The central limit theorem applies regardless of the distribution that produced the observed values as long as the sample size is large.

The two theorems, nevertheless, serve the same purpose. They allow probabilities to be calculated to evaluate the likelihood that a specific sample mean value occurs under specific conditions. Furthermore, as the sample size increases, the distinctions between the two approaches become less important. A t-distribution, therefore, is most useful when the sample size is small, usually less than 30.

A single population mean (one-sample t-test)

Frequently a sample is collected and a statistical test constructed to compare an observed mean value to a known or hypothetical mean (denoted μ_0). For instance, an experimental process employed to purify drinking water to be useful must not change the acidity of the treated water (maintain a neutral pH of 7.0). To assess the process, the mean of a sample of pH-values is compared to the hypothetical mean pH of 7.0.

The experimental process applied 24 times produces 24 independent and normally distributed observations. The 24 measured pH-values are:

Observation	1	2	3	4	5	6	7	8
pH-value (X)	5.95	7.39	6.88	6.54	6.50	6.73	6.69	6.95

Observation	9	10	11	12	13	14	15	16
pH-value (X)	7.58	6.62	6.96	6.90	6.93	6.32	7.22	6.36

Observation	17	18	19	20	21	22	23	24
pH-value (X)	6.54	6.67	7.25	6.94	7.21	6.83	6.80	6.59

The pH of each sample of treated water is measured ($x_1 = 5.95, x_2 = 7.39, \cdots, x_{24} = 6.59$) yielding a sample mean pH of $\bar{x} = 6.806$. The estimated variance is $S_X^2 = 0.134$ leading to an estimate of the standard deviation of the mean of $S_{\bar{X}} = \sqrt{0.134/24} = 0.075$ based entirely on these $n = 24$ sampled values. The question becomes: Is there evidence from the data that the experimental process fails to give a neutral pH? The null hypothesis (H_0) states that only random variation causes the 24 observed values to differ from pH $= 7.0$ or $\mu = \mu_0 = 7.0$. The alternative hypothesis (H_1) states that increased acidity occurred or $\mu < \mu_0 = 7.0$. Or, more simply, the difference between $\bar{x} = 6.806$ and $\mu_0 = 7$ is due to chance alone (H_0) or to systematic influences that lowered the pH-levels of some or all of the tested samples (H_1). In symbols, the two hypotheses are

$$H_0: \mu = \mu_0 = 7.0 \quad \text{versus} \quad H_1: \mu < \mu_0.$$

The choice between the null hypothesis H_0 (pH is neutral) and the alternative hypothesis H_1 (pH is acidic) is made using the sample mean $\bar{x}$, but not directly. Rather, $\bar{x}$ is converted to the test statistic $T = (\bar{x} - \mu_0)/S_{\bar{X}}$. The test statistic T varies from sample to sample depending on the values of the sample mean $\bar{x}$ and the sample variance S_X^2. The value T is itself a random variable that is described by a specific t-distribution when the null hypothesis is true $[E(\bar{X}) = \mu_0]$. Decisions are based on the value of T and not the mean $\bar{x}$, because the probability distribution of T is known (previous theorem and Table A.2) and accounts for the influence of the sampling variation associated with both estimated mean and estimated variance. Parallel to statistical tests based on the central limit theorem (Z—Chapter 5), extreme values of the T-statistic are either unlikely events (H_0 is true) or caused by a systematic difference between $\bar{x}$ and μ_0 (H_1 is true).

To assess the likelihood that the difference between the sample mean $\bar{x} = 6.806$ and a pH of 7 arose by chance, the level of significance is set to 0.05. In symbols, $P(Type\ I\ error) = \alpha = P(reject\ H_0: \mu_0 = 7 \mid \mu = 7) = 0.05$. Using Table A.2 gives $P(T \leq t_{0.05}) = P(T \leq -1.714 \mid H_0\ is\ true) = 0.05$ for $n = 24$ observations (degrees of freedom are $n - 1 = 23$). Therefore, values of T less than -1.714 form an $\alpha = 0.05$ critical region (critical point $= c = -1.714$). This particular test is called a *one-tail test* since the null hypothesis H_0 is rejected only if the observed T-value is small (found in the left tail). One tail of the t-distribution yields the critical region, which looks like

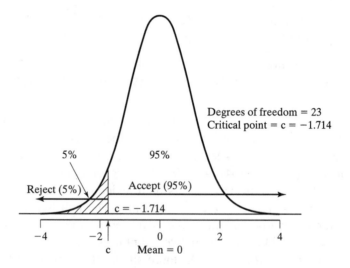

Degrees of freedom = 23
Critical point = $c = -1.714$

5%   95%

Reject (5%)   Accept (95%)

$c = -1.714$

-4   -2   0   2   4
          c Mean = 0

For a two-tail test, the critical region is constructed using both tails.

Now, the T-statistic is calculated from the observed data and the null hypothesis, yielding the value

$$T = \frac{\bar{x} - \mu_0}{S_{\bar{x}}} = \frac{6.806 - 7}{0.075} = -2.591.$$

The null hypothesis is rejected because the observed T-value falls within the critical region ($-2.591 < -1.714$). The test indicates that the mean pH of the population that generated the sample is likely less than 7, likely acidic.

A one-sample t-test used to compare a sample mean ($\bar{x}$) to a null hypothesis generated constant μ_0 follows a general pattern:

1. Define the random variable to be analyzed.
2. Select a null hypothesis ($\mu = \mu_0$).

3. Select an alternative hypothesis. It is one of three choices: $\mu \neq \mu_0$ (two-tail), $\mu > \mu_0$ (one-tail—right tail) or $\mu < \mu_0$ (one-tail—left tail).
4. Select a level of significance α ($\alpha = 0.05$ or $\alpha = 0.01$ are frequently chosen values).
5. Describe the critical region—the values of the T-statistic that lead to the rejecting H_0.

When decisions are made about the alternative hypothesis and the critical region (steps 1 through 5) without knowledge gained from the sample, the probability of a Type I error is known. It is the chosen level α. If information obtained from the sample influences decisions about steps 1 through 5, then the statistical test of a hypothesis depends in some way on these decisions and the probability of a Type I error is usually no longer known. The primary purpose of a t-test is to assess the difference between $\bar{x}$ and μ_0 with a known error rate (α). When the error rate is not known, the process is not of much use.

6. Calculate the test statistic T using the value μ_0 generated from a null hypothesis, the estimated mean ($\bar{x}$), and the estimated standard deviation of the sample mean ($S_{\bar{X}}$).
7. Reject H_0 or accept H_0 based on the resulting T-statistic and the predefined critical region.

The specific hypothesis testing pattern for the pH data is:

1. Define the random variable—the pH measurement.
2. Select the null hypothesis—H_0: $\mu = 7$.
3. Select an alternative hypothesis—H_1: $\mu < 7$ (one-tail).
4. Select the level of significance—$\alpha = 0.05$.
5. Describe the critical region—$T \leq -1.714$ (degrees of freedom = 23).
6. Calculate the T-statistic—$\mu_0 = 7$, $\bar{x} = 6.806$, and $S_{\bar{X}} = 0.075$, giving $T = -2.591$.
7. Reject H_0—the observed T is less than -1.714 implying that $\bar{x} = 6.806$ is sufficiently below a pH $= 7$ to infer that the water purifying process likely fails to maintain a neutral pH.

When the T-statistic is not found in the critical region, the phrase "accept H_0" does not mean that the null hypothesis is true. It means one of two things. The null hypothesis is true or the present sample is too small or too variable or both to determine that it is false (insufficient evidence). When it is stated that null hypothesis is "accepted," it means that no grounds exist to infer that the observed difference between $\bar{x}$ and μ_0 is due to systematic (nonrandom) influences. The phrase "accept H_0" loosely corresponds to the legal verdict given in court of "not guilty." When a jury announces its verdict as "not guilty" it means that the defendant is found to be innocent or the evidence is not sufficient to convict. A "not guilty" verdict does not distinguish between these two reasons for the jury's decision. Similarly, a statistical inference "accept H_0" also does not distinguish between a true null hypothesis and insufficient evidence to reject a false null hypothesis.

In court, the presumption of innocence is the "null hypothesis." The prosecutor must convince the jury that sufficient evidence exists to conclude that the presumption of innocence is false. The error rate associated with a jury falsely convicting an innocent defendant ("Type I error") is "beyond a reasonable doubt." Like the prosecutor in a courtroom, the burden of "proof" is on the statistical analysis to demonstrate the presumption that the observed difference due entirely to random variation (H_0) is not plausible. When sufficient evidence exists to show that the null hypothesis is clearly unlikely, the alternative hypothesis becomes attractive ("guilty"). Rejecting the null hypothesis simply means that random variation is not a likely explanation of the observed difference. But, unlike the courtroom, the exact probability of an error is known, since the probability of error (Type I) is predetermined.

EXAMPLE

Standards established by the National Institute of Occupational Safety and Health (NIOSH) limit the maximum permissible levels of toxic materials in the workplace. The standard (permissible exposure) to benzene in the oil refining industry is one part per million (ppm). An industrial hygienist at a specific oil company measured the benzene exposure levels (denoted X) of 20 workers to assess compliance to this standard. The 20 observations are (part of a data set containing approximately 90,000 benzene worker measurements[16]):

Observation	1	2	3	4	5	6	7	8	9	10
Benzene (ppm)	0.7	0.9	0.5	0.8	1.1	1.4	1.2	0.8	0.5	0.8

Observation	11	12	13	14	15	16	17	18	19	20
Benzene (ppm)	0.9	0.6	0.4	1.0	0.5	0.8	0.8	0.9	1.2	1.8

The sample mean value $\bar{x} = 0.880$ ppm gives an indication of compliance (<1 ppm). It is entirely possible, however, that random variation produced a mean value below 1.0. If this is the case, a sample mean of 0.880 is not evidence of a safe workplace environment. A t-test provides an evaluation of the hypothesis that the difference between the observed mean ($\bar{x} = 0.880$) and the standard ($\mu_0 = 1.0$) arose because of chance variation alone. The estimated variance based on the 20 sampled benzene measurements is $S_X^2 = 0.115$, making the estimated variance of the sample mean $S_{\bar{X}}^2 = S_X^2/n = 0.115/20 = 0.00577$ ($S_{\bar{X}} = 0.076$).

A null hypothesis postulates that the underlying mean exposure is 1.0 or H_0: $\mu = \mu_0 = 1.0$ and all 20 observed values differ from 1.0 only because of sampling variation. The alternative hypothesis postulates that the workplace environment is below the standard with respect to benzene exposure or H_1: $\mu = \mu_1 < 1.0$. This is a one-tail alternative hypothesis (the critical region is made up of only the left-tail of the t-distribution) since only low values of benzene levels lead logically to the inference that the workplace is below the standard. Selecting the level of significance $\alpha = 0.05$, the t-distribution with 19 degrees of freedom (Table A.2) determines the critical value $P(T \leq -t_{0.05}) = P(T \leq -1.729) = 0.05$. The critical region then consists of all T-values less than -1.729 (critical point $= c = -1.729$) and the level of significance (probability of a Type I error) is 0.05. The values that make up the T-statistic are $\mu_0 = 1.0$, $\bar{x} = 0.880$, and $S_{\bar{X}} = 0.076$, producing a test statistic of

$$T = \frac{\bar{x} - \mu_0}{S_{\bar{X}}} = \frac{0.880 - 1.0}{0.076} = -1.580.$$

The null hypothesis is accepted because the calculated test statistic T fails to be less than the critical point ($-1.720 < -1.580$). Based on the 20 sampled benzene measurements, the statistical analysis produces no strong evidence that the workplace level of benzene exposure is substantially below the NIOSH standard. Implicit in the application of this t-test analysis is the assumption or knowledge that the benzene measurements are sampled independently from the same normal distribution.   ∎

The three kinds of critical regions associated with a t-test are identified in detail in the following table:

	One-tail (left)	One-tail (right)	Two-tail
null hypotheses	$\mu = \mu_0$	$\mu = \mu_0$	$\mu = \mu_0$
alternative hypotheses	$\mu \leq \mu_0$	$\mu \geq \mu_0$	$\mu \neq \mu_0$
critical regions	$T \leq t_{1-\alpha}$	$T \geq t_{1-\alpha}$	$T \leq t_{1-\alpha/2}$ or $T \geq t_{1-\alpha/2}$
levels of significance (0.05)	$T \leq t_{0.05}$	$T \geq t_{0.95}$	$T \leq t_{0.025}$ or $T \geq t_{0.975}$
examples (degrees of freedom = 10)	$T \leq -1.812$	$T \geq 1.812$	$T \leq -2.228$ or $T \geq 2.228$

When an exact alternative hypothesis (H_1: $\mu = \mu_1$) is postulated, power calculations can be applied to a t-test along the same lines previously discussed (Chapter 5). However, the calculations are more complex and realistic alternative hypotheses yielding exact values of μ_1 are rarely available. In fact, the data are usually collected because μ_1 is unknown and is the focus of the analysis.

Constructing a confidence interval for μ (σ^2 unknown)

A sample of $n = 10$ women weighed at the end of their second trimester of pregnancy produced a mean weight gain of $\bar{x} = 7.030$ kilograms with an estimated variance of $S_X^2 = 1.210$. Additionally, it is known that the observed weights were sampled from an essentially normal distribution. The small sample size and the variability in weight gained during the first and second trimesters of pregnancy makes the observed mean subject to considerable sampling variation. The impact of this variation can be judged by constructing a confidence interval for the population mean weight gain μ based on its estimated mean $\bar{x}$ and the estimated variance S_X^2.

The construction of a 95% confidence interval employing an estimated variance S_X^2 starts with a t-distribution, specifically the probability $P(t_{0.025} \leq T \leq t_{0.975}) = 0.95$. From Table A.2 (degrees of freedom $= df = n - 1 = 9$), the percentile values of $t_{0.025}$ and $t_{0.975}$ are -2.262 and 2.262 making $P(-2.262 \leq T \leq 2.262) = 0.95$. Now, algebraically manipulating this probability, as before (Chapter 5), yields a likely (95%) range for possible values of the mean weight gained (μ), the mean of the population that generated the data.

Specifically, the confidence interval using both an estimated mean and variance is constructed from the relationship that

$$P(t_{0.025} \leq T \leq t_{0.975}) = P\left(-2.262 \leq \frac{\bar{X} - \mu}{S_{\bar{X}}} \leq 2.262\right)$$

$$= P(\bar{X} - 2.262 S_{\bar{X}} \leq \mu \leq \bar{X} + 2.262 S_{\bar{X}})$$

$$= P\left(\bar{X} - 2.262 \sqrt{\frac{S_X^2}{n}} \leq \mu \leq \bar{X} + 2.262 \sqrt{\frac{S_X^2}{n}}\right)$$

$$= P(\hat{A} \leq \mu \leq \hat{B}) = 0.95$$

giving the estimated lower and upper bounds of the $1 - \alpha = 0.95$ level confidence interval, denoted again $(\hat{A}, \hat{B})$. The creation of a confidence interval based in the t-distribution follows the same pattern discussed in detail for the normally distributed mean value (Chapter 5). The 95% confidence bounds estimated from $\bar{x} = 7.030$, $n = 10$, and $S_X^2 = 1.210$ are

$$\hat{A} = lower\ bound = 7.030 - 2.262\sqrt{1.210/10} = 6.243$$

and

$$\hat{B} = upper\ bound = 7.030 + 2.262\sqrt{1.210/10} = 7.817.$$

The confidence interval $(\hat{A}, \hat{B}) = (6.243, 7.817)$ indicates a range for likely values of μ and the precision of the second trimester sample mean weight gain ($\bar{x} = 7.030$) as an estimate of μ.

In general, $(1 - \alpha)$-confidence interval bounds ($\hat{A}$ and $\hat{B}$) imply that

$$P\left[\overline{X} - t_{1-\alpha/2}S_{\overline{X}} \leq \mu \leq \overline{X} + t_{1-\alpha/2}S_{\overline{X}}\right] = 1 - \alpha \qquad \text{note: } t_{\alpha/2} = -t_{1-\alpha/2}$$

or, in more detail,

$$P\left(\overline{X} - t_{1-\alpha/2}\sqrt{\frac{S_X^2}{n}} \leq \mu \leq \overline{X} + t_{1-\alpha/2}\sqrt{\frac{S_X^2}{n}}\right) = P(\hat{A} \leq \mu \leq \hat{B}) = 1 - \alpha.$$

The estimated interval endpoints $\hat{A}$ and $\hat{B}$ are respectively the lower and upper bounds of the $(1 - \alpha)\%$ confidence interval for μ when σ_X^2 is not known but estimated by S_X^2. Once again, the use of a t-distribution requires that the observations be sampled independently from the same normally distributed population but applies to any sample size.

The interpretation of a confidence interval based on the t-distribution is the same as the previously discussed interval where the variance σ^2 is known (Chapter 5). As with all confidence intervals, the lower and upper bounds ($\hat{A}$ and $\hat{B}$) are calculated from sampled observations and subject to sampling variation. Again, the estimated bounds $\hat{A}$ and $\hat{B}$ vary from sample to sample and the population mean μ does not.

Comparing two mean values from independent populations (two-sample t-test)

The possibility of a difference between two population mean values is usually investigated by taking a sample from each population. The population structure and notation for two sampled populations are summarized in Table 6.1.

The natural question arises: Are the population mean values (represented by μ_1 and μ_2) different ($\mu_1 \neq \mu_2$) or are they the same ($\mu_1 = \mu_2$)? If the

TABLE 6.1: Samples from two populations.

Populations	I	II
Population mean values	μ_1	μ_2
Population variances	σ_1^2	σ_2^2
Sample sizes	n_1	n_2
Sample means	$\overline{x}_1$	$\overline{x}_2$
Sample variances	S_1^2	S_2^2
Estimated variances of the mean	$S_{\overline{X}_1}^2 = \dfrac{S_1^2}{n_1}$	$S_{\overline{X}_2}^2 = \dfrac{S_2^2}{n_2}$

population mean values differ, this difference will likely but not necessarily be reflected by differences between the sample mean values. In addition, the two sample mean values will certainly differ, at least to some extent, because of the influence of sampling variation.

More formally, the difference between two sample means $\bar{x}_1$ and $\bar{x}_2$ will undoubtedly not equal zero for one of two reasons: The mean values differ (1) because of the sampling variation associated with the variable being investigated but, in fact, $\mu_1 = \mu_2$, or (2) because the two population mean values differ ($\mu_1 \neq \mu_2$).

Two properties of the estimated difference between sample mean values ($\bar{x}_1 - \bar{x}_2$) necessary to construct a two-sample t-test are:

Distribution: When the values sampled from populations I and II are normally distributed, the difference ($\bar{x}_1 - \bar{x}_2$) is also normally distributed (Chapter 3). If the samples from population I or population II do not consist of normally distributed observations, the central limit theorem implies that the difference ($\bar{x}_1 - \bar{x}_2$) has an approximate normal distribution when large numbers of observations are sampled from both populations. The quantity $\bar{x}_1 - \bar{x}_2$ is a sample mean value. It is an estimate of the mean difference.

Variance: If the two populations are independent, then the variance of the mean difference ($\bar{x}_1 - \bar{x}_2$) is

$$\sigma^2_{\bar{X}_1 - \bar{X}_2} = \sigma^2_{\bar{X}_1} + \sigma^2_{\bar{X}_2}$$

because $\sigma^2_{aX+bY} = a^2\sigma^2_X + b^2\sigma^2_Y$ (Chapters 3 and 8) and $a = 1$, $X = \bar{x}_1$, $b = -1$, and $Y = \bar{x}_2$.

A valid t-test to assess an observed difference between two sample mean values requires:

1. population I to be independent of population II and the two samples to consist of independently sampled observations,
2. the observations to be sampled from normally distributed parent populations, and
3. the variance to be the same for both populations sampled ($\sigma^2_1 = \sigma^2_2$), occasionally called *homoscedasticity*.

A typical null hypothesis states that no difference exists between the population mean values or H_0: $\mu_1 = \mu_2$. Any observed difference between the two sample mean values is then attributed to random variation. An alternative hypothesis states that the two populations have different mean values, H_1: $\mu_1 \neq \mu_2$. Illustrations of the null hypothesis and two possible alternative hypotheses are:

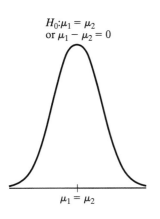
$H_0: \mu_1 = \mu_2$
or $\mu_1 - \mu_2 = 0$

$\mu_1 = \mu_2$

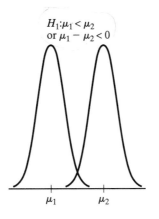
$H_1: \mu_1 < \mu_2$
or $\mu_1 - \mu_2 < 0$

μ_1 μ_2

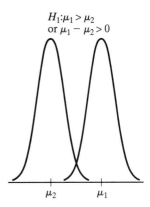
$H_1: \mu_1 > \mu_2$
or $\mu_1 - \mu_2 > 0$

μ_2 μ_1

A test statistic is

$$T = \frac{(\bar{x}_1 - \bar{x}_2) - (\mu_1 - \mu_2)}{S_{\bar{X}_1 - \bar{X}_2}}$$

and, as before, this T-statistic varies from sample to sample and this variation is described by a t-distribution with $(n_1 - 1) + (n_2 - 1) = n_1 + n_2 - 2$ degrees of freedom when the null hypothesis is true (for example, when $\mu_1 - \mu_2 = 0$).

Because

$$\sigma^2_{\bar{X}_1 - \bar{X}_2} = \sigma^2_{\bar{X}_1} + \sigma^2_{\bar{X}_2},$$

a natural estimate of the variance of the difference between two estimated mean values is

$$S^2_{\bar{X}_1 - \bar{X}_2} = S^2_{\bar{X}_1} + S^2_{\bar{X}_2} = \frac{S^2_1}{n_1} + \frac{S^2_2}{n_2}.$$

The estimated variances S^2_1 and S^2_2 are calculated from each sample in the usual way (Chapter 1).

Taking advantage of the equal variance requirement, a weighted average of the two estimated variances (one for each sampled population—S^2_1 and S^2_2) produces a single estimate of the common variance. The two estimated variances are weighted by $n_1 - 1$ and $n_2 - 1$ giving a weighted average or pooled estimate of the common variance ($\sigma^2_1 = \sigma^2_2 = \sigma^2$—requirement 3) of

$$S^2_{pooled} = \frac{(n_1 - 1)S^2_1 + (n_2 - 1)S^2_2}{(n_1 - 1) + (n_2 - 1)},$$

then

$$S^2_{\bar{X}_1 - \bar{X}_2} = \frac{S^2_{pooled}}{n_1} + \frac{S^2_{pooled}}{n_2} = S^2_{pooled} \left(\frac{1}{n_1} + \frac{1}{n_2} \right)$$

estimates the variability associated with the observed difference between two sample mean values. That is, the difference in mean values $\bar{x}_1 - \bar{x}_2$ has a normal distribution (requirement 2) with a variance estimated by $S^2_{\overline{X}_1-\overline{X}_2}$. The weights $n_1 - 1$ and $n_2 - 1$ are selected so that the expected-value of the weighted average is the common population variance. In symbols, $E(S^2_{pooled}) = \sigma^2$ when $\sigma^2_1 = \sigma^2_2 = \sigma^2$ (justification is given elsewhere[17]).

Using the pooled estimate of the variance, the test statistic to evaluate the difference between two sample mean values becomes

$$T = \frac{(\overline{x}_1 - \overline{x}_2) - (\mu_1 - \mu_2)}{S_{\overline{X}_1-\overline{X}_2}} = \frac{(\overline{x}_1 - \overline{x}_2) - (\mu_1 - \mu_2)}{\sqrt{S^2_{pooled}\left(\dfrac{1}{n_1} + \dfrac{1}{n_2}\right)}} = \frac{(\overline{x}_1 - \overline{x}_2) - 0}{S_{pooled}\sqrt{\dfrac{1}{n_1} + \dfrac{1}{n_2}}}.$$

The T-statistic, as noted, has a t-distribution with degrees of freedom $n_1 + n_2 - 2$ when the null hypothesis is true ($\mu_1 = \mu_2 = 0$). This two-sample version of the test statistic T is in principle the same as the one-sample version. The numerator is a sample mean $\overline{x}_1 - \overline{x}_2$ (subject to sampling variation) minus a theoretically generated population value $\mu_1 - \mu_2 = 0$ (not subject to sampling variation) and the estimated variance in the denominator accounts for the random variation of the estimate in the numerator.

For samples from nonnormal populations, a parallel test statistic can be constructed, which has an approximate normal distribution. If the variances σ^2_1 and σ^2_2 are known, then

$$Z = \frac{(\overline{x}_1 - \overline{x}_2) - (\mu_1 - \mu_2)}{\sqrt{\sigma^2_{\overline{X}_1-\overline{X}_2}}} = \frac{(\overline{x}_1 - \overline{x}_2) - (\mu_1 - \mu_2)}{\sqrt{\dfrac{\sigma^2_1}{n_1} + \dfrac{\sigma^2_2}{n_2}}}$$

and the test statistic Z has an approximate standard normal distribution ($\mu = 0$ and $\sigma^2_Z = 1$) for large samples selected from both populations (central limit theorem).

When both n_1 and n_2 are large and the variances σ^2_1 and σ^2_2 are unknown but not very unequal, generally little error occurs if S^2_1 and S^2_2 are used to estimate the variances necessary to calculate Z. Therefore, when sufficient numbers of observations are available the variance $\sigma^2_1/n_1 + \sigma^2_2/n_2$ is replaced by its estimate $S^2_1/n_1 + S^2_2/n_2$ and the test statistic becomes

$$Z = \frac{(\overline{x}_1 - \overline{x}_2) - (\mu_1 - \mu_2)}{\sqrt{\dfrac{S^2_1}{n_1} + \dfrac{S^2_2}{n_2}}},$$

which also has an approximate standard normal distribution. The test statistic Z is then used to assess the observed difference $(\overline{x}_1 - \overline{x}_2)$ when no difference exists between population means (H_0: $\mu_1 - \mu_2 = 0$). Strictly, the central limit theorem requires that the denominator of Z to be a fixed quantity that does not depend on the observed values. For large values of both n_1 and n_2, the test statistic Z, nevertheless, has an approximate normal distribution in most applied situations.

When n_1 and n_2 are both greater than 30 or so, the comparison of two means based on the t-distribution ($\sigma^2_{\overline{X}_1-\overline{X}_2}$ unknown but estimated by $S^2_{\overline{X}_1-\overline{X}_2}$) and the comparison based on the normal distribution (central limit theorem) become practically indistinguishable (again compare Table A.1 to Table A.2). From another perspective, the estimated variance $S^2_{\overline{X}_1-\overline{X}_2}$ becomes sufficiently precise so that the issue of whether the variance is known or unknown is relatively unimportant. As in the case of a one-sample t-test, the two sample t-test is most valuable when one or both of the sample sizes are small.

Two advantages exist when the sample sizes are equal or nearly equal:

1. The estimated variance $S^2_{\overline{X}_1-\overline{X}_2}$ is reduced when $n_1 = n_2$, increasing the value of T, which, in turn, increases the probability of detecting a difference between $\overline{x}_1$ and $\overline{x}_2$ when a difference exists (increased power). More technically, because the factor $(1/n_1 + 1/n_2)$ is smallest when $n_1 = n_2$, multiplying S^2_{pooled} by the smallest possible value for a fixed sample size $n = n_1 + n_2$ reduces the estimated variance $S^2_{\overline{X}_1-\overline{X}_2}$.

2. The comparison of two mean values requires the sampled populations to have the same variance (requirement 3). When the sample sizes are approximately equal ($n_1 \approx n_2$), the t-distribution that describes the possible values the test statistic T is relatively unaffected when the compared populations do not have equal variances.[18] In addition, the pooled and the unpooled variance estimates are approximately equal or

$$S^2_{\overline{X}_1-\overline{X}_2} = S^2_p \left(\frac{1}{n_1} + \frac{1}{n_2} \right) \approx \frac{S^2_1}{n_1} + \frac{S^2_2}{n_2}$$

regardless of the values of S^2_1 and S^2_2 when $n_1 \approx n_2$.

Thus, it is advantageous to sample equal numbers of observations from each population whenever it is possible.

EXAMPLE

The final grade in a statistics course was determined from an average of several test scores. In order to investigate the possibility of a difference between male (population I) and female (population II) students, the final scores for a sample of 67 students were classified into male (sample I) and female (sample II) categories:

Male (sample I)

85.6	54.8	82.3	91.5	98.8	83.7
90.4	87.2	65.2	94.2	91.7	86.5
85.5	96.0	82.8	87.6	93.7	94.2
75.0	80.9	87.2	87.0	90.6	85.9
98.9	93.7	98.5	88.6	84.2	91.4
69.1	83.0	48.3	94.3	96.9	74.3
92.8					

$n_1 = 37$ $\bar{x}_1 = 85.738$

$\sum (x_i - \bar{x}_1)^2 = 4655.587$

$S_1^2 = \sum (x_i - \bar{x}_1)^2 / (n_1 - 1) = 4655.587/36 = 129.322$

Female (sample II)

86.2	95.0	99.2	94.3	98.5
92.9	83.1	64.9	99.0	96.5
75.0	54.5	93.4	79.1	89.6
97.8	78.8	97.2	93.0	98.6
94.3	96.7	100.0	87.2	95.7
96.0	91.5	83.3	88.0	82.7

$n_2 = 30$ $\bar{x}_2 = 89.400$

$\sum (x_i - \bar{x}_2)^2 = 3294.300$

$S_2^2 = \sum (x_i - \bar{x}_2)^2 / (n_2 - 1) = 3293.300/29 = 113.597$

Next, the null hypothesis is

> H_0: no difference exists between final scores of male and
> female students ($\mu_1 = \mu_2$)

and the alternative hypothesis is

> H_1: a difference exists ($\mu_1 \neq \mu_2$, two-tail alternative).

The degrees of freedom are $n_1 + n_2 - 2 = 37 + 30 - 2 = 65$. Setting $\alpha = 0.05$ gives a two-tail critical region of $T \leq t_{0.025} = -1.997$ or $T \geq t_{0.975} = 1.997$.
   An estimate of the common population variance σ^2 is

$$ S_{pooled}^2 = \frac{36(129.322) + 29(113.597)}{65} = 122.306. $$

The test statistic T used to assess the observed mean difference $\bar{x}_1 - \bar{x}_2 = 85.738 - 89.400 = -3.662$ becomes

$$T = \frac{85.738 - 89.400}{\sqrt{122.306 \left(\dfrac{1}{37} + \dfrac{1}{30} \right)}} = \frac{-3.662}{2.717} = -1.348$$

and T does not fall within the critical region $(-1.997 < -1.348)$. The analysis, therefore, fails to provide sufficient evidence to reject the null hypothesis that no difference exists between the test scores of male and female students. Random variation remains a plausible explanation of the observed difference. Four assumptions were made: Male and female scores are (1) independently sampled from (2) independent and (3) normally distributed populations with (4) the same variance $(\sigma_1^2 = \sigma_2^2 = \sigma^2)$. ∎

Constructing a confidence interval for $\mu_1 - \mu_2$ (σ_1^2 and σ_2^2 unknown)

To construct 95% confidence interval bounds for the difference between population means $\mu_1 - \mu_2$, based on the difference between sample means $\bar{x}_1 - \bar{x}_2$, the starting point is again the t-distribution where

$$P(t_{0.025} \leq T \leq t_{0.975}) = 0.95. \qquad \text{(Table A.2)}$$

Substituting $\left[(\bar{X}_1 - \bar{X}_2) - (\mu_1 - \mu_2) \right] / S_{\bar{X}_1 - \bar{X}_2}$ for T and, as before, algebraically manipulating this probability statement (Chapter 5) gives

$$P\left[(\bar{X}_1 - \bar{X}_2) - t_{0.975} S_{\bar{X}_1 - \bar{X}_2} \leq (\mu_1 - \mu_2) \leq (\bar{X}_1 - \bar{X}_2) + t_{0.975} S_{\bar{X}_1 - \bar{X}_2} \right] = 0.95.$$

As always, $t_{0.025} = -t_{0.975}$.

The 95% confidence interval for the difference in population mean scores for the male and female students estimated from the corresponding sample means and variance (previous example) are

$$\hat{A} = lower\ bound = (\bar{x}_1 - \bar{x}_2) - t_{0.975} S_{\bar{X}_1 - \bar{X}_2}$$
$$= (85.738 - 89.400) - 1.997(2.717) = -9.089 \quad \text{and}$$
$$\hat{B} = upper\ bound = (\bar{x}_1 - \bar{x}_2) + t_{0.975} S_{\bar{X}_1 - \bar{X}_2}$$
$$= (85.738 - 89.400) + 1.997(2.717) = 1.764$$

where again $\bar{x}_1 - \bar{x}_2 = -3.662$ and $S_{\bar{X}_1 - \bar{X}_2} = 2.717$. Thus, a likely range of the "true" difference in mean scores ($\mu_1 - \mu_2$) is reflected by the confidence interval $(-9.089, 1.764)$. The fact that the estimated interval contains zero indicates that a difference of zero is a plausible candidate for the underlying difference between population mean values. From this perspective, the confidence interval and the hypothesis test agree. Both approaches show no persuasive statistical evidence of a systematic difference between male and female students based on a sample of 67 test scores.

Significance probability—*p*-value

It enhances a statistical analysis to summarize the result from a hypothesis test with more than the statement "reject H_0" or "accept H_0." This simple yes/no statement contains little information on the strength of the data to either support or not support the null hypothesis. A popular summary of a test of hypothesis is a quantity formally called the *significance probability* or, less formally, the *p-value*. A *p*-value is defined as the probability of obtaining a more extreme value of the test statistic than the one observed, when the null hypothesis is true. The *p*-value is a quantitative statement of the likelihood that the observed result occurred strictly by chance alone. The probability calculated (1/70) in the tea-drinking example (Chapter 5) is a significance probability. It is the probability that the outcome (eight correct) resulted from only guessing—a null hypothesis.

For the one-tail test, the *p*-value is typically
P(test statistic ≥ observed value | H_0 is true) or
P(test statistic ≤ observed value | H_0 is true).
For the two-tail test, the *p*-value is typically
P(test statistic ≤ − (observed value) | H_0 is true) +
P(test statistic ≥ observed value | H_0 is true) where *observed value > 0*.

A significance probability indicates the degree of circumstantial evidence supporting the null hypothesis rather than the dichotomous choice of "accept H_0" or "reject H_0." The smaller the *p*-value, the less likely it becomes that the null hypothesis is true. A significance probability measures the plausibility of the null hypothesis in light of sampling variation.

EXAMPLE

The T-statistic calculated from the male/female test scores is $T = -1.348$ which leads to accepting H_0: $\mu_1 = \mu_2$. Additionally, the *p*-value associated with a two-tail alternative hypothesis is

$$p\text{-}value = P(T \leq -1.348 \mid H_0\text{: } \mu_1 = \mu_2)$$
$$+ P(T \geq 1.348 \mid H_0\text{: } \mu_1 = \mu_2),$$

which is the probability of observing a more extreme value of T than the one obtained, when no difference exists between the populations that produced the male and female test scores. Specifically, the p-value is $0.09 + 0.09 = 0.18$ when T equals -1.348. A significance probability of 0.18 indicates that in about 18 times out of 100 a result more extreme than $T = -1.348$ or $T = 1.348$ would occur by chance alone when $\mu_1 = \mu_2$. Reporting a significance probability indicates the "weight-of-the-evidence" for the null hypothesis H_0. ∎

The significance probabilities in this text are not derived from Tables A.1–A.5 in the appendix but are exact values found with computer algorithms. Approximate values, of course, can be found in published tables. For example, the t-probabilities associated with 65 degrees of freedom, like most t-probabilities associated with large sample sizes, are not usually given in tables but they can be accurately approximated using the standard normal distribution. For the male/female test score data, the t-distribution based on 65 degrees of freedom hardly differs from the standard normal distribution given in Table A.1. Specifically, $P(|T| \geq 1.348) = 0.182$ (exactly) $\approx P(|Z| \geq 1.348) = 0.178$ (approximate).

EXAMPLE

The T-statistic associated with the null hypothesis that the level of benzene in a specific oil refinery is not systematically below the compliance standard set by NIOSH for benzene levels (1 ppm) is $T = -1.580$. The one-tail significance probability is p-value $= P(T \leq -1.580 \,|\, H_0 \ true) = 0.07$. Instead of simply stating "the null hypothesis is accepted," the moderately small p-value of 0.07 produces a suspicion that the data support the conjecture that the workplace exposure to benzene is safely below the exposure standard of 1.0 ppm. ∎

Presumably the "p" in p-value stands for probability but, perhaps more to the point, the "p" should stand for plausibility since the p-value directly measures the plausibility of the null hypothesis. Less seriously, the "p" could stand for publication or promotion.

A p-value is readily related to a test of hypothesis. The relationship between a p-value and an α-level test of hypothesis is

$$\text{if the } p\text{-value} \geq \alpha, \text{ then } H_0 \text{ is accepted, and}$$

$$\text{if the } p\text{-value} \leq \alpha, \text{ then } H_0 \text{ is rejected.}$$

Although inferences drawn from the magnitude of a p-value are by and large an informal process that involves nonstatistical issues, the following is one possible scale:

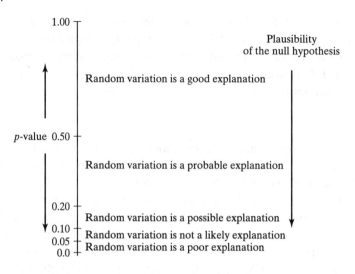

Two mean values from nonindependent populations (dependent *t*-test)

Two nonindependent populations arise, for example, from a "before–after" experiment. A series of experimental units (mice, people, trees, etc.) are measured at the beginning of an experiment ("baseline") then treated in a special way and measured again some time later. The same individual is measured both at the beginning and the end of the experiment. Since the same individual is measured twice, the two measurements are not independent. For example, in evaluating an experimental diet, a woman who weighs 100 pounds before a diet will weigh about 100 pounds after the diet period. The before and after measures are predictably similar, even if the diet has a substantial effect. Data from two nonindependent populations are typically sampled as a series of matching pairs.

The sample structure and notation are:

Sample	Before measurements	After measurements	Differences
1	x_1	y_1	$d_1 = x_1 - y_1$
2	x_2	y_2	$d_2 = x_2 - y_2$
.	.	.	.
.	.	.	.
.	.	.	.
n	x_n	y_n	$d_n = x_n - y_n$
Mean values	$\bar{x}$	$\bar{y}$	$\bar{d} = \bar{x} - \bar{y}$

Little new exists when the analysis of two nonindependent samples is based on the n differences within each pair of measurements. If $x_1, x_2, \cdots, x_n$ and $y_1, y_2, \cdots, y_n$ are normally distributed samples, then the differences $d_i = x_i - y_i$ and the mean difference $\bar{d} = \bar{x} - \bar{y}$ are also normally distributed. As before, the mean difference $\bar{d}$ has a normal distribution since a mean made up of normally distributed components is normally distributed (Chapter 3). For large samples ($n > 30$ or so) from nonnormal distributions, the mean difference $\bar{d}$ typically has an approximate normal distribution (central limit theorem). In both cases, the null hypothesis is

$$H_0: \mu_{before} = \mu_{after} \qquad \text{(no before/after effect, also denoted}$$
$$\mu_d = \mu_{before} - \mu_{after} = 0).$$

Less formally, the null hypothesis states that all observed differences within pairs of matching observations are due entirely to random variation.

Possible alternative hypotheses are:

$$H_1: \mu_{before} < \mu_{after} \quad \text{or} \quad \mu_d < 0 \text{ (one-tail)} \quad \text{or}$$
$$H_1: \mu_{before} > \mu_{after} \quad \text{or} \quad \mu_d > 0 \text{ (one-tail)} \quad \text{or}$$
$$H_1: \mu_{before} \neq \mu_{after} \quad \text{or} \quad \mu_d \neq 0 \text{ (two-tail)}.$$

The alternative hypothesis dictates, as always, the choice between a one-tail and a two-tail critical region.

When the n sampled differences (d_i-values) are normally distributed, a one-sample t-test ($\bar{x}$ versus μ_0) directly applies. The test statistic comparing $\bar{d}$ to $\mu_d = 0$ becomes

$$T = \frac{\bar{d} - 0}{S_{\bar{D}}}$$

where the estimated variance of the mean $\bar{d}$ is, once again,

$$S_{\bar{D}}^2 = \frac{S_D^2}{n} = \frac{\sum(d_i - \bar{d})^2/(n-1)}{n}.$$

This test statistic T, like the previous one-sample t-test, has a t-distribution with $n - 1$ degrees of freedom when the measured variables have normal distributions and the null hypothesis is true. When the assumption of normality is suspect, the mean value $\bar{d}$ has an approximately normal distribution for large values of n regardless of the distribution of the x-values and y-values (central limit theorem) and normal probabilities (Table A.1) are used in place of the t-distribution probabilities (Table A.2). As already noted, no practical difference typically exists between these two approaches (T or Z) for $n > 30$.

EXAMPLE

To study the physiological impact of meditation, a large number of individuals (200^{+}) were measured for a variety of biochemical substances before and after one hour of meditation. The levels of one of these chemical substances measured in the blood of 11 individuals before and then after meditation are (Figure 6.2):

Individual	1	2	3	4	5	6	7	8	9	10	11
before: x_i	73.1	43.8	91.3	70.1	88.3	111.4	93.0	78.4	61.2	85.9	63.2
after: y_i	80.3	50.2	96.3	69.4	84.3	101.4	96.4	83.2	60.1	89.7	70.4
before−after: d_i	−7.2	−6.4	−5.0	0.7	4.0	10.0	−3.4	−4.8	1.1	−3.8	−7.2

The null and alternative hypotheses are

$$H_0:\ \mu_d = \mu_{before} - \mu_{after} = 0 \qquad \text{versus} \qquad H_1:\ \mu_d = \mu_{before} - \mu_{after} \neq 0$$

where μ_{before} represents the sampled population mean before meditation and μ_{after} represents the sampled population mean after meditation. A level of significance $\alpha = 0.05$ gives $T \leq t_{0.025} = -2.228$ and $T \geq t_{0.975} = 2.228$ (degrees

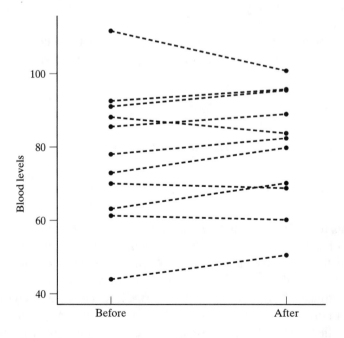

FIGURE 6.2: A graphic display of the before−after data from the meditation experiment.

of freedom are $n - 1 = 10$), forming a two-tail critical region. The following quantities are calculated from the data to test the null hypothesis of no meditation effect:

$$\bar{d} = -2.000 \quad \text{and} \quad S_D^2 = 29.238 \qquad \text{giving}$$

$$S_{\bar{D}}^2 = 29.238/11 = 2.658 \quad (S_{\bar{D}} = 1.630).$$

The T-statistic becomes

$$T = \frac{\bar{d} - 0}{S_{\bar{D}}} = \frac{-2.000}{1.630} = -1.227.$$

The null hypothesis is, therefore, not rejected ($-2.228 < -1.227$). The inference is made that no substantial evidence exists that meditation influences the blood levels of the specific chemical measured. The p-value is $P(T \leq -1.227 \mid H_0 \text{ true}) + P(T \geq 1.227 \mid H_0 \text{ true}) = 0.124 + 0.124 = 0.25$. In words, the probability of observing a more extreme value of the T-statistic than the observed value of -1.227, in either a positive or negative direction, is 0.25 when meditation has no effect. Thus, random variation remains a probable explanation for the observed difference ($\bar{d} = -2.0$). To reiterate, the p-value is the probability that a more extreme result could have occurred by chance alone.

A confidence interval constructed from the difference between two sample mean values when the sampled populations are not independent is no different from the previously discussed confidence intervals. In symbols, a $(1 - \alpha)$-level confidence interval $(\hat{A}, \hat{B})$ based on $\bar{d}$ and $S_{\bar{D}}$ has estimated bounds

lower bound $= \hat{A} = \bar{d} - t_{1-\alpha/2} S_{\bar{D}}$ and *upper bound* $= \hat{B} = \bar{d} + t_{1-\alpha/2} S_{\bar{D}}$.

For the meditation data, the confidence interval $(\hat{A}, \hat{B})$ is $-2.000 \pm 2.228(1.630)$ yielding a 95% confidence interval of $(-5.633, 1.633)$. ∎

Goodness-of-fit

A question fundamental to the application of a t-test or construction of a confidence interval is: Does the variable sampled have a normal distribution or even an approximate normal distribution? Often the first step in deciding on the direction of an analytic approach is to investigate this question (normal or nonnormal data?). Less formally, the question is: How well does the data "fit" a normal distribution? The answer clearly dictates subsequent analytic decisions. A simple graphic comparison of two cumulative distributions is frequently sufficient to decide if the observations are likely to have been sampled from a normal distribution. The following graphic technique is only one of many possible approaches.

Goodness-of-fit: comparing cumulative distributions

To graphically compare a normal distribution to a distribution of sample data, two sets of cumulative probabilities are necessary: one based on the theoretical normal distribution and one based on the sampled data.

The probability that a value sampled from a normal distribution is less than or equal to a specified value x_i is, as before,

$$P_i = F(x_i) = P(X \leq x_i) = P(Z \leq z_i).$$

This cumulative probability can be calculated using a computer program or found in tables such as Table A.1. It does not depend on the data or the sample size. It is entirely theoretical.

The parallel cumulative probability estimated from the data is

$$\hat{P}_i = \frac{the\ number\ of\ observations \leq x_i}{n} = \frac{i}{n},$$

where $x_1, x_2, \cdots, x_n$ is an ordered sample of n independent observations. This cumulative probability is based on the sampled data only. The estimated cumulative probability is simply the proportion of observed values that are less than or equal to the ith-ordered observation producing an estimated cumulative probability $\hat{P}_i$ for each of the n sampled values. Such an estimated probability is a special case of the relative cumulative frequency (Chapter 1).

Goodness-of-fit is measured by the correspondence of these two cumulative probabilities; the theoretically derived normal cumulative probabilities are compared to the sample estimated cumulative probabilities. Specifically, the probabilities P_i are compared to the probabilities $\hat{P}_i$ at each observed value x_i. If the theoretically and the empirically derived probabilities are similar ("good-fit"), reason exists to believe that a normal distribution is an effective description of the data. Conversely, if these two cumulative probabilities substantially differ ("lack-of-fit"), using an analytic technique that requires normally distributed data potentially produces misleading results, especially for small sample sizes. A plot of P_i against $\hat{P}_i$, called a *probability plot*, is a graphic display of the correspondence between these two sets of cumulative probabilities.

EXAMPLE

The comparison of theoretical and empirical cumulative probabilities is illustrated with a sample of 20 observations thought to be normally distributed. An ordered sample of data (x_i-values), in terms of standardized values $z_i = (x_i - \bar{x})/S_X$, is contained in Table 6.2, along with the cumulative probabilities P_i and $\hat{P}_i$.

TABLE 6.2: Goodness-of-fit: Normal distribution?

i	x_i	z_i	P_i	$\hat{P}_i$
1	0.18	−1.49	0.068	0.05
2	1.15	−1.21	0.113	0.10
3	1.22	−1.19	0.117	0.15
4	1.67	−1.06	0.145	0.20
5	1.84	−1.01	0.156	0.25
6	2.32	−0.87	0.192	0.30
7	2.98	−0.68	0.248	0.35
8	3.15	−0.63	0.264	0.40
9	5.09	−0.07	0.472	0.45
10	5.36	0.01	0.504	0.50
11	5.36	0.01	0.504	0.55
12	5.47	0.04	0.516	0.60
13	5.57	0.07	0.528	0.65
14	5.85	0.15	0.560	0.70
15	5.85	0.15	0.560	0.75
16	6.23	0.26	0.603	0.80
17	6.78	0.42	0.663	0.85
18	7.96	0.76	0.776	0.90
19	9.93	1.33	0.908	0.95
20	10.41	1.47	0.929	1.00

The 20 theoretical cumulative probabilities P_i are based on a standard normal distribution (Table A.1). For the first observation $z_1 = -1.49$, the corresponding cumulative normal probability is $P_1 = 0.068$ ($P_1 = P(Z \le -1.49) = 0.068$ from tables such as A.1 or a computer program). For the same observation, the sample cumulative probability is $\hat{P}_1 = 0.05$ ($\hat{P}_1 = 1/n = 1/20 = 0.05$). For the second observation, $z_2 = -1.21$ yields $P_2 = 0.113$ (theoretical) and $\hat{P}_2 = 2/20 = 0.10$ (empirical). The other 18 pairs of theoretical and empirical probabilities are similarly calculated and compared. The cumulative probabilities P_i and $\hat{P}_i$ given in Table 6.2 are plotted in Figure 6.3. The points $(P_i, \hat{P}_i)$ will likely form an approximate straight line (slope = 1.0 or 45° angle) when the population sampled is normally distributed ("good-fit") and will likely deviate from this line where the data fail to be accurately described by a normal probability distribution ("lack-of-fit"). Although a number of ways exist to formally assess these deviations, Rupert Miller of Stanford University, a well-known statistician, said, "if a deviation from normality cannot be spotted on a probit plot [probability plot], it is not worth worrying about." ■

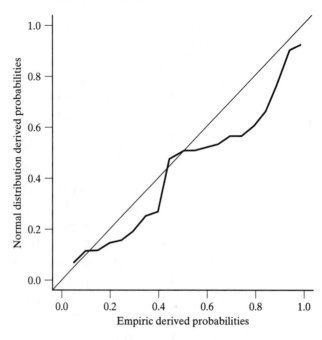

FIGURE 6.3: Comparison of P_i and $\hat{P}_i$ (is the data normally distributed?).

A single population proportion: $\hat{p}$ versus p_0

Parallel to comparing a sample mean value $\bar{x}$ to a postulated mean μ_0, it is equally possible to compare a sample proportion $\hat{p}$ to a postulated proportion p_0 using the same hypothesis testing strategy. Like $\bar{x}$, $\hat{p}$ is an estimated quantity subject to sampling variation and, like μ_0, p_0 is a fixed quantity generated from theoretical considerations.

The null hypothesis is

$$H_0: p = p_0$$

and the alternative hypothesis is

$$H_1: p \neq p_0 \qquad \text{(could also be a one-tail alternative hypothesis).}$$

The fact that $\hat{p}$ can be viewed as a special kind of a mean value (Chapter 4) implies that

$$Z = \frac{\bar{x} - \mu_0}{\sigma_{\bar{X}}} = \frac{\hat{p} - p_0}{\sigma_{\hat{p}}} = \frac{\hat{p} - p_0}{\sqrt{p_0(1 - p_0)/n}}$$

has an approximate normal distribution when n is large (central limit theorem—Chapter 3). The test statistic Z reflects the difference $(\hat{p} - p_0)$ but transformed to have a known probability distribution, namely an approximate standard normal distribution when the null hypothesis is true ($p = p_0$). As before, the level of significance of the test is a selected probability α. The critical region for a $(1 - \alpha)$-level two-tail test of the null hypothesis then becomes $Z \leq -z_{1-\alpha/2}$ or $Z \geq z_{1-\alpha/2}$ ($z_{1-\alpha/2}$ comes from Table A.1). This approach is approximate. Nevertheless, for sample sizes n larger than 30 and p in the neighborhood of 0.5, the distribution of the test statistic Z has an approximate normal distribution, producing accurate results (Table 4.3).

When testing a proportion $\hat{p}$, the null hypothesis determines its variance where $\sigma_{\hat{p}}^2 = p_0 (1 - p_0)/n$. The variance of $\hat{p}$ ($\sigma_{\hat{p}}^2$) is not a random variable and fulfills the requirement of the central limit theorem that the variance is known rather than estimated. Since the parent distribution of the sampled values that generate $\hat{p}$ is not normally distributed and the variance is not estimated, a test of a proportion does not involve a t-distribution.

EXAMPLE

It is frequently claimed that the white pieces have an advantage in a chess match (white moves first). If this claim is correct, persons playing the white pieces should win more than 50% of the games played (disregarding drawn games). A series of tournament matches can be classified as a win for white or a win for black. Such data from 630 tournament matches are:

	White wins	Black wins	Total
observed numbers	334	296	630
estimated proportions ($\hat{p}$)	0.530	0.470	1.0
expected numbers	315	315	630
expected probabilities (p_0)	0.5	0.5	1.0

The question is whether evidence from these matches supports the contention that players with the white pieces have an advantage. In other words, does the observed proportion indicate more than a random fluctuation from 0.50? Define p as the probability of winning when playing the white pieces, then the null hypothesis becomes

$$H_0\colon p = p_0 = 0.5 \text{ (white has no advantage)}$$

versus the alternative hypothesis

$$H_1\colon p > p_0 = 0.5 \text{ (white has an advantage)}.$$

The estimate $\hat{p}$ is transformed to the test statistic

$$Z = \frac{\hat{p} - p_0}{\sqrt{\dfrac{p_0(1 - p_0)}{n}}} = \frac{\hat{p} - 0.5}{\sqrt{\dfrac{(0.5)(0.5)}{630}}} = \frac{\hat{p} - 0.5}{0.020},$$

which has an approximate standard normal distribution when $p = 0.5$ (H_0 is true—$\hat{p}$ differs from 0.5 by chance alone). Selecting a level of significance $\alpha = 0.05$ creates a critical region of $Z \geq z_{0.95} = 1.645$ (H_0 is rejected for all values $Z \geq 1.645$—one-tail). In symbols, the probability of a Type I error is $\alpha = P(Z \geq 1.645 \mid p = 0.5) = 0.05$. The value of the test statistic is

$$z = \frac{0.530 - 0.5}{0.020} = 1.540$$

and does not fall into the critical region ($1.540 < 1.645$). The null hypothesis H_0 is accepted at the 5% level. The analysis of 630 matches fails to supply sufficient evidence to declare that white pieces have a definite advantage in tournament chess.

The hypothesis test indicates that it is not unlikely (probability greater than 0.05) to observe a value of $\hat{p}$ more than 1.540 standard deviations above the hypothetical value 0.5 when white has no advantage, but how unlikely? The significance probability is p-value $= P(\hat{p} \geq 0.530 \mid p = 0.5) = P(Z \geq 1.540 \mid p = 0.5) = 0.07$. Instead of simply stating "the null hypothesis is accepted," a p-value of 0.07 hints that white may have a slight advantage. ∎

Another sample size calculation

Suppose, for example, the standard treatment of a specific disease is effective in 20% of the cases. A new and more costly treatment will be included if it is as effective. A question arises: How many patients need to be tested to accurately assess whether the efficacy of adding the new procedure reaches a level of 40%? This question translates into determining the sample size (denoted again n_0) necessary to detect this increase. Expressed more statistically, a sample size is desired so that a decision can be made about the effectiveness of combining both treatments with specific Type I and Type II error rates. For example, a typical choice is $\alpha = 0.05$ and $\beta = 0.05$. The null hypothesis is H_0: $p = p_0 = 0.20$ (the new treatment has no additional effect) and the alternative hypothesis is H_1: $p = p_1 = 0.40$ (the new treatment has the specified additional effect) where p represents the underlying probability that a patient responds to the treatment.

Employing the normal distribution to approximate the binomial distribution (Chapter 4) furnishes an effective approach to finding the necessary sample size. Therefore, when $p_0 = 0.20$ (H_0 is true) and $\hat{p}$ estimates the observed proportion who respond, the variance of $\hat{p}$ is $variance\,(\hat{p}) = p_0(1 - p_0)/n_0 = 0.20(0.80)/n_0$. Assuming the null hypothesis $p = p_0 = 0.20$ is true, the test statistic Z is

$$Z = \frac{\hat{p} - p_0}{\sqrt{p_0(1 - p_0)/n_0}} = \frac{\hat{p} - 0.20}{\sqrt{(0.20)(0.80)/n_0}}$$

and the value Z has an approximate standard normal distribution. The calculation of the critical value c (critical region is $\hat{p} \geq c$) is then

$$\alpha = P(\text{Type I error}) = P(Z \geq 1.645 \mid p = 0.20)$$

$$= P\left(\frac{\hat{p} - 0.20}{\sqrt{(0.20)(0.80)/n_0}} \geq 1.645\right)$$

$$= P(\hat{p} \geq 0.20 + 1.645\sqrt{0.16/n_0}) = 0.05.$$

The critical region is all observed values of $\hat{p}$ greater than $c = 0.20 + 1.645\sqrt{0.16/n_0}$. The sample size n_0 is unknown at this point.

A Type II error occurs when $\hat{p}$ is not in the critical region ($\hat{p} \leq c$) when $p = p_1 = 0.40$ (H_1 is true) or

$$\beta = P(\text{Type II error}) = P(\hat{p} \leq c \mid p = 0.40)$$

$$= P(\hat{p} \leq 0.20 + 1.645\sqrt{0.16/n_0} \mid p = 0.40)$$

$$= P\left(Z \leq \frac{0.20 + 1.645\sqrt{0.16/n_0} - 0.40}{\sqrt{(0.4)(0.6)/n_0}}\right) = 0.05.$$

Therefore,

$$\frac{0.20 + 1.645\sqrt{0.16/n_0} - 0.40}{\sqrt{0.24/n_0}} = -1.645 \qquad \text{since}$$

$$\beta = P(Z \leq -1.645) = 0.05$$

and solving for n_0 gives

$$n_0 = \frac{\left[1.645\sqrt{0.16} + 1.645\sqrt{0.24}\right]^2}{(0.20 - 0.40)^2} = 53.564 \text{ (use 54 patients)}.$$

The calculation shows that the selected error rates of $\alpha = \beta = 0.05$ are achieved when 54 patients are tested with the combined treatments and the estimate $\hat{p}$ is used to choose between $p_0 = 0.20$ and $p_1 = 0.40$.

If Type I and Type II errors are set at $\alpha = 0.01$ and $\beta = 0.01$, then

$$n_0 = \frac{\left[2.326\sqrt{0.16} + 2.326\sqrt{0.24}\right]^2}{(0.20 - 0.40)^2} \qquad z_{0.99} = 2.326$$

$$= 107.144 \text{ (use 108 patients)}.$$

To meet these more stringent conditions, the sample size must be doubled.

The general expression for calculating a sample size (n_0) to compare an estimated proportion to a fixed value ($\hat{p}$ versus p_0) with selected Type I and Type II error rates α and β is

$$n_0 = \frac{\left[z_{1-\alpha}\sqrt{p_0(1-p_0)} + z_{1-\beta}\sqrt{p_1(1-p_1)}\right]^2}{(p_0 - p_1)^2}$$

where p_0 is defined by the null hypothesis and p_1 is defined by the alternative hypothesis. This expression is not substantially different from the previous sample size expression (Chapter 5) except in the case of assessing a proportion the variances are determined by H_0 and H_1.

EXAMPLE

Chevalier de Mèrè played two gambling games, one involving a single die and the other involving a pair of dice (Chapter 2). As the story goes, he found that the second game produced more losses than wins. It turns out that the probability of winning is 0.491.

A sample size calculation sheds some light on this story. Formally, a relevant question becomes, how many games would have to be played to determine, with specific error rates (α and β), that the probability of winning is 0.491 and not 0.5? Setting the error rates to $\alpha = 0.05$ and $\beta = 0.10$, then the number of games (sample size) necessary is

$$
\begin{aligned}
n_0 &= \frac{\left[z_{0.95}\sqrt{p_0(1-p_0)} + z_{0.90}\sqrt{p_1(1-p_1)}\right]^2}{(p_0 - p_1)^2} \\
&= \frac{\left[1.645\sqrt{(0.500)(0.500)} + 1.282\sqrt{(0.491)(0.509)}\right]^2}{(0.500 - 0.491)^2} = 26{,}428
\end{aligned}
$$

where $p_0 = 0.5$ and $p_1 = 0.491$. Not surprisingly, a huge number of games ($n_0 = 26{,}428$) is necessary to detect accurately that the second dice game is a loser ($p < 0.5$), because p_1 hardly differs from p_0.   ∎

The difference between two proportions: ($\hat{p}_1$ versus $\hat{p}_2$)

A class of 310 law students was randomly divided into two groups. Each group listened to the same tape recording of a trial concerning a drunk-driving case. Group 1 was shown a picture of an attractive, well-groomed defendant while group 2 was shown a picture of an ugly, slovenly-dressed defendant (adapted from a report in *Newsweek*). Each student decided independently whether the defendant was not guilty or guilty. A table summarizing the results is

Group	Not guilty	Guilty		Total	Proportion
group 1 (well groomed)	$x_1 = 85$	$n_1 - x_1 = 70$	$n_1 = 155$		$\hat{p}_1 = 85/155 = 0.548$
group 2 (slovenly)	$x_2 = 67$	$n_2 - x_2 = 88$	$n_2 = 155$		$\hat{p}_2 = 67/155 = 0.432$
Total	$x_1 + x_2 = 152$	$n - (x_1 + x_2) = 158$	$n = 310$		$\hat{p} = 152/310 = 0.490$

The data were collected to examine the possibility of a systematic difference between the proportions of not guilty verdicts. Statistically, the question becomes

$$P(not\ guilty\ |\ group\ 1) = P(not\ guilty\ |\ group\ 2)? \qquad \text{or} \qquad p_1 = p_2?$$

and is naturally addressed by comparing sample estimates $\hat{p}_1$ and $\hat{p}_2$. The estimate $\hat{p}_1$ is the proportion of students in group 1 who concluded that the defendant was not guilty ($\hat{p}_1 = 85/155 = 0.548$) and the estimate $\hat{p}_2$ is similarly the proportion of students in group 2 who concluded the defendant was not guilty ($\hat{p}_2 = 67/155 = 0.432$). These two proportions are used to create a test statistic that becomes the basis to decide whether the observed difference $\hat{p}_1 - \hat{p}_2 = 0.548 - 0.432 = 0.116$ indicates that the pictures of the defendant influenced the choice between not guilty and guilty verdicts ($p_1 - p_2 \neq 0$).

The null hypothesis is that no difference exists between the two groups or

$$H_0: p_1 = p_2 = p \qquad \text{(the pictures have no influence)}$$

versus the alternative hypothesis that a difference exists or

$$H_1: p_1 \neq p_2 \qquad \text{(the pictures have an influence)}.$$

Similar to comparing mean values $\bar{x}_1$ and $\bar{x}_2$ from nonnormal populations, the central limit theorem provides a theoretical distribution to compare $\hat{p}_1$ and $\hat{p}_2$ when the sample sizes for both groups are large. A t-test is again not appropriate because the parent populations sampled are not normally distributed. The parent populations yield binary observations (not guilty coded 1 and guilty coded 0).

To apply the central limit theorem, the variance of the difference between two proportions is needed. Using the same reasoning that yielded the variance of the difference between two sample mean values gives

$$\sigma^2_{\hat{p}_1 - \hat{p}_2} = \sigma^2_{\hat{p}_1} + \sigma^2_{\hat{p}_2} = \frac{p_1(1 - p_1)}{n_1} + \frac{p_2(1 - p_2)}{n_2}.$$

Taking advantage of the null hypothesis ($p_1 = p_2 = p$), the expression for $\sigma^2_{\hat{p}_1 - \hat{p}_2}$ becomes

$$\sigma^2_{\hat{p}_1 - \hat{p}_2} = \frac{p(1 - p)}{n_1} + \frac{p(1 - p)}{n_2} = p(1 - p)\left(\frac{1}{n_1} + \frac{1}{n_2}\right)$$

where $p = P(not\ guilty)$ when the pictures have no influence. Since the proportion p is unknown, an estimate of p comes from the combining (a weighted average) the estimates $\hat{p}_1$ and $\hat{p}_2$ or

$$\hat{p} = \frac{n_1 \hat{p}_1 + n_2 \hat{p}_2}{n_1 + n_2} = \frac{x_1 + x_2}{n_1 + n_2}$$

where x_1 is the number of not guilty verdicts in the first group (well groomed) and x_2 is the number not guilty verdicts in the second group (slovenly). The weights are the sample sizes n_1 and n_2 in each group. Specifically, the estimate of p from the law school experiment is

$$\hat{p} = \frac{155(0.548) + 155(0.432)}{155 + 155} = \frac{85 + 67}{155 + 155} = \frac{152}{310} = 0.490.$$

The estimate $\hat{p}$ is the proportion of law students who arrived at a not guilty verdict, disregarding any influence of the pictures of the defendant. The null hypothesis states that the pictures have no influence, so p is estimated using all the collected data (combining all 310 observations). Estimates necessary to perform a statistical test are almost always calculated as if the null hypothesis is true.

Now, the test statistic (both n_1 and n_2 must be large)

$$Z = \frac{(\hat{p}_1 - \hat{p}_2) - (p_1 - p_2)}{\sigma_{\hat{p}_1 - \hat{p}_2}} = \frac{\hat{p}_1 - \hat{p}_2 - 0}{\sigma_{\hat{p}_1 - \hat{p}_2}}$$

has an approximate standard normal distribution (central limit theorem) when the null hypothesis is true ($p_1 = p_2 = p$). Setting the level of significance α at 0.05, the two-tail critical region becomes $Z \le z_{0.025} = -1.960$ and $Z \ge z_{0.975} = 1.960$. The test statistic Z calculated from the verdicts of the 310 law students is

$$Z = \frac{(\hat{p}_1 - \hat{p}_2) - (p_1 - p_2)}{\sqrt{\hat{p}(1 - \hat{p})\left(\frac{1}{n_1} + \frac{1}{n_2}\right)}} = \frac{(0.548 - 0.432) - 0}{\sqrt{(0.490)(0.510)\left[\frac{1}{155} + \frac{1}{155}\right]}} = 2.045.$$

The null hypothesis of no difference between p_1 and p_2 ($p_1 - p_2 = 0$) is rejected at the 5% level ($1.960 < 2.045$). The significance probability is p-value $= P(Z \leq -2.045) + P(Z \geq 2.045) = 0.020 + 0.020 = 0.04$.

In general, this test of the equality of two proportions works well for large samples (both n_1 and $n_2 \geq 30$) when p is not extremely close to 0 or 1 (Table 4.3). This same statistical test is discussed again in a different context in the next chapter.

Contrasting the *T*-test and the *Z*-test approach

Table 6.3 contrasts the T-approach and the Z-approach for comparing two statistical summaries calculated from samples from two independent populations (two-sample test).

TABLE 6.3: Comparison of the two-sample T-statistic and Z-statistic.

	T-approach	Z-approach
1. parent populations	normally distributed	large variety of possibilities
2. sample selections	observations must be independent	observations must be independent
3. sample sizes	any sample size	large: usually n_1 and $n_2 > 30$ or so
4. variances	equal ($\sigma_1^2 = \sigma_2^2$)	should not be very different
5. estimated variances	pooled from sample estimates	not necessarily pooled
6. degrees of freedom	$n_1 + n_2 - 2$	not relevant
7. statistical issues	difference in two mean values	difference in two mean values or proportions
8. distributions	exact t-distribution	approximate normal distribution
9. critical regions	from a t-distribution	from a normal distribution
10. significance probabilities	from a t-distribution	from a normal distribution

GLOSSARY: STATISTICAL HYPOTHESIS TESTING

Statistical hypothesis.   A conjecture concerning the structure of a probability distribution.

Null hypothesis (H_0).   A conjecture postulating that observed deviations from a fixed value are due only to the random variation associated with the variable under investigation.

Test statistic.   A random variable constructed to assess the null hypothesis in terms of a probability.

Alternative hypothesis (H_1).   A conjecture postulating that observed deviations from a fixed value are due to a systematic effect associated with the variable under investigation.

Level of significance (α).   An error rate set by the investigator measured in terms of the probability of incorrectly rejecting the null hypothesis when the null hypothesis is true; denoted $P(reject\ H_0 \mid H_0\ is\ true)$.

Critical region.   The set of all values of the test statistic that lead to rejecting the null hypothesis.

P(Type I error).   The probability of incorrectly rejecting the null hypothesis when the null hypothesis is true; denoted $\alpha = P(reject\ H_0 \mid H_0\ is\ true)$ and is another term for the level of significance.

P(Type II error).   The probability of incorrectly rejecting the alternative hypothesis when the alternative hypothesis is true; denoted $\beta = P(reject\ H_1 \mid H_1\ is\ true)$.

Power ($1 - \beta$).   The probability of correctly rejecting the null hypothesis when the alternative hypothesis is true; denoted $1 - \beta = P(reject\ H_0 \mid H_1\ is\ true)$.

Two-tail statistical test.   A statistical test for which the critical region comprises both large and small values of the test statistic.

One-tail statistical test.   A statistical test for which the critical region comprises either large or small values of the test statistic but not both possibilities.

Significance probability (p-value).   The probability of observing a more extreme value of the test statistic than the value observed, when the null hypothesis is true.

Summary of Two-Sample Analyses

I: $X_1, X_2, X_3, \cdots X_{n_1}$ (n_1 observations)

II: $Y_1, Y_2, Y_3, \cdots Y_{n_2}$ (n_2 observations)

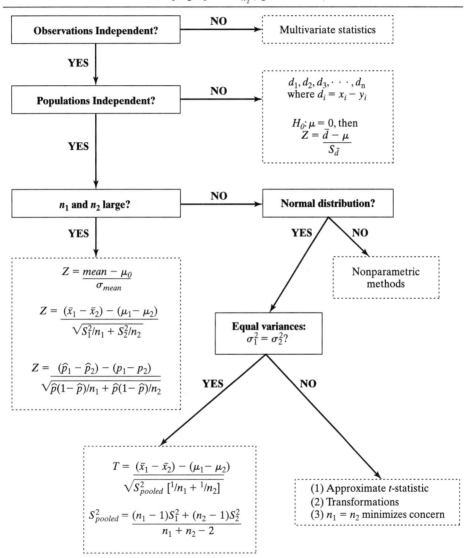

Observations Independent? — NO → Multivariate statistics

YES ↓

Populations Independent? — NO →

$d_1, d_2, d_3, \cdots, d_n$
where $d_i = x_i - y_i$

$H_0: \mu = 0$, then
$$Z = \frac{\bar{d} - \mu}{S_{\bar{d}}}$$

YES ↓

n_1 and n_2 large? — NO → **Normal distribution?**

YES ↓   YES ↙   NO ↘ Nonparametric methods

$$Z = \frac{mean - \mu_0}{\sigma_{mean}}$$

$$Z = \frac{(\bar{x}_1 - \bar{x}_2) - (\mu_1 - \mu_2)}{\sqrt{S_1^2/n_1 + S_2^2/n_2}}$$

$$Z = \frac{(\hat{p}_1 - \hat{p}_2) - (p_1 - p_2)}{\sqrt{\hat{p}(1 - \hat{p})/n_1 + \hat{p}(1 - \hat{p})/n_2}}$$

Equal variances:
$\sigma_1^2 = \sigma_2^2$?

YES ↙   NO ↘

$$T = \frac{(\bar{x}_1 - \bar{x}_2) - (\mu_1 - \mu_2)}{\sqrt{S_{pooled}^2\,[^1/n_1 + {}^1/n_2]}}$$

$$S_{pooled}^2 = \frac{(n_1 - 1)S_1^2 + (n_2 - 1)S_2^2}{n_1 + n_2 - 2}$$

(1) Approximate t-statistic
(2) Transformations
(3) $n_1 = n_2$ minimizes concern

One day three statisticians went deer hunting in the Maine woods. As they came over a rise, in front of them was a large and magnificent buck. The first hunter raised his gun and fired, missing to the left. Immediately the second hunter fired, missing to the right. The third hunter then lowered his rifle and exclaimed, "We got him."

PROBLEM SET 6

1. Consider the following data on the additional hours of sleep gained by 10 patients who participate in an experiment with a newly developed drug. Determine whether these data justify the claim that this drug produces additional sleep. Each participant was randomly assigned to the drug (active pill) or a placebo (inactive pill) the first week. Then one week later, each patient was given the other kind of pill. The results below are the hours of sleep on the drug minus the hours of sleep on the placebo.

Patient	Hours gained	Patient	Hours gained
1	0.7	6	3.4
2	−1.1	7	3.7
3	−0.2	8	0.8
4	−1.2	9	1.8
5	−0.1	10	2.0

What null hypothesis and alternative hypothesis would you suggest? Test the null hypothesis against the alternative at the 5% level of significance. Assume that the hours of sleep are normally distributed for the individuals taking either the active or placebo drug.

2. The following measurements of blood viscosity were made on laboratory mice:

$$3.29, 3.91, 4.64, 3.55, 3.67, 4.18, 3.74, 3.03, 4.61, 3.84.$$

Test the hypothesis that the mean blood viscosity of these mice was sampled from a normal distribution with mean $\mu = 3.95$ against the alternative hypothesis that the mean is not 3.95 ($\alpha = 0.05$).

Suppose a sample of 16 wild honey bees was collected. Wing widths were measured and the sample mean was $\bar{x} = 4.50$ mm with estimated variance $S^2 = 0.0784$ mm^2. Only one wing measurement is taken per bee creating a sample of $n = 16$ observations from a normal distribution.

3. Find the 90% confidence interval for μ.
4. Find the 99% confidence interval for μ.
5. Give an interpretation (in words) of these two confidence intervals.
6. Why not measure both wings producing a sample of size $= 32$?

In a sample of 1600 twin live births, 1100 were found to be dizygotic (fraternal) and the remainder monozygotic (identical) twins.

7. Is the proportion of monozygotic twins different from that of dizygotic twins? Select $\alpha = 0.05$.
8. Find the 95% confidence interval for the probability that a live twin birth will be monozygotic.

Assume it is known that 20% of the trees affected by a pest are defoliated. A parasite of the pest was introduced into an area with 400 trees known to be infested with the eggs of this pest. Sixty of these trees were defoliated.

9. Is there evidence that the "treated" 400 trees were subject to a different probability (different from 20%) of being defoliated? Select $\alpha = 0.05$.

10. Of the 100 numbers thought to be randomly selected, 42 were odd and 58 were even numbers. Is this significantly different from an expected 50:50 split?

11. Middle-aged white male executives who belonged to a running club were compared to a control group who did little or no exercise. Their heart rates after 6 minutes on a treadmill are given below. Test for evidence of a difference assuming the treadmill data are normally distributed with the same variance for both groups; select $\alpha = 0.05$.

Group	Six-minute treadmill heart rate (beats per minute)
runners ($n = 10$)	99, 119, 122, 111, 115, 113, 103, 100, 78, 100
control ($n = 10$)	120, 130, 108, 129, 115, 111, 127, 102, 118, 140

12. Sudden infant death syndrome (SIDS) is also known as "sudden unexplained death," "crib-death," or "cot death" and is the major cause of death in the post-neonatal period, with a peak between 2 and 4 months. It is particularly perplexing as it occurs in infants who are apparently healthy.

A study was done on a variety of the maternal and post partum variables that might be associated with SIDS. Ninety white female SIDS birth weights were compared with ninety white female control birth weights. Is there evidence of a difference between the mean birth weights of the two groups at $\alpha = 0.01$? Assume that birth weights in both groups are normally distributed with the same variance.

	Controls	SIDS
sample sizes	$n_1 = 90$	$n_2 = 90$
sample means	$\bar{x}_1 = 3440\,g$	$\bar{x}_2 = 3010\,g$
sample standard deviations	$S_1 = 550\,g$	$S_2 = 523\,g$

13. The following data were adapted from a study of twins. On the basis of this study, can it be concluded that the mean age of mothers who give birth to dizygotic twins is greater than the mean age of mothers who give birth to monozygotic twins? Assume that the maternal ages were sampled from normal distributions with the same variance; set $\alpha = 0.01$.

	Monozygotic twins	Dizygotic twins
numbers of twin deliveries	$n_1 = 718$	$n_2 = 1112$
sample means	$\bar{x}_1 = 27.09$ years	$\bar{x}_2 = 30.23$ years
sample standard deviations	$S_1 = 7.51$ years	$S_2 = 6.42$ years

14. In an experimental study of the longevity of *Drosophila melanogaster* (fruit fly), 270 male adults and 275 female adults were raised at a certain larval density and observed until the death of the last member in each group. The mean lifetime for the males was found to be $\bar{x}_1 = 43.2$ days with a standard deviation $S_1 = 9.1$ days. The corresponding figures for the females were $\bar{x}_2 = 37.5$ days and $S_2 = 8.8$ days. Would you conclude that the male *Drosophila* has a greater longevity than the female? Assume that the survival times were sampled from normal distributions with the same variances for both males and females.

15. Twenty-three out of 50 treated mice gave a positive response to a specific antigen test. Of the 50 controls, there were 10 positive responses. Is there evidence of a difference? Calculate the significance probability (*p*-value).

16. When DDT was banned, new pesticides were introduced without thorough investigation of their effects on the environment. Toxaphene is one such pesticide.* It appears to cause a vitamin C deficiency in fish which leads to stunted growth and skeletal fragility. Calculate the significance probability (*p*-value) from the following data.

Two common species of freshwater fish were raised in the presence of the same concentration of Toxaphene. In species A, 15% of the 200 fish had fractured spines. Seventy of the 300 fish of species B were similarly affected. Test the hypothesis that skeletal fragility in the form of fractured spines occurs with different frequencies in these two species.

A classic study[†] of the relationship between cancer of the lung and smoking habits was carried out in England using data from a series of hospitals. The number of smokers and nonsmokers among lung cancer patients and a control group of patients with other diseases is given in the following table:

Disease group	Smokers	Nonsmokers	Total
lung cancer patients	1418	47	1465
control patients	1345	120	1465
Total	2763	167	2930

17. Is the proportion of smokers in the cancer group significantly different from that in the controls? Give *a p*-value.

Suppose the prevalence of lung cancer in the general population was $P(C) = 1.55$ per 10,000.

18. Estimate $P(C \mid S)$ and $P(C \mid \bar{S})$ directly from the table. What is the ratio of these probabilities? Are these answers usable? Sensible?

---

*The Environmental Protection Agency (EPA) began proceedings to cancel the registration for Toxaphene in 1977. In late 1982, the EPA ordered its cancellation, but allowed over 10 million pounds to be used between 1983 and 1986 (*Science*).

†*Source*: R. Doll, and R. B. Hill. "A study of the etiology of carcinoma of the lung," *British Medical Journal.*

19. Estimate $P(C \mid S)$ and $P(C \mid \overline{S})$ using the given prevalence of lung cancer or $P(C \mid S) = ?$ and $P(C \mid \overline{S}) = ?$

20. Calculate the ratio of these two estimates, that is, relative risk $= P(C \mid S)/P(C \mid \overline{S})$.

Note: These data are of historical interest in the identification of smoking as a cause of lung cancer. However, the study design is not perfect. A bias called Berkson's Fallacy involves the unrepresentativeness of hospital patients compared to the general population. In this case, we know smoking is associated with other diseases (emphysema, heart disease, etc.) so the control patients probably are more likely to be smokers than the general population.

CHAPTER 7

Chi-Square Analysis

Another fundamentally important probability distribution is the *chi-square probability distribution*. Like the normal distribution and the *t*-distribution, the chi-square distribution describes the likelihood of the occurrence of specific values of a test statistic calculated from sample data. The specific test statistic and the probability distribution are new but a chi-square analysis employs the same terminology and basic hypothesis testing strategy previously discussed (Chapters 5 and 6).

The chi-square probability distribution is defined by the following theorem:

if $Z_1, Z_2, \cdots, Z_m$ are m independent and normally distributed random variables each with mean $= 0$ and variance $= 1$, then the sum of the m squared Z-values,

$$X^2 = Z_1^2 + Z_2^2 + \cdots + Z_m^2,$$

has a chi-square distribution with m degrees of freedom.

Each chi-square distribution is a member of a family of probability distributions identified by an associated number of degrees of freedom (denoted *df*). Like the *t*-distribution, the degrees of freedom completely define the shape and properties of each chi-square distribution. The number of degrees of freedom is the defining parameter of the chi-square distribution and depends on the number of independent values in the sum (denoted *m*) that make up the chi-square statistic (denoted X^2). Three chi-square distributions each identified by its degrees of freedom (parameters $= df = 1$, 2, and 3) are:

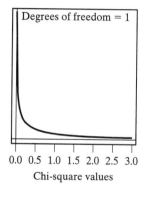

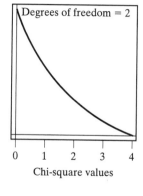

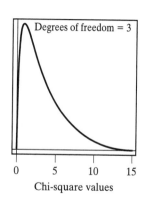

For most chi-square analyses these values $(Z_1, Z_2, \cdots, Z_m)$ are not independent. This lack of independence is dealt with by adjusting the degrees of freedom. The details of the adjustment are discussed throughout the chapter.

Figure 7.1 displays a typical chi-square probability distribution. The plotted percentiles are (3.94, 6.74, 9.34, 12.55, and 18.31) with corresponding probabilities (0.05, 0.25, 0.50, 0.75, and 0.95) or $P(X^2 \leq 3.94) = 0.05$, $P(X^2 \leq 6.74) = 0.25$, $P(X^2 \leq 9.34) = 0.50$, $P(X^2 \leq 12.55) = 0.75$ and $P(X^2 \leq 18.31) = 0.95$. The dotted line displays (Figure 7.1) the normal distribution with $\mu = 10$ and $\sigma_X^2 = 20$, included for contrast.

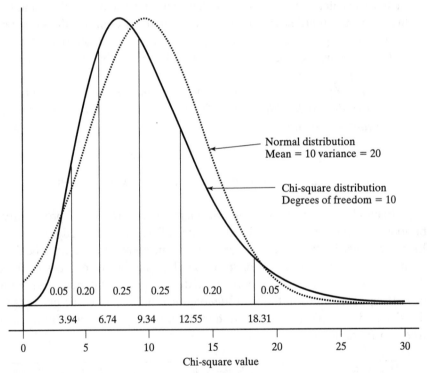

FIGURE 7.1: A typical chi-square distribution (degrees of freedom $= 10$) with selected percentiles.

The chi-square distribution is asymmetric but as the number of degrees of freedom increases, it becomes more symmetric and ultimately similar in shape to the normal distribution. A chi-square variable is never negative since it is a sum of a series of squared values. The mean (expected value) of a chi-square probability distribution equals its degrees of freedom $[E(X^2) = df$ when $df > 2]$ and its variance is two times the degrees of freedom ($\sigma_{X^2}^2 = 2df$ when $df > 4$). For example, the mean of a chi-square distribution with 10 degrees of freedom is 10 with a variance of 20 (Figure 7.1). A few probabilities for selected chi-square distributions are given in Table A.3. For example, Table A.3 shows

$$
\begin{aligned}
P(X^2 \le 7.815) &= 0.95 & degrees\ of\ freedom &= df = 3, \\
P(X^2 \le 1.145) &= 0.05 & degrees\ of\ freedom &= df = 5, \\
P(X^2 \ge 16.013) &= 0.025 & degrees\ of\ freedom &= df = 7, \\
P(X^2 \le 10.851) &= 0.05 & degrees\ of\ freedom &= df = 20, \\
P(X^2 \ge 37.566) &= 0.01 & degrees\ of\ freedom &= df = 20, \\
P(X^2 \le 79.334) &= 0.50 & degrees\ of\ freedom &= df = 80.
\end{aligned}
$$

In general, $P(X^2 \le \chi^2_{1-\alpha}) = 1 - \alpha$ where the percentile values $\chi^2_{1-\alpha}$ are calculated with a computer program or found in statistical tables such as Table A.3.

The principal role of the chi-square probability distribution in statistical analysis is to provide a summary of a series of independent and normally distributed test statistics. Each member of the series is standardized by subtracting its mean and dividing by its standard deviation, creating a series of normally distributed values each with a mean value of zero and a variance of one (Chapter 4). These values are squared and the sum forms a single overall summary test statistic with a chi-square distribution.

EXAMPLE

An example of combining a series of independent and normally distributed variables into a chi-square summary statistic shows that the sample variance S_X^2 multiplied by a specific constant has a chi-square distribution and leads to the construction of a confidence interval. Specifically,

when the sample $x_1, x_2, x_3, \cdots, x_n$ are n independent and normally distributed sample values (mean $= \mu$ and variance $= \sigma_X^2$), then each value

$z_i = \dfrac{x_i - \mu}{\sigma_X}$ has a standard normal distribution (mean $= 0$ and variance $= 1$),

$z_i^2 = \left[\dfrac{x_i - \mu}{\sigma_X}\right]^2$ has a chi-square distribution with one degree of freedom, and

$X^2 = \sum z_i^2 = \dfrac{1}{\sigma_X^2} \sum (x_i - \mu)^2$ has a chi-square distribution with

n degrees of freedom.

The last two steps come directly from the theorem describing the chi-square probability distribution.

If the mean μ is replaced by its estimate $\bar{x}$, then

$$X^2 = \frac{1}{\sigma_X^2} \sum (x_i - \bar{x})^2 = (n-1) \frac{S_X^2}{\sigma_X^2}$$

has a chi-square distribution with $n-1$ degrees of freedom. As mentioned, the adjustment of the degrees of freedom ($n-1$ not n) is due to the lack of independence between the x_i-observations and the mean value $\bar{x}$. Therefore, the sample variance S_X^2 has a chi-square distribution with $n-1$ degrees of freedom when multiplied by the constant $(n-1)/\sigma_X^2$. That is, a chi-square probability distribution with $n-1$ degrees of freedom describes the impact of sampling variation on the estimated variance S_X^2. ■

Confidence interval for the variance σ_X^2

In symbols, when a variable X^2 has a chi-square distribution, then

$$P\left(\chi_{\alpha/2}^2 \leq X^2 \leq \chi_{1-\alpha/2}^2\right) = 1 - \alpha$$

where $\chi_{\alpha/2}^2$ and $\chi_{1-\alpha/2}^2$ represent the $\alpha/2^{th}$- and $(1-\alpha/2)^{th}$-percentiles of a chi-square distribution. For example, the percentiles $\chi_{0.025}^2 = 3.247$ and $\chi_{0.975}^2 = 20.483$ give $P(3.247 \leq X^2 \leq 20.483) = 0.95$ for a chi-square distributed variable X^2 with 10 degrees of freedom (Table A.3).

Specifically, for $X^2 = (n-1)S_X^2/\sigma_X^2$, the chi-square distribution yields

$$P\left[\chi_{\alpha/2}^2 \leq \frac{(n-1)S_X^2}{\sigma_X^2} \leq \chi_{1-\alpha/2}^2\right] = 1 - \alpha.$$

With a bit of algebraic manipulation (Chapter 5), this probability statement produces confidence interval bounds $(\hat{A}, \hat{B})$ for the population variance σ_X^2, which are estimated from the sample variance S_X^2. The estimated bounds of the $(1-\alpha)\%$ confidence interval are

$$\hat{A} = lower\ bound = \frac{(n-1)S_X^2}{\chi_{1-\alpha/2}^2} \quad and \quad \hat{B} = upper\ bound = \frac{(n-1)S_X^2}{\chi_{\alpha/2}^2}$$

because

$$P\left[\frac{(n-1)S_X^2}{\chi_{1-\alpha/2}^2} \leq \sigma_X^2 \leq \frac{(n-1)S_X^2}{\chi_{\alpha/2}^2}\right] = 1 - \alpha.$$

As usual, the estimated confidence interval bounds $(\hat{A}, \hat{B})$, constructed from the sample estimated variance S_X^2, provide a likely range of values for the population variance σ_X^2 as well as an indication of the precision of the estimate S_X^2.

EXAMPLE

A sample of $n = 10$ women were weighed after the second trimester of pregnancy (Chapter 6). Their mean weight gain was $\bar{x} = 7.030$ kilograms and the
corresponding 95% confidence interval for the mean value μ, estimated by $\bar{x}$, was
(6.243, 7.817). The sample variance estimated from the same data is $S_X^2 = 1.210$
and, like $\bar{x}$, is subject to sampling variation. It too is based on the same $n = 10$
observations. A confidence interval for σ_X^2 constructed from the estimate S_X^2
effectively displays the impact of sampling variation on this estimated value.
The necessary chi-square percentiles (Table A.3) are

$$\chi^2_{0.025} = 2.700 \quad \text{and} \quad \chi^2_{0.975} = 19.023$$

since the degrees of freedom are $n - 1 = 10 - 1 = 9$. The estimated 95%
confidence interval bounds become

$$\hat{A} = lower\ bound = \frac{9(1.210)}{19.023} = 0.572 \quad \text{and}$$

$$\hat{B} = upper\ bound = \frac{9(1.210)}{2.700} = 4.033.$$

The 95% confidence $(\hat{A}, \hat{B}) = (0.572, 4.033)$ produces the expected result that,
like $\bar{x}$, the estimated variance (1.210) is not very precise (wide confidence interval) due primarily to the small sample of only 10 women. The application of the
chi-square distribution to construct a confidence interval requires the data to be
independently sampled from an at least approximate normal distribution.   ■

Chi-square analysis of tables

The simplest table (table with two cells)

The chi-square theorem applies to a single normally distributed z-value ($m = 1$).
Therefore, a variable with a standard normal distribution, when it is squared, has
a chi-square distribution. For example, when a sample mean $\bar{x}$ is compared to a
postulated value μ_0 (Chapter 5) and the test statistic

$$Z = \frac{\bar{x} - \mu_0}{\sigma_{\bar{X}}}$$

has a standard normal distribution ($\mu = 0$ and $\sigma_Z^2 = 1$), then the quantity

$$Z^2 = \frac{(\bar{x} - \mu_0)^2}{\sigma_{\bar{X}}^2}$$

has a chi-square distribution with one degree of freedom ($df = 1$). The probability associated with a two-tail test of hypothesis using a standard normal variable Z is identical to the probability associated using the variable Z^2. For example,

$$P(Z \leq -1.960) + P(Z \geq 1.960) = 0.025 + 0.025 = 0.05 \qquad \text{Table A.1}$$

or

$$P[Z^2 \geq (1.960)^2] = P(Z^2 \geq 3.841) = 0.05. \qquad \text{Table A.3.}$$

Because test statistics Z and Z^2 yield the identical probabilities associated with a two-tail test, it makes little difference which test statistic is used.

The same pattern applies to an estimated proportion. When the null hypothesis is $H_0: p = p_0$ and the alternative hypothesis is $H_1: p \neq p_0$, a test statistic, as before (Chapter 6), is

$$Z = \frac{\hat{p} - p_0}{\sqrt{\dfrac{p_0(1 - p_0)}{n}}}$$

and the value Z has an approximate standard normal distribution for large values of n (central limit theorem) when $p = p_0$. The squared value

$$Z^2 = \frac{(\hat{p} - p_0)^2}{\left[\dfrac{p_0(1 - p_0)}{n}\right]},$$

then has an approximate chi-square distribution with one degree of freedom. In terms of significance probabilities, these two approaches (Z or Z^2) are again identical.

EXAMPLE

In certain genetic situations (simple Mendelian inheritance), when two heterozygotic individuals mate (Aa $\times$ Aa), the expected proportion of offspring with one or two dominant genes (A) is 3/4 ($p_0 = 3/4$). Data from 64 heterozygotic matings are:

	AA, Aa individuals	aa individuals	Total
observed frequencies (f)	$f = 40$	$n - f = 24$	64
observed proportions ($\hat{p} = f/n$)	$\hat{p} = 0.625$	$1 - \hat{p} = 0.375$	1.0

Do these data support the conjecture that $p = 3/4$? For a level of significance $\alpha = 0.05$, values $Z^2 \geq 3.841$ (Table A.3—degrees of freedom $= 1$) form a critical region. The chi-square test statistic is

$$Z^2 = \frac{(\hat{p} - 3/4)^2}{\left[\dfrac{(3/4)(1/4)}{64}\right]} = \frac{(0.625 - 0.75)^2}{0.00293} = 5.333.$$

The null hypothesis is, therefore, rejected at level $\alpha = 0.05$ because 5.333 is in the critical region ($3.841 < 5.333$). This chi-square test is exactly equivalent to using two-tails of a normal distribution where Z would be $\sqrt{5.333} = 2.309$ with critical values -1.960 and 1.960 ($\sqrt{3.841} = 1.960$). The p-values are necessarily identical, $P(X^2 \geq 5.333 \,|\, p = 0.75) = 0.02$ (Table A.3) or $P[Z^2 \geq (2.309)^2] = P(Z \leq -2.309) + P(Z \geq 2.309) = 0.01 + 0.01 = 0.02$ (Table A.1). The test statistic Z^2 applied to evaluate a proportion, however, leads to a general class of chi-square tests used to assess relationships within more extensive tables.   ∎

One-way classification (table with k cells)

A sample of n observations classified by the presence or absence of a characteristic (denoted C and $\overline{C}$) is summarized in Table 7.1.

The chi-square assessment of a sample proportion involves three probabilities: (1) the unknown underlying population probability, represented by p, that is the subject of the investigation, (2) the probability generated by a conjecture of what p might be, represented by p_0, and (3) the estimated probability (estimate of p), represented by $\hat{p}$. The probabilities p and p_0 are fixed values and the estimate $\hat{p}$ is, like all estimates, subject to sampling variation.

TABLE 7.1: A one-way classification ($k = 2$ cells) of a sample of n observations by the presence or absence of a characteristic.

	C = present	$\overline{C}$ = absent	Total
observed numbers	f_1	f_2	n
observed proportions	$\hat{p} = f_1/n$	$1 - \hat{p} = \hat{q} = f_2/n$	1.0
population proportions	p	$1 - p = q$	1.0
postulated proportions	p_0	$1 - p_0 = q_0$	1.0
expected numbers	$F_1 = np_0$	$F_2 = nq_0$	n

Specifically, for the Mendelian inheritance data, Table 7.1 becomes

	C = AA/Aa	$\overline{C}$ = aa	Total
observed numbers (f)	40	24	64
observed proportions ($\hat{p}$)	0.625	0.375	1.0
population proportions (p)	unknown	unknown	1.0
postulated proportions (p_0)	0.75	0.25	1.0
expected numbers (F)	48	16	64

An alternative form of the test statistic Z^2 is

$$Z^2 = \frac{(\hat{p} - p_0)^2}{\left[\dfrac{p_0(1 - p_0)}{n}\right]} = \frac{(f_1 - np_0)^2}{np_0} + \frac{(f_2 - nq_0)^2}{nq_0}$$

$$= \frac{(f_1 - F_1)^2}{F_1} + \frac{(f_2 - F_2)^2}{F_2} = X^2$$

and is often called the *Pearson chi-square statistic* after the early statistician Karl Pearson (b. 1857) who developed the chi-square analysis (Box 7.1).

Box 7.1. Chi-square Statistic

$$Z^2 = \frac{(\hat{p} - p_0)^2}{\left[\dfrac{p_0(1 - p_0)}{n}\right]} = \frac{(f_1 - np_0)^2}{np_0(1 - p_0)} = \frac{(f_1 - np_0)^2}{n} \times \left[\frac{1}{p_0} + \frac{1}{1 - p_0}\right]$$

$$= \frac{(f_1 - np_0)^2}{np_0} + \frac{(f_1 - np_0)^2}{n(1 - p_0)} = \frac{(f_1 - np_0)^2}{np_0} + \frac{(f_2 - nq_0)^2}{nq_0}$$

$$= \frac{(f_1 - F_1)^2}{F_1} + \frac{(f_2 - F_2)^2}{F_2} = X^2. \qquad (q_0 = 1 - p_0)$$

Note: $(f_1 - np_0)^2 = (-f_1 + np_0)^2 = (n - f_1 - n + np_0)^2$
$$= [f_2 - n(1 - p_0)]^2 = (f_2 - nq_0)^2$$

To repeat, the normal distribution-based test statistic Z applied to a proportion ($p = p_0$) gives results identical to the Pearson chi-square expression applied to a simple two category table. For the genetic example, $f_1 = 40$, $F_1 = 0.75(64) = 48$, $f_2 = 24$, and $F_2 = 0.25(64) = 16$, giving the previous result,

$$X^2 = \frac{(40 - 48)^2}{48} + \frac{(24 - 16)^2}{16} = 5.333$$

and again X^2 is a single observation from a chi-square distribution with one degree of freedom when the underlying proportion p is 0.75.

An extension of the Pearson chi-square analysis of a two-category table yields one of the most used statistical tools. The extended chi-square statistic is designed to test hypotheses about a series of counts represented by f_i and is

$$X^2 = \frac{(f_1 - F_1)^2}{F_1} + \frac{(f_2 - F_2)^2}{F_2} + \cdots + \frac{(f_k - F_k)^2}{F_k}$$

$$= \sum \frac{(f_i - F_i)^2}{F_i} = \sum \frac{(observed\ i^{th}\text{-}count - expected\ i^{th}\text{-}count)^2}{expected\ i^{th}\text{-}count}$$

and $i = 1, 2, 3, \cdots, k$ where k counts f_i are each contrasted to k expected values F_i. The test statistic X^2 has an approximate chi-square distribution with $df =$ degrees of freedom when each observed f_i-value is a random deviation from each expected F_i-value. A specific value for the degrees of freedom is determined by the situation that generates the F_i-counts.

The sample frequencies $f_1, f_2, \cdots, f_k$ often result from counts contained in a table and the corresponding expected cell frequencies $F_1, F_2, \cdots, F_k$ are generated by a null hypothesis. The k differences $(f_i - F_i)$ compare each observed cell frequency f_i to its theoretically generated expected value F_i and are summarized with a single chi-square test statistic. Such a test statistic makes it possible to calculate the probability that a more extreme set of differences resulted strictly from random variation. Identical to the previous test statistics, the null hypothesis is rejected when the probability of observing a particular result by chance alone is small, leading to the inference that the hypothesis that some or all the generated expected values are not plausible.

A *one-way table* is created by categorizing data based on a single random variable and counting the number of observations that fall into each category. The five-year-old children classified by their body weights is an example of a one-way table (Chapter 1—Table 1.2). When a Pearson chi-square test is applied to a one-way table with k categories, there are $k-1$ and not k degrees of freedom associated with the chi-square test statistic because the cell frequencies are not independent. Effectively only $k-1$ independent categories exist. The sample size n is fixed (not random) which means that all the independent information in the table is contained in $k-1$ cells because the kth-value must be such that the sum of all k frequencies equals the total number of observations n. The kth-frequency is predicted exactly from the $k-1$ other frequencies. The lack of independence in a one-way table requires reducing the number of degrees of freedom by one and employing a chi-square distribution with $k-1$ degrees of freedom (an illustration follows).

The reduction in the degrees of freedom was seen in the previous genetic example illustrating a chi-square test statistic applied to a binary outcome (dominant versus recessive genetic characteristics). The genetic data are contained in a one-way table with two categories ($k = 2$) but the chi-square test statistic has $k - 1 = 2 - 1 = 1$ degree of freedom. Only one cell provides independent information, summarized by a single random variable ($\hat{p}$, Z, Z^2, or X^2).

Situations where data are classified into a table always involve some degree of nonindependence. When a Pearson chi-square test statistic is applied, the degrees of freedom are always less than the number of cells in the table. It is not possible to give a completely rigorous explanation of the degrees of freedom without considerable use of mathematics but the determination of the degrees of freedom associated with most chi-square analyses follows a simple pattern.

EXAMPLE

From a volume of *Who's Who*, which reports both the date of birth and date of death of famous people, individuals can be classified into two categories: those who died less than six months before their birthday and those who died less than six months after their birthday. For a total of 348 individuals, the one-way table ($k = 2$) is

	Before	After	Total
number of persons (f_i)	148	200	348
expected values (F_i)	174	174	348
differences ($f_i - F_i$)	−26	26	0

If there is no relationship between the date of birth and date of death, then the expected proportion of deaths six months before and six months after one's birthday is $p_0 = 0.5$. The observed proportion of those who died after their birthday is $\hat{p} = 200/348 = 0.575$.

When $p_0 = 0.5$ (H_0), the observed frequencies (148 and 200) randomly differ from the expected before/after counts (174 and 174) where $np_0 = n(1 - p_0) = nq_0 = 348(0.5) = 174$. The comparisons of these two null hypothesis generated frequencies (F_i) to the two observed frequencies (f_i) are summarized by

$$X^2 = \frac{(148 - 174)^2}{174} + \frac{(200 - 174)^2}{174} = 7.770.$$

The test statistic X^2 has a chi-square distribution with one degree of freedom, when the observed differences (−26 and 26) are due entirely to chance. The p-value is $P(X^2 \geq 7.770 \mid p = 0.5) = 0.01$.

A more detailed analysis frequently produces additional insight into the distribution of observed data tabulated into a table. A one-way table classifying the same 348 birth/death observations by individual months of death before and after a birthday (displayed in Figure 7.2) describes more completely the distribution of death dates relative to an individual's birthday:

	Months before						Months after						
	6	5	4	3	2	1	1	2	3	4	5	6	Total
number of persons (f_i)	25	23	25	25	27	23	42	40	32	35	30	21	348
expected values (F_i)	29	29	29	29	29	29	29	29	29	29	29	29	348
differences ($f_i - F_i$)	−4	−6	−4	−4	−2	−6	13	11	3	6	1	−8	0

If date of birth is unrelated to date of death, then the probability of dying in any particular month is 1/12 (approximate). The expected value, again assuming no relationship between date of birth and date of death, is then $np_0 = 348(1/12) = 29$ deaths for each of the 12 months. The chi-square test statistic contrasting the observed frequencies (first row of the table) to the theoretically generated frequencies (second row of the table) is

$$X^2 = \sum \frac{(f_i - F_i)^2}{F_i} = \frac{(25 - 29)^2}{29} + \frac{(23 - 29)^2}{29} + \frac{(25 - 29)^2}{29}$$
$$+ \cdots + \frac{(21 - 29)^2}{29} = 18.069.$$

The test statistic X^2 is a single summary of the 12 comparisons and has a chi-square distribution with $k - 1 = 12 - 1 = 11$ degrees of freedom when the observed numbers of deaths are strictly random deviations from the expected number of 29. The p-value is $P(X^2 \geq 18.069 \,|\, p_0 = 1/12) = 0.08$.

The analysis of the more extensive 12-category table shows less evidence of a systematic relationship than the analysis of the two-category table but continues to hint at some nonrandomness among the 348 individuals sampled, particularly the first two months after a birthday (Figure 7.2) where the deviations (13 and 11) are relatively large. Geometrically, this chi-square analysis is a formal evaluation of the deviations of the observed counts per month (dashed line) from a null hypothesis-generated horizontal line (expected counts $= F_i = 29$). ∎

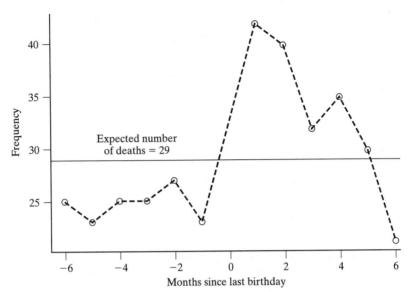

FIGURE 7.2: The distribution of individuals classified by the number of months their deaths occurred before or after their birthday.

EXAMPLE

Austrian monk Gergor Mendel (b. 1823) published the results of a large series of experiments (1866) that are undoubtedly the beginning of the theory of genetics. His classic experiments consisted of raising ornamental sweet peas (*Pisum sativum*) to determine the frequencies of different kinds of seed and plant characteristics among the offspring from specific parental matings. Six of Mendel's many experiments produced the following data:

	Characteristics	Total (n)	$AA/Aa(f_1)$	$aa(f_2)$
1.	seed: shape	7324	5474	1850
2.	seed: color	8023	6022	2001
3.	plant: pod shape	1181	882	299
4.	plant: pod color	580	428	152
5.	plant: flower position	858	651	207
6.	plant: stem length	1064	787	277

Today, it is known that a mating of two heterozygotic individuals ($Aa \times Aa$) produces three kinds of offspring, represented by AA, Aa, and aa. The probabilities of these three kinds of offspring are 0.25, 0.50, and 0.25, respectively. In Mendel's time, this fact was not known and, furthermore, Mendel could not directly distinguish between the AA and the Aa kinds of offspring.

A chi-square analysis of each of the six experiments provides a comparison of Mendel's observed results to those that would have occurred if the ratio of the two kinds of offspring was exactly 3:1. Specifically, the degree of correspondence between the two observed counts (f_1 and f_2) and specific theoretical frequencies of AA/Aa and aa offspring (F_1 and F_2) can be investigated.

For the first experiment, the two theoretically generated frequencies ($p_0 = 0.75$) are

$$F_1 = np_0 = 7324(0.75) = 5493 \qquad \text{and}$$

$$F_2 = n(1 - p_0) = 7324(0.25) = 7324 - 5493 = 1831$$

producing a 3:1 ratio ($5493/1831 = 3$, exactly). The corresponding observed frequencies are $f_1 = 5474$ and $f_2 = 1850$. The chi-square test statistic is

$$X_1^2 = \frac{(5474 - 5493)^2}{5493} + \frac{(1850 - 1831)^2}{1831} = 0.263$$

and X_1^2 has an approximate chi-square distribution with one degree of freedom yielding a p-value of $P(X_1^2 \geq 0.263 \,|\, \textit{the expected values are correct}) = 0.61$. The phrase "the expected values are correct" means that the differences between observed and expected values (± 19) are due entirely to the random variation associated with the sampled observations. A significance probability of 0.61 confirms the conjecture of a 3:1 ratio.

The same chi-square analysis applied to the other five experiments are

$$X_2^2 = 0.015 \text{ yielding a } p\text{-value of } 0.90,$$

$$X_3^2 = 0.064 \text{ yielding a } p\text{-value of } 0.80,$$

$$X_4^2 = 0.451 \text{ yielding a } p\text{-value of } 0.50,$$

$$X_5^2 = 0.350 \text{ yielding a } p\text{-value of } 0.55, \text{ and}$$

$$X_6^2 = 0.607 \text{ yielding a } p\text{-value of } 0.44.$$

Each of the six experiments shows no evidence of a substantial deviation from the 3:1 ratio. All p-values are large (smallest $= 0.44$). ∎

Since a chi-square test statistics consists of a sum of squared values, then a sum of chi-square statistics also consists of a sum of squared values. The new sum contains more values but nevertheless remains a sum of squared normally distributed values. The resulting sum also has a chi-square distribution when the values combined are independent and all observed and expected values differ only by chance. The degrees of freedom are equal to the sum of the degrees of freedom of the component chi-square statistics.

For Mendel's sweet pea data, the combined chi-square statistic is

$$X^2 = X_1^2 + X_2^2 + \cdots + X_6^2 = 0.263 + 0.015 + 0.063$$
$$+ 0.451 + 0.350 + 0.607 = 1.750$$

and the summary test statistic X^2 has a chi-square distribution with six degrees of freedom when $p_0 = 0.75$ for all six experiments. The p-value summarizing the likelihood associated with all six experiments combined is $P(X^2 \geq 1.750 \,|\, 3{:}1 \; ratio) = 0.94 \; (df = 6)$. Once again, absolutely no evidence exists that Mendel's data do not "fit" the theoretical 3:1 ratio. In fact, it has been suggested that the "fit" is too good to be true. This suggestion is based on the fact that a certain amount of variation should exist in any sampled data and Mendel's data appear to lack this natural random variation. More analytically, it is argued that a chi-square statistic as small or smaller than 1.750 occurring by chance alone is unlikely $(1 - 0.94 = 0.06)$. Although chi-square tests based on the left tail of the distribution are rare, a small probability such as p-value $= P(X^2 \leq 1.750 \,|\, p_0 = 0.75) = 0.06$, perhaps, indicates a bias in collecting the sweet pea data, causing an extremely close and, therefore, a somewhat unlikely correspondence between observed and expected frequencies.

Two-way classification (2 by 2 table)

Testing the equality of two proportions ($p_1 = p_2$?) is another situation where using the chi-square test statistic is identical to employing a standardized normal value Z (Chapter 6). The two test statistics are

$$Z = \frac{\hat{p}_1 - \hat{p}_2}{\sqrt{\hat{p}(1 - \hat{p}) \left(\dfrac{1}{n_1} + \dfrac{1}{n_2} \right)}}$$

and

$$Z^2 = \frac{(\hat{p}_1 - \hat{p}_2)^2}{\hat{p}(1 - \hat{p}) \left(\dfrac{1}{n_1} + \dfrac{1}{n_2} \right)}.$$

When n_1 and n_2 are both large and p_1 and p_2 are not close to 0 or 1, the central limit theorem applies (Chapter 4). Therefore, when p_1 equals p_2 (null hypothesis), again Z has an approximate standard normal distribution and Z^2 necessarily has an approximate chi-square distribution with one degree of freedom.

EXAMPLE

As part of a large study of attitudes in rural America, a sample of 130 individuals was collected independently in a small Texas community and asked whether they approve or disapprove of stricter handgun regulations. The same individuals were also classified by two income levels (low and high). The data displayed in a 2 by 2 table are

	$A =$ approve	$\overline{A} =$ disapprove	Total
$B =$ low income	$f_{11} = 18$	$f_{12} = 48$	$n_1 = 66$
$\overline{B} =$ high income	$f_{21} = 42$	$f_{22} = 22$	$n_2 = 64$
Total	$m_1 = 60$	$m_2 = 70$	$n = 130$

The notation f_{ij} again represents the frequency of individuals contained in the $(i, j)^{\text{th}}$-cell (Chapter 3).

A null hypothesis postulates that the same proportion of individuals approve of stricter handgun regulations in both income categories. In other words, estimates $\hat{p}_1 = f_{11}/n_1 = 18/66 = 0.273$ (low income) and $\hat{p}_2 = f_{21}/n_2 = 42/64 = 0.656$ (high income) differ only because of the sampling variation. Formally, the null hypothesis states that the two proportions are the same or

$$H_0: p_1 = p_2 = p$$

and the alternative hypothesis states that the two proportions are systematically different or

$$H_1: p_1 \neq p_2 \quad \text{(two-tail alternative)}.$$

Selecting $\alpha = 0.01$ creates the critical region $Z^2 \geq 6.635$ because Z^2 has an approximate chi-square distribution with one degree of freedom when $p_1 = p_2 = p$. The specific value of the test statistic Z^2 is

$$Z^2 = \frac{(\hat{p}_1 - \hat{p}_2)^2}{\hat{p}(1 - \hat{p})\left(\frac{1}{n_1} + \frac{1}{n_2}\right)} = \frac{(0.273 - 0.656)^2}{(0.462)(0.538)\left(\frac{1}{66} + \frac{1}{64}\right)} = 19.231$$

where $\hat{p} = 60/130 = 0.462$ is the proportion of those interviewed who approved of stricter handgun regulation regardless of their income status.

The null hypothesis is rejected ($6.635 < 19.231$). The p-value is $P(X^2 \geq 19.231 \mid p_1 = p_2 = p) < 0.001$. The computer calculated significance probability is 0.000012 but it is more realistic to state the level simply as less than 0.001. To do otherwise gives a false sense of accuracy. Remember the chi-square statistic is approximate (central limit theorem) and undoubtedly the data are subject to various sources of biases and inaccuracies of measurement so that a p-value is never extremely accurate. As Professor Paulos of Temple University writes, "71.38416743321 percent of statistics are made up on the spot." ∎

Box 7.2. Computational Formula

Let f_{ij} represent the frequency in the $(i, j)^{\text{th}}$-cell and n_i and m_j represent the sums of the rows and columns of the table where $i = 1, 2$, and $j = 1, 2$, then

$$Z^2 = \frac{(\hat{p}_1 - \hat{p}_2)^2}{\hat{p}(1 - \hat{p})\left(\dfrac{1}{n_1} + \dfrac{1}{n_2}\right)} = \frac{(f_{11}/n_1 - f_{21}/n_2)^2}{\left(\dfrac{m_1}{n}\right)\left(\dfrac{m_2}{n}\right)\left(\dfrac{1}{n_1} + \dfrac{1}{n_2}\right)}$$

$$= \frac{(n_2 f_{11} - n_1 f_{21})^2/(n_1 n_2)^2}{\dfrac{m_1 m_2}{n^2}\left(\dfrac{n}{n_1 n_2}\right)} = \frac{(n_2 f_{11} - n_1 f_{21})^2}{\dfrac{1}{n}(m_1 m_2 n_1 n_2)}$$

$$= \frac{[(f_{21} + f_{22})f_{11} - (f_{11} + f_{12})f_{21}]^2}{\dfrac{1}{n}(n_1 n_2 m_1 m_2)} = \frac{n(f_{11}f_{22} - f_{12}f_{21})^2}{n_1 n_2 m_1 m_2} = X^2.$$

The quantity X^2 (or Z^2) is equally expressed in a compact and often used computational form, which is

$$X^2 = Z^2 = \frac{n(f_{11}f_{22} - f_{12}f_{21})^2}{n_1 n_2 m_1 m_2}. \qquad \text{Box 7.2.}$$

For the Texas community data, again,

$$X^2 = \frac{130[18(22) - 48(42)]^2}{(66)(64)(60)(70)} = 19.231.$$

Yet another form of the same test statistic results from applying the Pearson chi-square expression, $X^2 = \sum\sum (f_{ij} - F_{ij})^2/F_{ij}$. The expected values are:

$$F_{11} = n_1 \hat{p} = 66(0.462) = 30.46,$$
$$F_{12} = n_1(1 - \hat{p}) = 66(0.538) = 35.54,$$
$$F_{21} = n_2 \hat{p} = 64(0.462) = 29.54, \text{ and}$$
$$F_{22} = n_2(1 - \hat{p}) = 64(0.538) = 34.46$$

using $\hat{p} = 60/130 = 0.462$ generated from the null hypothesis that no difference exists between low and high-income respondents. Tabulated into a 2 by 2 table, the expected "data" are:

	$A =$ approve	$\overline{A} =$ disapprove	Total
$B =$ low income	$F_{11} = 30.46$	$F_{12} = 35.54$	$n_1 = 66$
$\overline{B} =$ high income	$F_{21} = 29.54$	$F_{22} = 34.46$	$n_2 = 64$
Total	$m_1 = 60$	$m_2 = 70$	$n = 130$

For these expected values, the hypothesis that $p_1 = p_2 = p$ is exactly true; thus, from the table of expected counts, $\hat{p}_1 = 30.46/66 = \hat{p}_2 = 29.54/64 = \hat{p} = 60/130 = 0.462$. The chi-square test statistic comparing the four observed and expected values is once again

$$X^2 = (18 - 30.46)^2/30.46 + (48 - 35.54)^2/35.54 + (42 - 29.54)^2/29.54$$
$$+ (22 - 34.46)^2/34.46$$
$$= 5.098 + 4.370 + 5.257 + 4.506 = 19.231.$$

The three chi-square tests differ only in form.

A fourth and identical version of the chi-square test comes from noting that the test of the equality of the "row" proportions yields the same chi-square test statistic as the test of equality of the "column" proportions. If opinions on gun control are unrelated to income, then income is equally unrelated to opinions on gun control (Chapter 2). For the Texas survey data, $\hat{P}_1 = 18/60 = 0.300$ is the proportion of low-income individuals among those who approve of stricter handgun control and $\hat{P}_2 = 48/70 = 0.686$ is the proportion of low-income individuals among those who disapprove of stricter handgun control ("column" proportions). Again, the test statistic is

$$Z^2 = \frac{(\hat{P}_1 - \hat{P}_2)^2}{\hat{P}(1 - \hat{P})\left(\dfrac{1}{m_1} + \dfrac{1}{m_2}\right)} = \frac{(0.0.300 - 0.686)^2}{(0.508)(0.492)\left(\dfrac{1}{60} + \dfrac{1}{70}\right)} = 19.231$$

where $\hat{P} = 66/130 = 0.508$ is an estimate of the proportion of low-income individuals regardless of their attitude toward handgun control. As illustrated, the identical chi-square analysis always emerges whether the "row" proportions ($\hat{p}_i$) or the "column" proportions ($\hat{P}_j$) are compared.

The number of degrees of freedom associated with the analysis of a 2 by 2 table is one, since only one cell of a 2 by 2 table provides independent information. For a specific set of marginal values, knowledge of one interior value of a 2 by 2 table determines the remaining three interior values by subtraction. These three nonindependent frequencies are, in a sense, redundant (completely predictable). Furthermore, the fact that the Pearson chi-square statistic X^2 has four components but is identical to a single value Z^2 (or Z) also indicates that only one independent variable is involved in the analysis of a 2 by 2 table. From either point of view, the chi-square statistic X^2 has one degree of freedom when applied to the usual analysis of a 2 by 2 table.

The accuracy of the chi-square analysis (accurate p-value) applied to tabular data depends on the central limit theorem. This fact is occasionally forgotten, particularly when the computational form of the chi-square statistic is used. A rule of thumb, frequently applied to assure that the large sample requirement of the central limit theorem is fulfilled, is to use a chi-square analysis only when all expected cell frequencies exceed five ($F_i > 5$). Although this rule is probably too strict, it serves as a guideline.

Two-way classification (2 by c table)

Data classified by a binary variable and by several levels of another categorical variable produce a 2 by c table of counts (c denotes the number of columns in the table). For example, smokers and non-smokers classified by five socio-economic levels produce a 2 by 5 table (Table 7.2).

A useful null hypothesis states that all socioeconomic levels have the same proportion of smokers ($p_1 = p_2 = p_3 = p_4 = p_5 = p$). Thus, the five estimated proportions $\hat{p}_j = f_{1j}/m_j$ (last row of Table 7.2) differ only because of sampling variation, which is another way of stating that smoking status is unrelated to socioeconomic status. In symbols, $P(smoker \mid social\ class) = P(smoker) = p$. A test of this hypothesis is sometimes called a *test of homogeneity*. Utilizing the entire data set, the most precise estimate of the proportion of smokers is $\hat{p} = n_1/n = 179/585 = 0.306$ when socioeconomic status has no influence on the likelihood of smoking. Under a "no influence" hypothesis, the expected number of smokers and nonsmokers in each socioeconomic class are estimated

TABLE 7.2: (a) A sample of 585 individuals classified by smoking exposure (2 levels) and socioeconomic status (5 levels).

	I (low)	II	III	IV	V (high)	Total
smokers	$f_{11} = 17$	$f_{12} = 76$	$f_{13} = 34$	$f_{14} = 32$	$f_{15} = 20$	$n_1 = 179$
nonsmokers	$f_{21} = 40$	$f_{22} = 195$	$f_{23} = 88$	$f_{24} = 53$	$f_{25} = 30$	$n_2 = 406$
Total	$m_1 = 57$	$m_2 = 271$	$m_3 = 122$	$m_4 = 85$	$m_5 = 50$	$n = 585$
proportion smokers	$\hat{p}_1 = 0.298$	$\hat{p}_2 = 0.280$	$\hat{p}_3 = 0.279$	$\hat{p}_4 = 0.376$	$\hat{p}_5 = 0.400$	$\hat{p} = 0.306$

TABLE 7.2: (b) (continued). The expected number of individuals classified by smoking exposure (2 levels) and socioeconomic status (5 levels).

	I (low)	II	III	IV	V (high)	Total
smokers	$\hat{F}_{11}=17.44$	$\hat{F}_{12}=82.92$	$\hat{F}_{13}=37.33$	$\hat{F}_{14}=26.01$	$\hat{F}_{15}=15.30$	$n_1=179$
nonsmokers	$\hat{F}_{21}=39.56$	$\hat{F}_{22}=188.08$	$\hat{F}_{23}=84.67$	$\hat{F}_{24}=58.99$	$\hat{F}_{25}=34.70$	$n_2=406$
Total	$m_1=57$	$m_2=271$	$m_3=122$	$m_4=85$	$m_5=50$	$n=585$
proportion smokers	$\hat{p}_1=0.306$	$\hat{p}_2=0.306$	$\hat{p}_3=0.306$	$\hat{p}_4=0.306$	$\hat{p}_5=0.306$	$\hat{p}=0.306$

by applying this estimated proportion to the column totals, where

$$\hat{F}_{1j} = m_j \hat{p} = m_j(0.306) \quad (smokers) \quad \text{and}$$
$$\hat{F}_{2j} = m_j - \hat{F}_{1j} \quad (nonsmokers),$$

gives 10 null hypothesis generated expected values (Table 7.2).

For example, the expected frequencies for socioeconomic level III are $\hat{F}_{13} = 122(0.306) = 37.33$ (smokers) and $\hat{F}_{23} = 122 - 37.33 = 84.67$ (nonsmokers) and the corresponding observed values are $f_{13} = 34$ and $f_{23} = 122 - 34 = 88$. The expected values $\hat{F}_{ij}$ conform perfectly to the null hypothesis for all five social classes or $P(smoker \,|\, social\ class) = P(smoker) = 0.306$ for the five socioeconomic classes (last row). For example, $\hat{p}_3 = 37.33/122 = 0.306$.

The Pearson chi-square statistic summarizing the 10 differences $f_{ij} - \hat{F}_{ij}$ provides an evaluation of the hypothesis of homogeneity. Specifically, the chi-square test statistic is

$$X^2 = \frac{(17 - 17.44)^2}{17.44} + \frac{(76 - 82.92)^2}{82.92} + \cdots + \frac{(30 - 34.70)^2}{34.70} = 5.346.$$

The test statistic X^2 has an approximate chi-square distribution with $c - 1$ degrees of freedom when the two categorical variables used to construct the 2 by c table are unrelated. Therefore, the smoking/social class data provide little evidence that these two variables are related since the p-value is $P(X^2 \geq 5.346 \,|\, no\ association) = 0.25$ calculated from a chi-square distribution with $c - 1 = 5 - 1 = 4$ degrees of freedom. Random variation remains a plausible explanation of the differences among the five $\hat{p}_j$-values.

Along the same lines as a 2 by 2 table, the cell counts once again are not independent. A 2 by c table produces a chi-square test statistic with $2c$ components but $c - 1$ degrees of freedom. Because each of the two rows must sum to the row marginal frequencies, only $c - 1$ cells in each row contain independent information. Additionally, each column must also sum to the column marginal frequency, so only one of the two frequencies in each of the $c - 1$

columns provides independent information. Therefore, only $c - 1$ independent cell frequencies exist in 2 by c table. For the special case of a 2 by 2 table, $c = 2$ yields $c - 1 = 2 - 1 = 1$ degree for freedom, as before.

The *Brandt-Snedecor form* of the Pearson chi-square statistic applied to a 2 by c table is

$$X^2 = \sum\sum \frac{(f_{ij} - \hat{F}_{ij})^2}{\hat{F}_{ij}} = \frac{1}{\hat{p}(1 - \hat{p})} \sum_{j=1}^{c} m_j(\hat{p}_j - \hat{p})^2 \qquad \text{See Box 7.3}$$

providing a direct comparison of the c estimated proportions (one from each column of the table) with the single null hypothesis generated proportion $\hat{p}$.

Box 7.3. The Brandt-Snedecor Form

Using the notation $\hat{q} = 1 - \hat{p}$ and $\hat{q}_j = 1 - \hat{p}_j$, then

$$X^2 = \sum\left[\frac{(f_{1j} - m_j\hat{p})^2}{m_j\hat{p}}\right] + \sum\left[\frac{(f_{2j} - m_j\hat{q})^2}{m_j\hat{q}}\right]$$

$$= \sum\left[\frac{m_j(\hat{p}_j - \hat{p})^2}{\hat{p}}\right] + \sum\left[\frac{m_j(\hat{q}_j - \hat{q})^2}{\hat{q}}\right]$$

$$= \sum m_j(\hat{p}_j - \hat{p})^2 \left(\frac{1}{\hat{p}} + \frac{1}{\hat{q}}\right) \qquad \text{since} \quad (\hat{p}_j - \hat{p})^2 = (\hat{q}_j - \hat{q})^2$$

$$= \frac{1}{\hat{p}\hat{q}} \sum m_j(\hat{p}_j - \hat{p})^2.$$

This contrast reflects directly the degree of homogeneity among the c-levels (columns) of a 2 by c table but is no more than a compact version of the classic Pearson expression. Illustrated by the smoking data, once again

$$X^2 = \frac{1}{(0.306)(0.694)}[57(0.298 - 0.306)^2 + 271(0.280 - 0.306)^2$$

$$+ \cdots + 50(0.400 - 0.306)^2]$$

$$= 5.346.$$

Independence of two categorical variables (*r* by *c* table)

A sample of observations is sometimes classified by two categorical variables (denoted A and B) to address the question of whether these variables are related.

By related it is meant that knowledge about the level of variable A predicts, at least to some extent, the frequency of observations at a specific level of variable B and vice versa. Three relevant *two-way tables* made up of r rows (levels of A) and c columns (levels of B) are displayed in Table 7.3. The observed frequency contained in the $(i, j)^{\text{th}}$-cell is once again denoted by f_{ij}. As before, the row and column totals (n_i and m_j) are the *marginal frequencies* (Chapter 3).

The joint occurrence of the two variables A and B is described by the joint probability distribution (probabilities p_{ij}—Table 7.3). To assess the degree of association, the two categorical variables are postulated (null hypothesis) to be unrelated (independent). This conjecture means that the variables used to construct the table have entirely separate influences on the counts recorded in each cell of the table (f_{ij}-values). Independence of two categorical variables causes the joint probabilities to be completely determined by the two sets of marginal probabilities (Chapter 3) and no need exists for a two-way table. From another point of view, independence means that no information is contained in the cells of the table that is not available from the marginal values.

The null hypothesis of independence is

H_0: categorical variable A and categorical variable B are independent

and the alternative hypothesis is

H_1: categorical variable A and categorical variable B are related in some way or simply

H_1: categorical variable A and categorical variable B are not independent.

A direct consequence of the null hypothesis is that the joint probabilities p_{ij} can be calculated from the row and column marginal probabilities or $p_{ij} = p_i q_j$ where p_i represents the probability a random observation belongs to the ith-row category and q_j represents the probability a random observation belongs to the jth-column category (Chapter 3).

When the row and column categorical variables are independent (H_0 is true), an estimate of cell frequency (denoted F_{ij}) is

$$\hat{F}_{ij} = n\hat{p}_i\hat{q}_j = n\left(\frac{n_i}{n}\right)\left(\frac{m_j}{n}\right) = \frac{n_i m_j}{n}.$$

This estimate of the $(i, j)^{\text{th}}$-cell frequency F_{ij} is simply the ith-row marginal total n_i multiplied by the jth-column marginal total m_j divided by the total number of observations n. Not surprisingly, this estimate is not influenced by the observed

TABLE 7.3: Classification of observations with respect to the categorical variables A (rows) and B (columns) displayed in three relevant r by c tables.

Observed frequencies (f_{ij})

A/B	1	$\cdots$	j	$\cdots$	c	Total
1	f_{11}	$\cdots$	f_{1j}	$\cdots$	f_{1c}	n_1
$\vdots$						
i	f_{i1}	$\cdot$	f_{ij}	$\cdots$	f_{ic}	n_i
$\vdots$						
r	f_{r1}	$\cdots$	f_{rj}	$\cdots$	f_{rc}	n_r
Total	m_1	$\cdots$	m_j	$\cdots$	m_c	n

Joint probabilities (p_{ij})

A/B	1	$\cdots$	j	$\cdots$	c	Total
1	p_{11}	$\cdots$	p_{1j}	$\cdots$	p_{1c}	p_1
$\vdots$						
i	p_{i1}	$\cdot$	p_{ij}	$\cdots$	p_{ic}	p_i
$\vdots$						
r	p_{r1}	$\cdots$	p_{rj}	$\cdots$	p_{rc}	p_r
Total	q_1	$\cdots$	q_j	$\cdots$	q_c	1

Expected frequencies (F_{ij})

A/B	1	$\cdots$	j	$\cdots$	c	Total
1	F_{11}	$\cdots$	F_{1j}	$\cdots$	F_{1c}	n_1
$\vdots$						
i	F_{i1}	$\cdot$	F_{ij}	$\cdots$	F_{ic}	n_i
$\vdots$						
r	F_{r1}	$\cdots$	F_{rj}	$\cdots$	F_{rc}	n_r
Total	m_1	$\cdots$	m_j	$\cdots$	m_c	n

cell frequencies. The Pearson chi-square statistic contrasting the observed and expected frequencies is then

$$X^2 = \sum_{all\ cells} \frac{(f_k - \hat{F}_k)^2}{\hat{F}_k} = \sum_{i=1}^{r}\sum_{j=1}^{c} \frac{(f_{ij} - \hat{F}_{ij})^2}{\hat{F}_{ij}} = \sum_{i=1}^{r}\sum_{j=1}^{c} \frac{(f_{ij} - n\hat{p}_i\hat{q}_j)^2}{n\hat{p}_i\hat{q}_j}$$

$$= \sum\sum \frac{\left(f_{ij} - \frac{n_i m_j}{n}\right)^2}{\left(\frac{n_i m_j}{n}\right)}.$$

As with the 2 by 2 and 2 by c tables, determination of the degrees of freedom requires a bit of care because the f_{ij}-values are again not independent even when the categorical variables A and B are independent. In each row, $r - 1$ cells are free to vary since one cell in each row is fixed because the cell frequencies sum to a specific row marginal frequency (n_i). Similarly, one value in each column is fixed since the cell frequencies in each column must also sum to a specific column marginal frequency (m_j). Therefore, $r - 1$ rows, each with $c - 1$ values, yield a total of $(r - 1)(c - 1)$ cells that provide independent information. The quantity $(r - 1)(c - 1)$ is simply the number of remaining cells after one row and one column are deleted from a r by c table. Therefore, a chi-square test statistic computed from an r by c table to assess the independence of two categorical variables has rc components but $(r - 1)(c - 1)$ degrees of freedom.

EXAMPLE

A sample of $n = 1065$ individuals classified by four age and five income levels gives the following 4 by 5 table (part of a community study of lung cancer[19]):

Age levels	1(low)	2	3	4	5(high)	Total
			Income levels			
35–44	34(42.2)	138(126.3)	59(58.7)	38(39.2)	19(21.6)	288
45–54	36(42.0)	125(125.8)	61(58.5)	41(39.1)	24(21.6)	287
55–64	39(37.1)	104(110.9)	53(51.6)	37(34.4)	20(19.0)	253
65+	47(34.7)	100(103.9)	44(48.3)	29(32.3)	17(17.8)	237
Total	156	467	217	145	80	1065

The number of expected individuals in each of the 20 age/income categories, estimated as if the categorical variables age and income are independent, are the values in parentheses. For example, the estimated frequency of individuals ages 45–54 with income level three is $\hat{F}_{23} = (287)(217)/1065 = 58.5$. The corresponding observed frequency is $f_{23} = 61$. Note that, $\sum_j f_{ij} = \sum_j \hat{F}_{ij} =$

n_i, $\sum_i f_{ij} = \sum_i \hat{F}_{ij} = m_j$ and $\sum_i \sum_j f_{ij} = \sum_i \sum_j \hat{F}_{ij} = \sum_j m_j = \sum_i n_i = n$ (n = total number of observed values). That is, both tables of observed and expected values have identical marginal frequencies.

To formally assess the differences between observed and expected values, age and income categories are postulated as independent (H_0: $p_{ij} = p_i q_j$) for individuals 35 years and older. The alternate hypothesis is that an association exists between age and income levels (H_1: $p_{ij} \neq p_i q_j$ for some or all the cells in the table). The degrees of freedom are $(r - 1)(c - 1) = (4 - 1)(5 - 1) = 12$ making the critical region $X^2 \geq 21.026$ at a level of significance of $\alpha = 0.05$. The chi-square test statistic is

$$X^2 = \sum_{i=1}^{4} \sum_{j=1}^{5} \frac{(f_{ij} - n\hat{p}_i\hat{q}_j)^2}{n\hat{p}_i\hat{q}_j} = \frac{(34 - 42.2)^2}{42.2} + \cdots + \frac{(17 - 17.8)^2}{17.8} = 10.449.$$

The summary chi-square test statistic $X^2 = 10.449$ is less than 21.026, so the hypothesis of independence of age and income is not rejected. In addition, the significance probability associated with this chi-square test is p-value $= P(X^2 \geq 10.449 \,|\, H_0$ is true$) = 0.58$. The chi-square analysis provides no persuasive evidence that age is related to income using these data. More extreme deviations from the expected values are rather likely to occur by chance alone (probability $= 0.58$). ■

In the analysis of a 2 by 2 table, the test of independence produces nothing new because

$$X^2 = \frac{(f_{11} - n\hat{p}_1\hat{q}_1)^2}{n\hat{p}_1\hat{q}_1} + \frac{(f_{21} - n\hat{p}_2\hat{q}_1)^2}{n\hat{p}_2\hat{q}_1} + \frac{(f_{12} - n\hat{p}_1\hat{q}_2)^2}{n\hat{p}_1\hat{q}_2} + \frac{(f_{22} - n\hat{p}_2\hat{q}_2)^2}{n\hat{p}_2\hat{q}_2}$$

$$= \frac{n(f_{11}f_{22} - f_{12}f_{21})^2}{n_1 n_2 m_1 m_2}$$

with degrees of freedom $(r - 1)(c - 1) = (2 - 1)(2 - 1) = 1$. Also in the analysis of a 2 by c table, the test of homogeneity is the same as applying a test of independence and the degrees of freedom are $(r - 1)(c - 1) = (2 - 1)(c - 1) = c - 1$. A constant proportion of observations at all the levels of another variable is a special kind of independence making the test for homogeneity a special case of the more general chi-square test of independence.

Goodness-of-fit

Occasionally a basic analytic strategy involves simply comparing the observed frequencies of a variable generated from a sample of data to expected frequencies generated from a specific theory. A statistical test used in this context is called a *goodness-of-fit test* but only differs slightly from the previously discussed chi-square tests applied to tabular data.

Symbolically, the data and expected values for a goodness-of-fit test are:

Categories	1	2	$\cdots$	k	Total
observed frequencies (f)	f_1	f_2	$\cdots$	f_k	$\sum f_i = n$
theoretical probabilities (P)	P_1	P_2	$\cdots$	P_k	$\sum P_i = 1.0$
theoretical frequencies (F)	$F_1 = nP_1$	$F_2 = nP_2$	$\cdots$	$F_k = nP_k$	$\sum F_i = n$
estimated frequencies ($\hat{F}$)	$\hat{F}_1 = n\hat{P}_1$	$\hat{F}_2 = n\hat{P}_2$	$\cdots$	$\hat{F}_k = n\hat{P}_k$	$\sum \hat{F}_i = n$

The chi-square test statistic $X^2 = \sum(f_i - \hat{F}_i)^2/\hat{F}_i = \sum(f_i - n\hat{P}_i)^2/n\hat{P}_i$ has an approximate chi-square distribution. The degrees of freedom are $df = k - 1 - b$ where k represents the number of comparisons (f_i versus $\hat{F}_i$) and b equals the number of independent estimates made from the data to establish the theoretical frequencies. That is, to estimate the k expected frequencies (again denoted $\hat{F}_1, \hat{F}_2, \cdots, \hat{F}_k$). Using the data to generate the theoretical values ($\hat{F}_i$) introduces a degree of non-independence. But, as before, adjusting the degrees of freedom produces the appropriate chi-square distribution.

EXAMPLE

The human ABO blood system consists of four distinct blood types called A, B, AB, and O. A specific Mendelian pattern of inheritance dictates that the occurrence of each of these blood types is a simple function of the frequency of genes A (denoted p), B (denoted q), and O (denoted r and $p+q+r = 1.0$). To verify this relationship for the ABO human blood groups, a geneticist collected $n = 105$ individual blood types (Table 7.4, first row).

When the gene frequencies p, q, and r are known ($p = 0.3$, $q = 0.1$, and $r = 0.6$), the theoretical (expected) frequency of each blood type can be calculated directly from genetic theory (Table 7.4—second row). The expected values are the four frequencies $F_i = nP_i$ generated as if the genetic theory is "correct" (Table 7.4—third row). For example, $P_1 = p^2 + 2pr = 0.3^2 + 2(0.3)(0.6) = 0.450$ and the expected number of A-type individuals is $F_1 = nP_1 = 105(0.450) = 47.250$. A justification for the expression that gives the P_i-values (row 2) can be found in most books on human genetics. The observed frequency is $f_1 = 40$. "Correct," in this context, means again that the differences between the observed and the theoretical values occurred by chance alone. To evaluate formally the conjecture that the data conform to the genetic theory, a chi-square goodness-of-fit test applies.

A level of significance set at $\alpha = 0.01$ creates the critical region $X^2 \geq 13.277$ ($df = k - b - 1 = 4 - 0 - 1 = 3$). No estimates are made from the data

TABLE 7.4: The observed and estimated frequencies of A, B, AB, and O individuals.

	A-type	B-type	AB-type	O-type	Total
observed frequencies f	$f_1 = 40$	$f_2 = 20$	$f_3 = 7$	$f_4 = 38$	105
theoretical probabilities P	$P_1 = p^2 + 2pr$	$P_2 = q^2 + 2qr$	$P_3 = 2pq$	$P_4 = r^2$	1.0
theoretical frequencies F	$F_1 = 105(0.450)$ $= 47.250$	$F_2 = 105(0.13)$ $= 13.650$	$F_3 = 105(0.06)$ $= 6.300$	$F_4 = 105(0.36)$ $= 37.800$	105
estimated frequencies $\hat{F}$	$\hat{F}_1 = 105(0.377)$ $= 39.587$	$\hat{F}_2 = 105(0.186)$ $= 19.533$	$\hat{F}_3 = 105(0.071)$ $= 7.448$	$\hat{F}_4 = 105(0.366)$ $= 38.443$	105

so $b = 0$. The chi-square test statistic comparing f_i (observed) to F_i (theoretical) frequencies is

$$X^2 = \sum_{i=1}^{4} \frac{(f_i - F_i)^2}{F_i} = \frac{(40 - 47.250)^2}{47.250} + \cdots + \frac{(38 - 37.800)^2}{37.800}$$

$$= 4.145.$$

The p-value is $P(X^2 \geq 4.145 \,|\, theory\ is\ \text{``correct''}) = 0.25$. The genetic hypothesis is not rejected. A goodness-of-fit test does not prove the theory but rather indicates that the theoretical values closely correspond to the observed frequencies, a good "fit."

When the gene frequencies p, q, and r are not known (the more typical case), they must be estimated from the data. It is then necessary to reduce the degrees of freedom by two. One degree of freedom is subtracted for each estimated independent gene frequency. The third estimated gene frequency is not independent because it is determined by subtraction ($\hat{r} = 1 - \hat{p} - \hat{q}$). Specifically, two estimates make $b = 2$ and $k - 1 - b = 4 - 1 - 2 = 1$ degree of freedom identifies the chi-square distribution appropriate to assess the "fit" of these data to the genetic theory. This reduction in the degrees of freedom is necessary because generally estimated frequencies correspond more closely to the observed data than theoretically generated values, a kind of the nonindependence. To compensate for the increased similarity between the theoretical but estimated frequencies ($\hat{F}_i$-values) and the observed frequencies (f_i-values), the degrees of freedom are reduced by the number of independent estimates made (specifically, $b = 2$), producing the parameter of the appropriate chi-square distribution.

Estimated values of the three ABO-gene frequencies are $\hat{p} = 0.257$, $\hat{q} = 0.138$, and $\hat{r} = 1 - \hat{p} - \hat{q} = 0.605$. These estimates produce the expected values $\hat{F}_i$ (Table 7.4—fourth row) based on the genetic theory. For example, the theoretical proportion of A-type individuals is $\hat{P}_1 = (0.257)^2 + 2(0.257)(0.605) = 0.377$ and $\hat{F}_1 = n\hat{P}_1 = 105(0.377) = 39.587$. Again, the observed frequency is $f_1 = 40$. No other estimates produce a smaller chi-square value.

The chi-square comparison of these four theoretically generated but estimated frequencies to the four observed frequencies is

$$X^2 = \sum_{i=1}^{4} \frac{(f_i - \hat{F}_i)^2}{\hat{F}_i} = \frac{(40 - 39.587)^2}{39.587} + \cdots + \frac{(38 - 38.433)^2}{38.433} = 0.047.$$

The test statistic X^2 has an approximate chi-square distribution with one degree of freedom $(k - 1 - b = 4 - 1 - 2 = 1)$ when the genetic theory "correctly" reflects these ABO-data. The p-value is $P(X^2 \geq 0.048 \,|\, \textit{"correct" theory}) = 0.83$ confirming that chance variation would very likely cause more extreme deviations than the obviously close correspondence between the expected and the observed frequencies of the four types of individuals.   ■

Some remarks about a chi-square test

1. When expected cell frequencies are small, applying an approximate chi-square test statistic X^2 may produce inaccurate significance probabilities. The source of this inaccuracy goes back to the central limit theorem, which requires moderate or large sample sizes to guarantee that all estimated proportions have an approximate normal distribution. A widely used rule (already mentioned) to minimize the impact from small counts requires all cell frequencies in a table to have expected values greater than five. The important point, however, is that the accuracy of the approximate Pearson chi-square test statistic depends on the distribution of the collected observations within a table and does not apply to all situations.

2. For a table that results from adding several heterogeneous samples, a chi-square test can be deceptive. For example, the relative frequency of a variable labeled A in Table I is 0.9 and in Table II is 0.7, and variables A and B are independent (exactly)

Table I	A	$\overline{A}$	Total
B	9	1	10
$\overline{B}$	81	9	90
Total	90	10	100

$$X_I^2 = 0$$

Table II	A	$\overline{A}$	Total
B	49	21	70
$\overline{B}$	21	9	30
Total	70	30	100

$$X_{II}^2 = 0$$

but for the combined table

Table I + II	A	$\overline{A}$	Total
B	58	22	80
$\overline{B}$	102	18	120
Total	160	40	200

$$X^2_{I+II} = 4.688 \qquad (p\text{-value} = 0.03)$$

the variables A and B are strongly associated.

The heterogeneity between Tables I and II causes the significantly large value of the chi-square statistic observed in the combined values (the sum of the Tables I and II; Table I + II). The combined table appears to involve only variables A and B when in fact, a third variable related to both A and B has an important influence but is not identified in the combined table. It is the difference between the tables (I versus II) and not the relationship between variables A and B within each table that causes the large X^2-value found in the combined table. Such "hidden" variables are common in applied situations and require more sophisticated analytic approaches to identify the relationships among all three variables.

3. A chi-square test statistic (X^2) by itself is not a useful measure of association between two categorical variables. Chi-square values in general increase as the degrees of freedom increase, so without adjustment, a chi-square test statistic alone does not reflect the magnitude of an association. Sometimes the square root of the chi-square test statistic divided by the total number of observations sampled ($\sqrt{X^2/n}$) is used to measure the degree of association. There are, additionally, a large number of other ways to measure association between two categorical variables.[20]

4. Frequently a factor of $n/2$ is incorporated into a chi-square statistic applied to a 2 by 2 table. This correction factor improves the accuracy of probabilities derived from a normal distribution to approximate the probabilities from a discrete distribution (continuity correction factor—Chapter 4). The test statistic becomes

$$X^2_c = \frac{n(|f_{11}f_{22} - f_{12}f_{21}| - n/2)^2}{n_1 n_2 m_1 m_2} \qquad (c \text{ for corrected})$$

and its distribution is more accurately approximated by a chi-square probability distribution. The factor $n/2$ reduces the value of the uncorrected chi-square statistic so that if X^2_c falls in the critical region, then necessarily the larger uncorrected chi-square statistic must also fall into the critical region ($X^2_c < X^2$), called a *conservative test*. (The uncorrected test statistic is further to the right.) The price paid for using the more accurate test statistic X^2_c is reduced power. The use of this correction factor is equivocal and debate exists in the statistical literature on the appropriate balance between accuracy and power. The correction factor is most often recommended when the sample size is small. The issue is not of great consequence when the sample size is large because the correction then has little impact.

5. Occasionally, a chi-square distribution is encountered that involves a large number of degrees of freedom. The associated chi-square probabilities are typically not found in tables (such as Table A.3). The following expression provides an approximate chi-square value:

$$\chi^2_{1-\alpha} \approx \tfrac{1}{2}\left[\sqrt{2(df)-1}+z_{1-\alpha}\right]^2.$$

The value $\chi^2_{1-\alpha}$ is the approximate $(1-\alpha)^{\text{th}}$-percentile for a chi-square distribution with df = degrees of freedom and is based on $z_{1-\alpha}$, which is the corresponding percentile from the more available standard normal distribution (Table A.1). For example, the approximate 95th-percentile value from a chi-square distribution with $df = 500$ is

$$\chi^2_{0.95} \approx \tfrac{1}{2}\left[\sqrt{2(500)-1}+1.645\right]^2 = 552.842 \qquad (\text{exact value} = 553.127)$$

using the standard normal 95th-percentile, $z_{0.95} = 1.645$.

Conversely, an approximate (large sample size) probability can be found for a given chi-square value. Using the same approximate relationship between $\chi^2_{1-\alpha}$ and $z_{1-\alpha}$ gives

$$z_{1-\alpha} \approx \sqrt{2X^2} - \sqrt{2(df)-1}$$

and $P(X^2 \le \chi^2_{1-\alpha}) = P(Z \le z_{1-\alpha}) \approx 1-\alpha$ is an approximate chi-square probability again based on the standard normal distribution (Table A.1). Specifically, if $X^2 = 553.127$ from a chi-square distribution with 500 degrees of freedom, then

$$z_{1-\alpha} \approx \sqrt{2(553.127)} - \sqrt{2(500)-1} = 1.653$$

and $P(X^2 \le 553.17) = P(Z \le 1.653) = 0.951$ (exact = 0.95). This approximation is one of many possible and serves to illustrate the process in a simple case. Typically, such probabilities and percentiles are found with complex computer algorithms.

A LAST EXAMPLE

Early physicists demonstrated that under most conditions the counts of atomic particles emitted from radioactive material followed a Poisson probability distribution. It was postulated that each particle has an extremely small and constant probability of being emitted. In other words, atomic particles are emitted at random. It is also known that even a small piece of radioactive material is made up of a huge number of independent particles. These are exactly the two assumptions that generate a Poisson probability distribution (constant probability of a binary event and a large population producing a sample of such events—Chapter 4).

Data from physics experiments (circa 1900) recorded the number of particles emitted from various radioactive materials. From one of these experiments, the counts of the number of particles emitted each minute over a $n = 60$ minute period are:

Number of particles emitted per minute, x	0	1	2	3	4	5$^+$	Total
Number of times x particles were observed in one minute (f_x)	18	24	14	3	1	0	60

If a Poisson probability distribution describes the radioactive decay, then

$$p_x = P(X = x) = \frac{e^{-\lambda}\lambda^x}{x!} \qquad \text{(Appendix B.3).}$$

where p_x is the probability that x particles are emitted during a specific minute ($x = 0, 1, 2, 3, \cdots$).

The value of the Poisson parameter λ is not known and must be estimated from the data. An estimate of the expected value λ is $\bar{x}$, the observed mean number of particles emitted per minute, because the mean is $E(\overline{X}) = E(X) = \lambda$ for a Poisson distribution (Chapter 4). The observed mean number of particles emitted per minute is

$$\hat{\lambda} = \frac{(18)(0) + (24)(1) + (14)(2) + (3)(3) + (1)(4) + (0)(5)}{60} = \frac{65}{60} = 1.083.$$

To generate theoretical frequencies under the hypothesis that the particles emitted have a Poisson probability distribution, the estimated parameter $\hat{\lambda} = 1.083$ is used. The probabilities $\hat{p}_x$ are then

$$
\begin{aligned}
\hat{p}_0 &= e^{-\hat{\lambda}} &&= e^{-1.083} &&= 0.338 \\
\hat{p}_1 &= \hat{\lambda}e^{-\hat{\lambda}}/1! &&= 1.083e^{-1.083}/1 &&= 0.367 \\
\hat{p}_2 &= \hat{\lambda}^2 e^{-\hat{\lambda}}/2! &&= (1.083)^2 e^{-1.083}/2 &&= 0.199 \\
\hat{p}_3 &= \hat{\lambda}^3 e^{-\hat{\lambda}}/3! &&= (1.083)^3 e^{-1.083}/6 &&= 0.072 \\
\hat{p}_4 &= \hat{\lambda}^4 e^{-\hat{\lambda}}/4! &&= (1.083)^4 e^{-1.083}/24 &&= 0.019
\end{aligned}
$$

and $P(5 \text{ or more emissions}) = \hat{p}_{5+} = 1 - \hat{p}_0 - \hat{p}_1 - \hat{p}_2 - \hat{p}_3 - \hat{p}_4 = 0.005.$

For a Poisson distribution with $\hat{\lambda} = 1.083$, the estimated theoretical frequencies ($\hat{F}_i = n\hat{p}_i$) observed during 60 minutes become

Number of particles emitted per minute, x	0	1	2	3	4	5$^+$	Total
Number of times x particles are expected in one minute ($\hat{F}_x$)	20.31	22.00	11.92	4.30	1.17	0.31	60

For example, when $x = 2$, then $\hat{p}_2 = 0.199$ and $\hat{F}_2 = n\hat{p}_2 = 60(0.199) = 11.92$. The observed value is $f_2 = 14$. That is, during the hour of observation, two particles were emitted during a single minute 14 times and, based on a Poisson distribution, 11.92 are expected. The expected values $\hat{F}_3$, $\hat{F}_4$, and $\hat{F}_{5+}$ are less than five and are grouped so that $\hat{F}_{3+} = 4.30 + 1.17 + 0.31 = 5.78$ and $f_{3+} = 3 + 1 + 0 = 4$ reducing the table to four categories but increasing the accuracy of the chi-square analysis. There are now four cells each with an expected value greater than five ($k - 1 = 4 - 1 = 3$) and one estimate is made from the data ($\hat{\lambda} = 1.083$) at the cost of one-degree of freedom ($b = 1$) making the total degrees of freedom equal to two ($df = k - 1 - b = 4 - 1 - 1 = 2$). Setting $\alpha = 0.05$ creates a critical region of $X^2 \geq 5.991$. The chi-square test statistic is

$$X^2 = \sum \frac{(f_i - \hat{F}_i)^2}{\hat{F}_i} = \frac{(18 - 20.31)^2}{20.31} + \frac{(24 - 22.00)^2}{22.00}$$
$$+ \frac{(14 - 11.92)^2}{11.92} + \frac{(4 - 5.78)^2}{5.78} = 1.354$$

and has an approximate chi-square distribution with two degrees of freedom when the observed values f_i differ from the expected values $\hat{F}_i$ strictly because of sampling variation. The test statistic is not in the critical region ($1.354 < 5.991$), which leads to accepting the "Poisson hypothesis," since essentially no evidence exists to reject the Poisson distribution as a description of the emission of atomic particles from this radioactive substance ("good-fit"). In addition, sampling variation alone causes a larger value of the test statistic X^2 to occur about half the time (p-value $= P(X^2 \geq 1.351 \mid random\ emissions) = 0.51$), further strengthening the inference that radioactive particles are emitted at random. ∎

Test of variance

An alternative to the chi-square goodness-of-fit test is a *test of variance*. This different kind of chi-square goodness-of-fit approach is generated by measuring variability in two ways—from the data and under specific conditions. The sample variance estimates variability under all conditions. A second measure is constructed so that it estimates variability under specific conditions. The comparison of these two measures of variability provides a measure of the impact of the imposed conditions and is the basis of a test of variance.

An estimate of sample variability is, as always,

$$\text{sample variance} = S_X^2 = \frac{1}{n-1} \sum_{i=1}^{n} (x_i - \overline{x})^2$$

where x_i does not represent a cell frequency from a table but represents one of the n observed values. Under the hypothesis that the data are sampled from a Poisson distribution, the variance $\sigma_X^2 = \lambda$ is estimated by $\hat{\lambda} = \overline{x}$. The evidence for or against the Poisson hypothesis comes from comparing these two estimated variances, S_X^2 and $\overline{x}$.

As noted earlier in this chapter, the quantity

$$X^2 = (n-1)\frac{S_X^2}{\sigma_X^2}$$

has an approximate chi-square distribution with $n-1$ degrees of freedom when the sample variance estimates the variance represented by σ_X^2. The chi-square test of variance, therefore, consists of a ratio of two measures of variability (one observed and one theoretical). When these two measures are close to equal, the test statistic X^2 is close to $n-1$, which is the expected value (mean) of a chi-square probability distribution with $n-1$ degrees of freedom. Conversely, a large difference between S_X^2 and σ_X^2 produces evidence that the theory generated value for the variance σ_X^2 is not correct.

The chi-square distributed test statistic X^2 in the Poisson case (hypothesis) then becomes

$$X^2 = (n-1)\frac{S_X^2}{\overline{x}}$$

where $\sigma_X^2 = \lambda$ is replaced by its estimate $\hat{\lambda} = \overline{x}$. The test statistic X^2 has an approximate chi-square distribution with $n-1$ degrees of freedom when the two measures of variability differ only by chance (no systematic difference between $\overline{x}$ and S_X^2).

EXAMPLE

Returning to the example of radioactive decay where the variance $\sigma_X^2 = \lambda$, under the hypothesis that the counts follow a Poisson distribution, the estimated variance becomes $\hat{\lambda} = \overline{x} = 1.083$. The sample variance estimated from the 60 observed particle counts is $S_X^2 = 0.891$. The chi-square test statistic contrasting these two estimated variances (1.083 versus 0.891) becomes

$$X^2 = (59)\frac{0.891}{1.083} = 48.538$$

and has an approximate chi-square distribution with $n - 1 = 60 - 1 = 59$ degrees of freedom when $\bar{x}$ and S_X^2 estimate the same quantity, namely σ_X^2 (λ). As mentioned, the x_i-values are not cell frequencies but rather the number of particles observed each minute (a total of $n = 60$ values). For the radioactive decay data with a level of significance set at $\alpha = 0.05$, the critical region is $X^2 \geq 77.305$ because there are $n - 1 = 59$ degrees of freedom. The value of the test statistic $X^2 = 48.538$ again leads to accepting the hypothesis that the observed values are a random sample from a Poisson distribution (p-value $= P(X^2 \geq 48.538 \,|\, Poisson\ distribution) = 0.83$. ∎

A test of variance is particularly effective for exploring specific conjectures about the data when the sample size is small making a table an ineffective summary. Comparing estimates of variability calculated under differing conditions provides a statistic tool with numerous applications and, not surprisingly, is called an *analysis of variance*.[21]

One winter night during one of the many German air raids on Moscow in World War II, a distinguished Soviet professor of statistics showed up at the local air-raid shelter. He had never appeared there before, "There are seven million people in Moscow," he used to say. "Why should I expect them to hit me?" His friends were astonished to see him and asked what had happened to change his mind. "Look," he explained, "there are seven million people in Moscow and one elephant. Last night they got the elephant."

from *Against the Gods: The Remarkable Story of Risk* by Peter Bernstein, published by John Wiley and Sons.

PROBLEM SET 7

1.–3. Work problems 15, 16, and 17 of problem set 6 using a chi-square test statistic.

4. An *epidemic** of severe dysentery occurred on St. Martin Island in the Bay of Bengal at a time when the island was isolated from the mainland because of the monsoon season. Of the total population of 1300, there were 430 cases of dysentery in a 10-week period.

What conclusions would you draw from the table below concerning the association of age and the dysentery attack rate? Is age related to risk of dysentery?

Age	Population	Cases	Controls
<1	50	20	30
1 to 5	200	105	95
5 to 10	200	80	120
10 to 15	200	70	130
15 to 50	550	130	420
≥50	100	25	75
Total	1300	430	870

In a study[†] of lung cancer, researchers were interested in the relationship between income (economic level) and smoking exposure. Two hundred and seventy-two white males (age ≥ 55) were classified by current smoking patterns and five economic levels. The data are:

	Economic level					
	1 (low)	2	3	4	5 (high)	Total
never smoked	14	37	15	22	11	99
past smoker	7	22	12	7	3	51
≤1 pack/day	3	25	6	9	3	46
>1 pack/day	13	26	18	15	4	76
Total	37	110	51	53	21	272

5. Test the hypothesis that smoking habits are independent of economic level at ages 55 and over. Use the information in the following tables to compute the chi-square test statistic X^2.

---

*Adapted from: M. Rahaman, M. Khan, K. Aziz, M. Islam, and A. Kibriya,: "An outbreak of dysentery caused by *S. dysenteriae* type 1 on a coral island in the Bay of Bengal," *J. Infectious Disease*.

[†]*Source:* S. Brown, S. Selvin, W. Winkelstein: "Association of economic status with the occurrence of lung cancer," *Cancer*.

	Observed (f_{ij})					
Smoking	1 (low)	2	3	4	5 (high)	Total
never	14	37	15	22	11	99
past	7	22	12	7	3	51
<1 pack	3	25	6	9	3	46
>1 pack	13	26	18	15	4	76
Total	37	110	51	53	21	272

	Expected (F_{ij})					
never	13.47	40.04	18.56	19.29	7.64	99
past	6.94	20.62	9.56	9.94	3.94	51
<1 pack	6.26	18.60	8.62	8.96	3.55	46
>1 pack	10.34	30.74	14.25	14.81	5.87	76
Total		110	51	53	21	272

	$(f_{ij} - F_{ij})^2/F_{ij}$					
never	.021	0.230	0.684	0.381	1.474	2.790
past	.0005	0.092	0.621	0.868	0.223	1.805
<1 pack	1.70	2.200	0.799	0.000	0.086	4.780
>1 pack	.684	0.730	0.987	0.002	0.594	2.997
Total						$12.372 = X^2$

In order to adhere strictly to the rule that all expected values should exceed 5 ($F_{ij} > 5$) for all cells, you should pool some rows or columns (your choice).

6. What are your new degrees of freedom?
7. What is your new chi-square value (X^2)?
8. Does this change your conclusion?
9. Test the hypothesis that there is no difference in the distribution by ABO blood types among the following three sampled populations.*

Blood type	U.S.	Norwegian	Chinese
O	90	78	30
A	82	98	25
B	20	17	35
AB	8	7	10
Total	200	200	100

*Adapted from: Philip L. Carpenter, *Immunology and Serology.*

10. Using the treadmill data from problem number 1 in problem set 10, estimate the variance of the heart rates for the runners and the controls based on the 10 observations recorded for each group. Estimate the 95% confidence interval limits for the "true" underlying variances in each group (runners and controls) assuming that the treadmill data are normally distributed and independently sampled. Is there evidence of an important difference in variability between these two groups?

Use the following data to infer whether political party affiliation is related to sex:

	Democrat	Republican	Independent	Total
females	250	300	50	600
males	250	100	50	400
Total	500	400	100	1000

11. The table of expected values is:

	Democrat	Republican	Independent	Total
females	_____	_____	_____	600
males	_____	_____	_____	400
Total	500	400	100	1000

12. The table of observed deviations from the expected values, $X_i - E(X_i)$, is

	Democrat	Republican	Independent	Total
females	_____	_____	_____	0
males	_____	_____	_____	0
Total	0	0	0	0

13. What is the chi-square test statistic and the associated p-value?
14. With reference to problem number one of problem set 6, you calculated the following table of expected values:

Number ill out of three susceptibles (number of secondary cases)	Number of families	
	Expected	Observed
x	$\hat{p} = 0.34$	
0	71.874	95
1	111.078	80
2	57.222	50
3	9.826	25
Total	250.000	250

The hypothesis that measles is not infectious implies that there is a constant probability p of contracting the disease. If each susceptible case had the same chance p of getting measles, it is estimated by $\hat{p} = 0.34$. Test the hypothesis that measles are not communicable (i.e., $p = $ constant).

15. In a botany experiment the results of crossing two species of flowers gave the observed frequencies of four genotypes of 119, 45, 40, 12. Do these results support the theoretical frequencies specifying a 9:3:3:1 ratio?

To determine whether the distribution of the number of fish with obvious cancer growth in areas of highly polluted water is described by a Poisson distribution, a specific species of fish was sampled on 200 random days over a five-year period. The number of diseased fish was counted in each catch yielding the following results:

x	Number of catches with x diseased fish
0	23
1	60
2	50
3	40
4	20
5	3
6	3
7	1
8+	0
Total	200

16. Find the mean number of diseased fish per catch ($\overline{x} = \hat{\lambda}$).
17. Assess the goodness-of-fit using a chi-square statistic.
18. Assess the goodness-of-fit using a test of variance.

CHAPTER 8

Linear Regression

Data collected to study the relationship between a mother's weight gained during pregnancy (X) and her weight lost (Y) after delivery (in kilograms) are

	X	Y		X	Y		X	Y
1	15.5	3.8	7	12.9	10.3	13	26.0	12.0
2	8.7	5.4	8	7.8	7.5	14	9.7	7.2
3	16.6	8.2	9	−1.3	6.1	15	9.8	8.1
4	14.6	9.3	10	13.2	8.8	16	10.9	4.6
5	11.1	6.4	11	16.5	3.8	17	9.3	6.4
6	27.1	13.8	12	4.2	1.8	18	15.6	5.7

Figure 8.1 displays these 18 pairs of weight changes selected from a large (998 observations) perinatal database.[22]

The four estimated values ($\bar{x}$, $\bar{y}$, S_X^2 and S_Y^2) summarize the distributions of weight gained and lost but give no hint of the relationship between these two variables. The point $(\bar{x}, \bar{y}) = (12.678, 7.178)$ indicates the center of the observed values (Figure 8.1—denoted "+") but one point is only a start in the description of the xy-relationship.

Numerous choices exist to summarize the relationship between two variables. A common and perhaps the simplest choice is a straight line. As with a mean value, a straight line can be a good or an adequate or a poor summary. Again, as with a mean value, the evaluation of the usefulness of a line as a summary is a necessary part of an effective description of the relationship between two variables, such as weight gained and lost during pregnancy (dotted line). A method for choosing the straight line that best represents the data, as might be expected, is essential. To choose a "best" line, two concepts require definition and illustration, namely covariance and least squares estimation.

Covariance

In Chapter 7, the chi-square statistic is used to assess the association between pairs of categorical variables. A statistical summary called the *covariance* (denoted σ_{XY}) is fundamental to assessing the association between pairs of variables and,

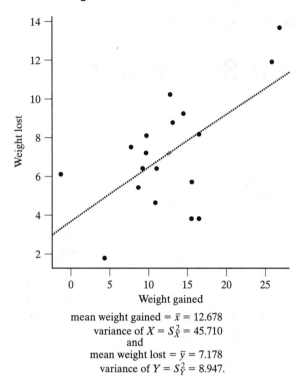

mean weight gained = $\bar{x} = 12.678$
variance of $X = S_X^2 = 45.710$
and
mean weight lost = $\bar{y} = 7.178$
variance of $Y = S_Y^2 = 8.947$.

FIGURE 8.1: Weight gained during pregnancy and weight lost after delivery.

furthermore, the members of these pairs can be either continuous or discrete measures and a tabular classification is not necessary. The covariance between two variables is defined by a sum of cross-product terms each weighted by a joint probability. The formal definition of the covariance between two discrete random variables X and Y is

$$covariance = \sigma_{XY} = \sum_{all\ x}\sum_{all\ y} p_{xy}[x - E(X)][y - E(Y)]$$

where $p_{xy} = P(X = x \text{ and } Y = y)$ represents the joint probability of the occurrence of a specific pair of observations (x, y).

The following is a specific application of the definition of a covariance:

Distribution of X		Distribution of Y	
$X = 0$	$P(X = 0) = p_0 = 0.5$	$Y = 1$	$P(Y = 1) = q_1 = 0.3$
$X = 1$	$P(X = 1) = p_1 = 0.5$	$Y = 2$	$P(Y = 2) = q_2 = 0.4$
		$Y = 3$	$P(Y = 3) = q_3 = 0.3$

$$E(X) = 0.5(0) + 0.5(1) = 0.5$$

$$\sigma_X^2 = 0.5(0 - 0.5)^2 + 0.5(1 - 0.5)^2 = 0.25$$

$$E(Y) = 0.3(1) + 0.4(2) + 0.3(3) = 2.0$$

$$\sigma_Y^2 = 0.3(1 - 2)^2 + 0.4(2 - 2)^2 + 0.3(3 - 2)^2 = 0.6.$$

The joint distribution (Chapter 3) of X and Y consists of six probabilities p_{ij} where

	$Y = 1$	$Y = 2$	$Y = 3$	Total
$X = 0$	$p_{11} = 0.20$	$p_{12} = 0.25$	$p_{13} = 0.05$	$p_0 = 0.5$
$X = 1$	$p_{21} = 0.10$	$p_{22} = 0.15$	$p_{23} = 0.25$	$p_1 = 0.5$
Total	$q_1 = 0.3$	$q_2 = 0.4$	$q_3 = 0.3$	1.0

The joint probability distribution of X and Y is not a sample but a hypothetical joint distribution that could possibly produce a sample.

The joint probabilities p_{ij} (the interior values in the table) are not computed from the individual probability distributions of X and Y. These joint probabilities reflect the likelihood that specific pairs of both X and Y occur simultaneously. If X and Y are independent, then and only then can the joint probabilities (interior values) be calculated from two separate probability distributions ($p_{xy} = p_x q_y$—Chapters 3 and 7).

The covariance of X and Y found by applying the definition is

$$\sigma_{XY} = \sum_{i=1}^{2} \sum_{j=1}^{3} p_{ij}[x_i - E(X)][y_j - E(Y)]$$

$$= 0.20(0 - 0.5)(1 - 2) + 0.25(0 - 0.5)(2 - 2) + 0.05(0 - 0.5)(3 - 2)$$

$$+ 0.10(1 - 0.5)(1 - 2) + 0.15(1 - 0.5)(2 - 2) + 0.25(1 - 0.5)(3 - 2)$$

$$= 0.15.$$

When $X = Y$, the expression for the covariance becomes the expression for the variance where

$$\sigma_{XX} = \sum p_{xx}[x - E(X)][x - E(X)] = \sum p_x[x - E(X)]^2 \quad \text{with } p_{xx} = p_x.$$

Thus, the variance of a random variable is a special case of a covariance.

Several properties associated with the concept of variance equally apply to the concept of covariance. For example, an estimate of the covariance between

X and Y (denoted S_{XY}) is

$$S_{XY} = \frac{\sum_{i=1}^{n}(x_i - \bar{x})(y_i - \bar{y})}{n - 1}$$

where n is the number of sampled pairs (x_i, y_i) of either discrete or continuous observations. This expression becomes the sample variance S_X^2 when $X = Y$. Also similar to the sample variance (Chapter 1), the following are properties of the estimated covariance:

1. A computational form is $S_{XY} = \left[\sum x_i y_i - \sum x_i \sum y_i/n\right]/(n-1)$.
2. Adding a constant to X or Y does not affect the covariance or $S_{X+c,Y+d} = S_{XY}$.
3. Multiplying X or Y by a constant multiplies the covariance by the same constant or $S_{aX,bY} = abS_{XY}$.

The justifications of properties 1, 2, and 3 follow arguments parallel to those given for the variance (Chapter 1).

EXAMPLE

A random sample of $n = 24$ pairs of values selected from the previously described joint distribution of X and Y yields

Pairs	1	2	3	4	5	6	7	8	9	10	11	12
x	0	1	0	1	0	0	1	0	1	1	0	1
y	1	3	1	1	2	3	2	2	3	2	2	3

Pairs	13	14	15	16	17	18	19	20	21	22	23	24
x	1	1	0	1	1	0	1	0	1	1	0	0
y	3	2	1	3	2	2	3	2	3	1	2	1

or summarized in a table

	$y = 1$	$y = 2$	$y = 3$	Total
$x = 0$	4 (0.17)	6 (0.25)	1 (0.04)	11 (0.46)
$x = 1$	2 (0.08)	4 (0.17)	7 (0.29)	13 (0.54)
Total	6 (0.25)	10 (0.42)	8 (0.33)	24 (1.00)

The values in the parentheses are estimates of the joint probabilities. For example, $\hat{p}_{22} = 4/24 = 0.17$, which is the estimate of the joint probability $p_{22} = 0.15$.

Then, calculated as usual,

$$\bar{x} = 0.542 \qquad S_X^2 = 0.259$$
$$\bar{y} = 2.083 \qquad S_Y^2 = 0.601$$

and the estimated covariance is

$$S_{XY} = \frac{\sum(x_i - \bar{x})(y_i - \bar{y})}{n-1} = \frac{3.917}{23} = 0.170.$$

These values are sample estimates of the previously given population values $[E(X) = 0.5, \sigma_X^2 = 0.25, E(Y) = 2.0, \sigma_Y^2 = 0.6$ and $\sigma_{XY} = 0.15]$. ∎

EXAMPLE

The birth weights (in pounds) of $n = 8$ pairs of identical twins are recorded, where X represents the weight of the firstborn and Y represents the weight of the second born twin:[2]

X	5.50	6.06	6.94	5.00	4.88	5.94	5.31	5.94
Y	5.06	6.00	6.75	5.06	4.75	5.50	5.00	4.88

$$n = 8 \quad \bar{x} = 5.693 \quad \bar{y} = 5.375$$

$$S_{XY} = \sum(x_i - \bar{x})(y_i - \bar{y})/(n-1)$$
$$= [(5.50 - 5.693)(5.06 - 5.375) + \cdots + (5.94 - 5.693)(4.88 - 5.375)]/7$$
$$= 2.783/7 = 0.398.$$

These twin data have a positive estimated covariance of $S_{XY} = 0.398$ but without additional statistical tools this value alone is not particularly meaningful. Linear regression (the rest of this chapter) and correlation analysis (Chapter 9) provide both the tools for a statistical assessment and a rich interpretation of a covariance as a summary of an association between two variables. ∎

The reason covariance measures the degree of association within pairs of observations is seen by the following argument:

The product of the terms $[x_i - E(X)]$ and $[y_i - E(Y)]$ produces either a positive or a negative value. The positive or negative values occur from four possible cases where

	$[x_i - E(X)] > 0$	$[x_i - E(X)] < 0$
$[y_i - E(Y)] > 0$	case I: $[x_i - E(X)][y_i - E(Y)] > 0$	case II: $[x_i - E(X)][y_i - E(Y)] < 0$
$[y_i - E(Y)] < 0$	case III: $[x_i - E(X)][y_i - E(Y)] < 0$	case IV: $[x_i - E(X)][y_i - E(Y)] > 0$

Cases I and IV occur when increased values of X are associated with increased values of Y or decreased values of X are associated with decreased values of Y, where an increase or decrease is measured relative to their corresponding expected values. Both cross-products are positive.

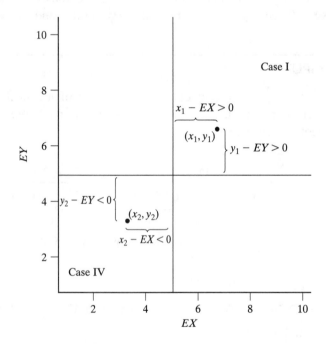

When cases I and IV dominate the sum of cross-products, the covariance is a positive value reflecting a *positive association*.

Cases II and III occur when increased values of X are associated with decreased values of Y or decreased values of X are associated with increased values of Y, again measured relative to their corresponding expected values. Both cross-products are negative.

Parallel to the positive case, when the sum of the cross-products is dominated by negative values (cases II and III), the covariance is a negative value, reflecting a *negative association*.

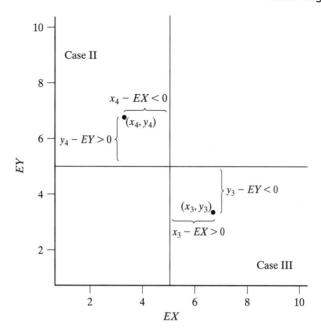

If X and Y are independent, then the covariance between X and Y is zero (Box 8.1). Perfect independence means that the positive and the negative weighted cross-product terms when added exactly cancel each other, producing a sum of zero. Unlike the previous two cases, the components that make up the covariance are balanced among the four cases (I, II, III and IV).

Box 8.1. Independence

independence implies $\sigma_{XY} = 0$

$$
\begin{aligned}
\sigma_{XY} &= \sum_i \sum_j p_{ij}[x_i - E(X)][y_j - E(Y)] \\
&= \sum_i \sum_j p_i q_j [x_i - E(X)][y_j - E(Y)] \qquad \text{since } p_{ij} = p_i q_j \\
&\quad \text{(independence)} \\
&= \sum_i \sum_j p_i[x_i - E(X)]q_j[y_j) - E(Y)] \\
&= \sum_i p_i[x_i - E(X)] \sum_j q_j[y_j - E(Y)] \\
&= \sum_i p_i[x_i - E(X)][(\sum q_j y_j) - E(Y)] \\
&= \sum_i p_i[x_i - E(X)][E(Y) - E(Y)] = 0.
\end{aligned}
$$

A positive covariance simply implies that similar observations are likely to occur together and, conversely, a negative covariance implies that dissimilar observations are likely to occur together. A covariance near zero implies that the magnitude of one member of a pair is not an indication of the magnitude of the other. Covariance, thus, summarizes (in a single number) the association within pairs of observations.

A positive covariance ($\sigma_{XY} > 0$) does not mean that when x is greater than $E(X)$, then y must be greater than $E(Y)$. That is, only cases I and IV occur within the sampled data. A positive covariance means that positive x-deviations generally occur with positive y-deviations and negative x-deviations with negative y-deviations. Some negative contributions to an overall positive covariance are always possible but they do not dominate the weighted sum. The same property holds for a negative covariance, which likely contains some positive contributions but the overall sum remains negative.

The variance of the sum $aX + bY$ involves the covariance of X and Y. Specifically,

$$\sigma^2_{aX+bY} = a^2\sigma^2_X + b^2\sigma^2_Y + 2ab\sigma_{XY}.$$

Similarly, the estimated variance of the sum $aX + bY$ is

$$S^2_{aX+bY} = a^2 S^2_X + b^2 S^2_Y + 2abS_{XY}, \qquad \text{See Box 8.2.}$$

substituting the sample estimates for the population values.

Box 8.2. Estimated Variance of $aX + bY$

$$
\begin{aligned}
S^2_{aX+bY} &= \frac{1}{n-1}\sum[(ax_i + by_i) - (a\bar{x} + b\bar{y})]^2 \\
&= \frac{1}{n-1}\sum[(ax_i - a\bar{x}) + (by_i - b\bar{y})]^2 \\
&= \frac{1}{n-1}\sum[(ax_i - a\bar{x})^2 + (by_i - b\bar{y})^2 + 2(ax_i - a\bar{x})(by_i - b\bar{y})] \\
&= \frac{1}{n-1}a^2\sum(x_i - \bar{x})^2 + b^2\sum(y_i - \bar{y})^2 + 2ab\sum(x_i - \bar{x})(y_i - \bar{y}) \\
&= a^2 S^2_X + b^2 S^2_Y + 2abS_{XY}
\end{aligned}
$$

A similar argument shows the expected property that $\sigma^2_{aX+bY} = a^2\sigma^2_X + b^2\sigma^2_Y + 2ab\sigma_{XY}$.

When X and Y are positively associated ($\sigma_{XY} > 0$), the sum $X + Y$ tends to produce more extreme values (increased variability) because large values of X are likely to occur with large values of Y and small values of X are likely to occur with small values of Y making extreme values of the sum $X + Y$ more likely. Conversely, when X and Y are negatively associated ($\sigma_{XY} < 0$), the sum $X + Y$ tends to produce less extreme values (reduced variability) because large values of X are likely balanced by small values of Y and small values of X are likely balanced by large values of Y making extreme values of the sum $X + Y$ less likely. The covariance directly accounts for the joint impact from the relationship between the two variables X and Y on the variance of the sum. A positive covariance increases and a negative covariance decreases the variability. When X and Y are independent, $\sigma_{XY} = 0$, then the variance of a sum is the sum of the variances or $\sigma^2_{aX+bY} = a^2\sigma^2_X + b^2\sigma^2_Y$ (Chapter 3).

Least squares estimation

A linear relationship between a numeric value denoted x and the expected value of a random variable, represented by the symbol $E(Y \mid x)$, is described by the expression

$$E(Y \mid x_i) = a + bx_i,$$

called a *linear regression equation*. All that is needed to describe this straight line are the two values a and b. Statisticians Yule and Kendall noted that "the term regression is not a particularly happy one from the etymological point of view, but it is so firmly embedded in statistical literature that we make no attempt to replace it by an expression which would more suitably express its essential properties."[13] They are referring to the fact that the word "regression" typically describes the act of moving backward to an earlier place, which has little to do with the statistical technique called *regression analysis*.

The basic elements of a linear regression equation are displayed in Figure 8.2. In this linear regression context, the value x is called the *predictor*, the *explanatory*,

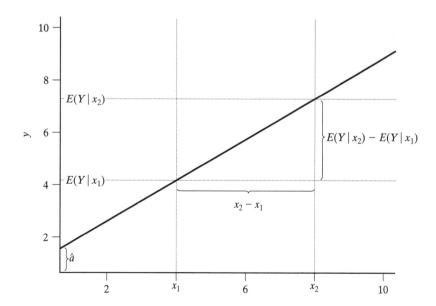

FIGURE 8.2: Linear regression.

or the *independent* variable and the value Y the *outcome*, the *response*, or the *dependent* variable.

The term independent applied to the value represented by x in a linear regression analysis has little to do with statistical independence between two events (Chapter 2). In fact, the relationship between x and Y is the primary issue in a regression analysis and when $E(Y \mid x_i) = a + bx_i$ the two variables are not independent in the probability sense. Quite the opposite is true. As long as b is not zero, the expected value Y is perfectly predicted by a value of x.

The value represented by a is the y-*intercept*. The y-intercept is the value of the dependent variable when $x = 0$ or $E(Y \mid x = 0) = a$. The *slope* (denoted b) of the regression line is the change in dependent variable divided by the corresponding change in the independent variable. Specifically, the slope of a regression line is given by

$$b = \frac{E(Y \mid x_i) - E(Y \mid x_j)}{x_i - x_j}.$$

A defining property of a linear relationship is that the slope is constant, which means that the expected change in Y divided by the corresponding change in x is the same for any two values of x. Therefore, a linear relationship is concisely characterized by the single value b.

Another useful but rather formal interpretation of the slope b derives from the following:

since $E(Y \mid x_i) = a + bx_i$ and $E(Y \mid x_i + 1) = a + b(x_i + 1)$,

then

$$E(Y \mid x_i + 1) - E(Y \mid x_i) = [a + b(x_i + 1)] - [a + bx_i] = b,$$

showing that the slope b is the expected change in the dependent random variable Y from a one-unit increase in the independent variable x.

Much like a sample mean that summarizes a sample of observations, a line summarizes a sample of pairs of observations, but which line? A sample consisting of eight pairs of observations (x_i, y_i) is displayed in Figure 8.3, called a *scatter diagram* or *scatterplot* as well as variety of other names. The lines labeled Line$_1$, Line$_2$, and Line$_3$ are among the huge number of possible candidates (actually infinite) for a single straight line that "best" summarizes the plotted points. A reasonable choice is to select the line "closest" to the observed data. Defining "closest," however, is not unequivocal and several definitions exist. The "closest" line might be the line for which the sum of the distances between the points and the line is zero, parallel to the definition of a sample mean value. This strategy fails to give a unique line because any line passing through the point $(\bar{x}, \bar{y})$ has this property (illustrated later on). An alternative approach that produces a unique line is to square the vertical distances between the data points and a line,

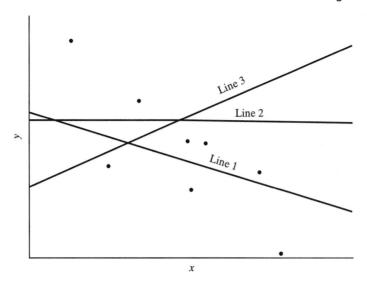

FIGURE 8.3: A small example of "data" and some possible representative lines.

then select the line that minimizes the sum of these squared differences. In this sense, the chosen line is "closest" to the data and is called the *least squares estimate*.

Least squares estimates

The sum of squared deviations (denoted L) of n observations y_i from a line $E(Y \mid x) = a + bx_i$ is represented by

$$L = \sum [y_i - E(Y \mid x_i)]^2 = \sum [y_i - (a + bx_i)]^2.$$

The least squares estimate of the line $E(Y \mid x_i) = a + bx_i$ results from choosing the parameter values of a and b (denoted $\hat{a}$ and $\hat{b}$) that make L as small as possible. Thus, the minimum value of L is $\sum [y_i - (\hat{a} + \hat{b}x_i)]^2$. The least squares estimates $\hat{a}$ and $\hat{b}$ directly yield the estimated regression line (denoted $\hat{y}_i$) and

$$\hat{y}_i = \hat{a} + \hat{b}x_i,$$

which is the only line that makes the quantity $\sum (y_i - \hat{y}_i)^2$ as small as possible.

The estimates $\hat{a}$ and $\hat{b}$ that minimize L are found by calculus techniques or some rather involved algebra (Appendix B.2). The process of minimizing the sum of the squared deviations of the observed values from a line (minimum L) leads to two equations, called the *normal equations*. They are

$$\sum [y_i - (\hat{a} + \hat{b}x_i)] = \sum (y_i - \hat{y}_i) = 0 \qquad \text{or} \qquad \sum y_i = n\hat{a} + \hat{b} \sum x_i$$

and

$$\sum[y_i - (\hat{a} + \hat{b}x_i)]x_i = \sum(y_i - \hat{y}_i)x_i = 0 \quad \text{or}$$

$$\sum x_i y_i = \hat{a}\left(\sum x_i\right) + \hat{b}\left(\sum x_i^2\right),$$

providing two equations with two unknowns. The least squares estimates $(\hat{a}, \hat{b})$ directly follow since $\sum y_i = n\hat{a} + \hat{b}\sum x_i$ yields $\hat{a} = \bar{y} - \hat{b}\bar{x}$ from the first normal equation and then substituting the value $(\bar{y} - \hat{b}\bar{x})$ into the second normal equation for $\hat{a}$ gives the value $\hat{b}$, or

$$\sum x_i y_i = (\bar{y} - \hat{b}\bar{x})\left(\sum x_i\right) + \hat{b}\left(\sum x_i^2\right)$$

and

$$\sum x_i y_i - \bar{y}\sum x_i = -\hat{b}\bar{x}\sum x_i + \hat{b}\sum x_i^2$$

or

$$\sum x_i y_i - \sum x_i \sum y_i/n = \hat{b}\left(\sum x_i^2 - \left(\sum x_i\right)^2/n\right)$$

or

$$\sum(x_i - \bar{x})(y_i - \bar{y}) = \hat{b}\sum(x_i - \bar{x})^2 \qquad \text{(Chapters 4 and 8)}$$

producing the least squares estimate $\hat{b}$ as

$$\hat{b} = \frac{\sum(x_i - \bar{x})(y_i - \bar{y})}{\sum(x_i - \bar{x})^2} = \frac{S_{XY}}{S_X^2}.$$

To summarize, the least squares estimates of a and b, which minimize L, are

$$\hat{a} = \bar{y} - \hat{b}\bar{x} \quad \text{and} \quad \hat{b} = \frac{S_{XY}}{S_X^2}.$$

Any values of the y-intercept or the slope other than $\hat{a}$ or $\hat{b}$ yield a larger value of L. For this reason, the estimates $\hat{a}$ and $\hat{b}$ produce a unique least squares estimate of the line, represented by $\hat{y}_i = \hat{a} + \hat{b}x_i$. The least squares estimates define an estimated line without requirements or assumptions about the data. The estimated line $\hat{y}_i$ minimizes L for any n pairs of numbers (x_i, y_i). It is certainly possible to use other criteria to establish an estimated line, such as minimizing $\sum|y_i - (a + bx_i)|$, but the least squares estimates are simple to compute and have rich statistical properties.

An intuitive justification of the least squares estimate of the slope b comes from viewing the estimate as a weighted average (Chapter 1) of individual estimated slopes. Each observation (x_i, y_i) yields an estimated slope because the quantity

$$\hat{B}_i = \left[\frac{y_i - \overline{y}}{x_i - \overline{x}}\right]$$

estimates the change in Y relative to the change in x for a line that goes through the point $(\overline{x}, \overline{y})$. An estimated slope results from combining these individual estimates using a weighted average of the n values $\hat{B}_i$ ($\hat{B}_1, \hat{B}_2, \cdots, \hat{B}_n$). The estimated slope becomes $\overline{b} = \sum w_i \hat{B}_i / \sum w_i$, but it remains to choose the weights.

When x_i is close to $\overline{x}$, even small amounts of variation in y_i have a relatively large impact on the slope of $\hat{B}_i$. As the distance $x_i - \overline{x}$ increases, variation in y_i has less and less influence. More technically,

$$variance(\hat{B}_i) = \frac{1}{(x_i - \overline{x})^2} variance(y_i - \overline{y})$$

because $\sigma^2_{aY} = a^2 \sigma^2_Y$ (Box 1.5). An estimate $\hat{B}_i$ based on a large deviation $x_i - \overline{x}$ is, therefore, a considerably more precise estimate of the slope than an estimate based on a smaller deviation. Points further from the mean are simply better indicators of the slope than points close to the mean. Because the precision of an estimated slope improves dramatically (impact of variability decreases) as the distance $(x_i - \overline{x})$ increases, a choice of weights reflecting the differing worth of each estimated slope $\hat{B}_i$ is the square of this distance. When weights $w_i = (x_i - \overline{x})^2$ are chosen, the weighted average $\overline{b} = \sum w_i \hat{B}_i / \sum w_i$ becomes

$$
\begin{aligned}
\overline{b} &= \frac{w_1 \hat{B}_1 + w_2 \hat{B}_2 + \cdots + w_n \hat{B}_n}{w_1 + w_2 + \cdots + w_n} \\
&= \frac{(x_1 - \overline{x})^2 \hat{B}_1 + (x_2 - \overline{x})^2 \hat{B}_2 + \cdots + (x_n - \overline{x})^2 \hat{B}_n}{(x_1 - \overline{x})^2 + (x_2 - \overline{x})^2 + \cdots + (x_n - \overline{x})^2} \\
&= \frac{(x_1 - \overline{x})(y_1 - \overline{y}) + (x_2 - \overline{x})(y_2 - \overline{y}) + \cdots + (x_n - \overline{x})(y_n - \overline{y})}{(x_1 - \overline{x})^2 + \cdots + (x_n - \overline{x})^2} \\
&= \frac{\sum (x_i - \overline{x})(y_i - \overline{y})}{\sum (x_i - \overline{x})^2} = \frac{S_{XY}}{S^2_X} = \hat{b}.
\end{aligned}
$$

This weighted average is exactly the least squares estimate derived from the normal equations.

The least squares estimate of the y-intercept can also be directly justified. The estimated slope based on any two values of x is

$$\hat{b} = \frac{\hat{y}_2 - \hat{y}_1}{x_2 - x_1}.$$

A special case is created by choosing two specific values $\hat{y}_2 = \bar{y}$ and $\hat{y}_1 = \hat{a}$, then the corresponding $x_2 = \bar{x}$ and $x_1 = 0$ give

$$\hat{b} = \frac{\bar{y} - \hat{a}}{\bar{x} - 0}$$

showing that $\hat{a} = \bar{y} - \hat{b}\bar{x}$. For both estimates $\hat{a}$ and $\hat{b}$, the least squares process leads to intuitive quantities for estimating the intercept and slope of a regression line.

The comparison of the observed values y_i to the values estimated from the least squares line $\hat{y}_i$ is central to regression analysis. The differences between y_i and $\hat{y}_i$ directly reflect the usefulness of the line as a summary. The value $\sum (y_i - \hat{y}_i)^2 = \sum [y_i - (\hat{a} + \hat{b}x_i)]^2$ measures how well the estimated values "fit" the data and is called the *residual sum of squares*. When the residual sum of squares is small, the estimated values $\hat{y}_i$ are, in general, similar to the values y_i. At one extreme, if $\sum (y_i - \hat{y}_i)^2 = 0$, then y_i is identical to $\hat{y}_i$ for all values of x_i and the estimated line exactly corresponds to the observed data. Conversely, large values of the residual sum of squares indicate a poor correspondence between at least some of the estimated and observed values. Figure 8.4 displays this property.

Like the total sum of squares associated with the sample mean $[\sum (x_i - \bar{x})^2$—Chapters 1 and 6], the residual sum of squares is at the center of the evaluation of the least squares estimate of a line as a summary of the sampled data.

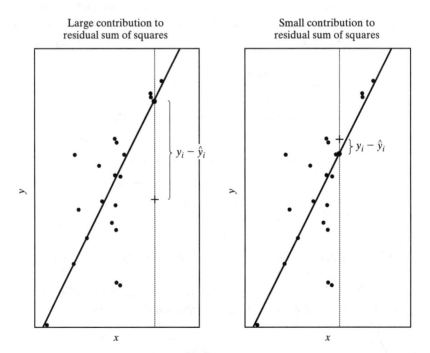

FIGURE 8.4: Two illustrations of the residual sum of squares.

Least squares estimates make the residual sum of squares as small as possible, guaranteeing the "best" summary straight line, but the "best" line is not necessarily an effective summary. Situations certainly arise where even the "best" straight line is next to useless for describing the relationship between two variables. An estimated straight line may be best of its kind (linear), however, the relationship within the data may not be linear or even near linear. A straight line may or may not be a good summary but, like a sample mean value, assessing the degree of usefulness is an essential part of the analysis.

Two properties of an estimated line (details again)

A notable property of the least squares estimated line $\hat{y}_i$ is that it always passes through the point $(\bar{x}, \bar{y})$ or if $x_i = \bar{x}$, then $\hat{y}_i = \bar{y}$ (Box 8.3).

Box 8.3. If $x_i = \bar{x}$, then $\hat{y}_i = \bar{y}$

question: $\hat{y}_i = ?$ when $x_i = \bar{x}$
answer: $\hat{y}_i = \hat{a} + \hat{b}x_i = \hat{a} + \hat{b}\bar{x} = (\bar{y} - \hat{b}\bar{x}) + \hat{b}\bar{x} = \bar{y}$

A second property of least squares line is that $\sum(y_i - \hat{y}_i) = 0$. The least squares estimated line, similar to the sample mean value, is the "middle" of the scatter of points (x_i, y_i) (Box 8.4).

Box 8.4. $\sum(y_i - \hat{y}_i) = 0$

$$\sum(y_i - \hat{y}_i) = \sum[y_i - (\hat{a} + \hat{b}x_i)] = \sum y_i - n\hat{a} - \hat{b}\sum x_i$$

Since $\hat{a} = \bar{y} - \hat{b}\bar{x}$, then

$$\sum y_i - n(\bar{y} - \hat{b}\bar{x}) - \hat{b}\sum x_i = \sum y_i - \sum y_i + \hat{b}\sum x_i - \hat{b}\sum x_i = 0.$$

For least squares estimation, the first normal equation requires that the sum be zero, or
$$\sum(y_i - \hat{y}_i) = \sum[y_i - (\hat{a} + \hat{b}x_i)] = 0.$$

corollary: the mean of the estimates $\hat{y}_i$ equals the mean of the observations y_i, or
$$mean(\hat{y}) = \frac{1}{n}\sum \hat{y}_i = \frac{1}{n}\sum y_i = \bar{y}$$

because $\sum(y_i - \hat{y}_i) = 0$, then $\sum y_i = \sum \hat{y}_i$.

A frequently encountered alternative form of the estimated regression line $\hat{y}_i = \hat{a} + \hat{b}x_i$ is

$$\hat{y}_i = \overline{y} + \hat{b}(x_i - \overline{x})$$

where the estimated y-intercept $\hat{a}$ is replaced by its estimate $\overline{y} - \hat{b}\overline{x}$.

EXAMPLE

Consider the four points (0, 1), (2, 5), (6, 5), and (8, 9) or

X	0	2	6	8
Y	1	5	5	9

The elements of a least squares estimated line are:

Observation	X	Y	$X - \overline{X}$	$Y - \overline{Y}$	$(X - \overline{X})^2$	$(X - \overline{X})(Y - \overline{Y})$
1	0	1	−4	−4	16	16
2	2	5	−2	0	4	0
3	6	5	2	0	4	0
4	8	9	4	4	16	16
sum	16	20	0	0	40	32

The estimated slope is $\hat{b} = 32/40 = 0.8$ and the estimated intercept is $\hat{a} = \overline{y} - \hat{b}\overline{x} = 5 - 0.8(4) = 1.8$, making the least squares estimated line $\hat{y}_i = 1.8 + 0.8x_i$. And,

Observation	X	Y	$\hat{Y}$	$Y - \hat{Y}$	$(Y - \hat{Y})^2$
1	0	1	$1.8 + 0.8(0) = 1.8$	−0.8	0.64
2	2	5	$1.8 + 0.8(2) = 3.4$	1.6	2.56
3	6	5	$1.8 + 0.8(6) = 6.6$	−1.6	2.56
4	8	9	$1.8 + 0.8(8) = 8.2$	0.8	0.64
sum	16	20	20	0	6.40

Figure 8.5 shows the "data" and the estimated line and the four deviations from the line ($d_1 = -0.8$, $d_2 = 1.6$, $d_3 = -1.6$, $d_5 = 0.8$). Figure 8.6 is a bit more complicated. The sum of squared deviations L for a range of values of the slope b and six selected values of the intercept a (1.0, 1.4, 1.8, 2.0, 2.4, and 2.8) are displayed. For example, when $a = 1.4$ and $b = 0.7$, the sum of squared

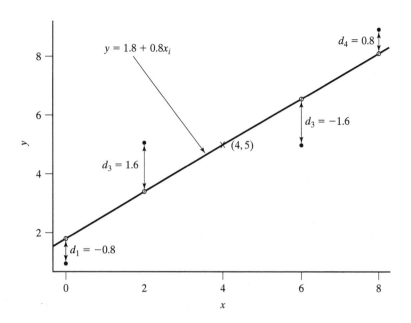

FIGURE 8.5: The least squares estimated line and deviations $d_i = (y_i - \hat{y}_i)$.

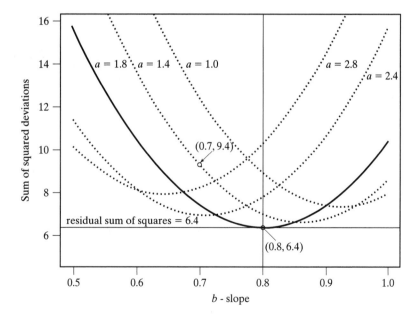

FIGURE 8.6: Values of the sum of squared deviations L for possible choices of the intercept a and slope b.

deviations L is 9.36 (marked on the plot as "o"). As required, the minimum among all possible candidates for the values a and b occurs when $\hat{a} = 1.8$ and $\hat{b} = 0.8$, producing the estimated line with the smallest possible residual sum of squares $L(minimum) = \sum(y_i - \hat{y}_i)^2 = 6.40$ (also marked on the plot).   ■

EXAMPLE

The following table contains the number of wins for each major league baseball team (Y) and the team's total payroll (x, in millions of dollars) for the year 1997. For example, the two highest payrolls (55.1 and 58.5 million dollars) are the teams in Baltimore and New York (Yankees), which are the teams that won the second and third highest number of games during the 1997 season. These data are not a sample. They are simply 28 pairs of numbers. A least squares estimated line, nevertheless, summarizes the relationship between the total amount a team pays its players and the total number of games won.

A straight line summarizing the relationship between wins and payroll has a slope $\hat{b} = 0.338$ with an intercept of $\hat{a} = 67.984$ and the least squares estimated line $\hat{y}_i = 67.984 + 0.338x_i$ predicts the total number of wins $\hat{y}_i$ for a cost of x_i million dollars (Figure 8.7). The slope of the regression line indicates that, on average, each win costs about one-third of a million dollars (338,000 dollars). The estimated line also indicates that to win half the games in a season ($y_0 = 162/2 = 81$), the team payroll should be 38.5 million dollars (if $x_0 = 38.456$, then $\hat{y}_0 = 67.984 + 0.338(38.456) = 81$).

American League			National League		
Team	Wins (Y)	Payroll (x)	Team	Wins (Y)	Payroll (x)
Baltimore	98	55.085	Atlanta	101	50.488
NY (Yankees)	96	58.500	Florida	92	47.738
Detroit	79	16.450	NY (Mets)	88	38.433
Boston	78	43.138	Montreal	78	18.454
Toronto	76	45.894	Philadelphia	68	35.503
Cleveland	86	54.122	Houston	84	32.930
Chicago (Cubs)	80	54.205	Pittsburgh	79	9.071
Milwaukee	78	21.420	Cincinnati	76	46.237
Minnesota	68	32.947	St. Louis	73	44.129
Kansas City	67	31.225	Chicago (Sox)	68	39.829
Seattle	90	39.421	San Francisco	90	33.465
Anaheim	84	29.197	Los Angeles	88	43.400
Texas	77	50.112	Colorado	83	42.852
Oakland	65	21.911	San Diego	76	34.692

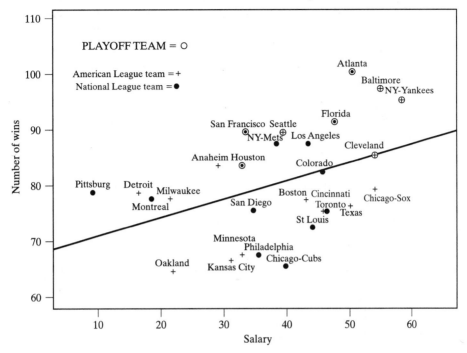

FIGURE 8.7: Number of wins and total team payroll in major league baseball (1997).   ■

Inference from a linear regression line

Up to this point, no assumptions have been made about the kind of data collected. The least squares estimates of the slope and intercept can be calculated from any n pairs of numbers (x_i, y_i), as mentioned. Specifically, the estimates $\hat{a}$ and $\hat{b}$ produce a summary line totally free of restrictions or assumptions.

To make statistical inferences about a sampled population based on an estimated regression line, a statistical structure is necessary. A statistical structure with five components provides a basis for estimating a line and assessing its effectiveness as a summary. The five components are:

1. The independent values x_i are fixed (not random variables).
2. The observed values $(y_1, x_1), (y_2, x_2), \cdots, (y_n, x_n)$ are n independently sampled pairs of observations.
3. For each value x_i, the value y_i is sampled from a normal distribution.
4. The variance of the dependent variable Y (denoted $\sigma^2_{Y|x}$) is the same for all x_i-values.
5. The regression line is linear or $E(Y \mid x_i) = a + bx_i$.

Collectively these five components are called the *simple linear regression model*. The word "simple" refers to the fact that the model relates a single x to a value Y and does not imply that the theory or application are simple. A statistical regression model is more than a statement of a mathematical expression (requirement 5). It is a broad description of the properties of the sampled population (requirements 1–5).

Requirements 3, 4, and 5 dictate that for each independent value x_i, there is a normal distribution describing the variability of the dependent variable Y. In symbols, for a specific x_i, the distribution of the Y-values is normal with mean $\mu_i = E(Y \mid x_i) = a + bx_i$ and variance $= \sigma^2_{Y \mid x}$. The regression model requires, therefore, that these mean values of normal distributions lie on a straight line. Furthermore, each sampled observation Y (each normal distribution) must have the same variance regardless of the value of the independent variable. These three requirements displayed geometrically produce the following plot.

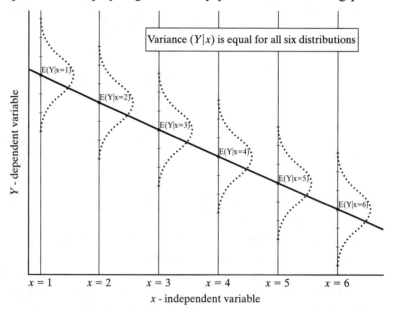

A sample of n independent pairs of observations $(x_1, y_1), (x_2, y_2), \cdots ,$ (x_n, y_n) makes it possible to estimate and assess the impact of random variation on such estimates as $\hat{a}$, $\hat{b}$, and $\hat{y}$ based on this statistical model, a process called *simple linear regression analysis*.

The regression model (requirements 1–5) provides one approach to the analysis of a sample of bivariate data but many alternatives exist. Some examples are: several independent variables might be relevant to understanding each value Y or the relationship between x and $E(Y \mid x)$ might not be linear or the x-values may be themselves subject to random variation or several separate lines might be appropriate. A good place to start, however, is the application of this simple linear regression model.

When the simple regression model requirements hold, deviations from the estimated line $(y_i - \hat{y}_i)$ arise only because of random variation among the observed y-values. The requirement of equal variances allows all such deviations to be combined regardless of the values of the independent variable x_i to form a single estimate of this variability. Such an estimate of the variance $\sigma^2_{Y|x}$ (denoted $S^2_{Y|x}$) is

$$S^2_{Y|x} = \frac{\sum(y_i - \hat{y}_i)^2}{n-2}.$$

The estimated variance $S^2_{Y|x}$ measures variability in much the same way as the sample variance $S^2_Y = \sum(y_i - \overline{y})^2/(n-1)$. The sample mean $\overline{y}$ is an estimate of the expected value $E(Y)$, just as $\hat{y}_i$ is an estimate of expected value $E(Y|x_i)$. The denominator of S^2_Y is $n-1$, reflecting a loss of one degree of freedom from the estimation of mean μ. The denominator of $S^2_{Y|x}$ is $n-2$, reflecting a loss of two degrees of freedom from the estimation of the mean values $E(Y|x_i)$, which involves two estimates, $\hat{a}$ and $\hat{b}$. Additionally, $S^2_{Y|x}$ plays a role similar to S^2_Y in the evaluation of the values estimated from the observed data because, like S^2_Y, it provides a measure of the sampling variation associated with the sampled population.

Statistician Joseph Fleiss noted:

> There was a statistician from Needham,
> Who was so bright, his clients would heed him.
> Yet his embarrassed confession
> Was that, in linear regression
> He'd never subtract the extra degree of freedom.

Aside: Parallel to estimating the slope and the intercept of a line, the estimated sample mean $(\overline{x})$ is the value that minimizes the quantity $L = \sum(x_i - \mu)^2$ where $x_1, x_2, \cdots, x_n$ is a sample of n independent observations (Chapter 1). The sample mean $\overline{x}$, therefore, is the least squares estimate of the population mean μ. Thus, the quantity $\sum(x_i - \overline{x})^2$ likely underestimates the true variability in the x-values because the choice of $\overline{x}$ as an estimate of μ makes L as small as possible. To estimate accurately the variability associated with the random variable X, since the quantity $\sum(x - \overline{x})^2$ is likely too small, the mathematics dictates that dividing by the smaller value $n - 1$ rather than n compensates for this downward bias making $S^2_X = \sum(x_i - \overline{x})^2/(n-1)$ an unbiased estimate of the population variance σ^2_X.

The same issue arises in the estimation of the variance $\sigma^2_{Y|x}$. The quantity $\sum(y_i - \hat{y}_i)^2$ also likely underestimates the true variability because it, too, is the minimum possible value. To form an unbiased estimate, it is divided by the smaller value $n - 2$ rather than n to estimate accurately the variability associated

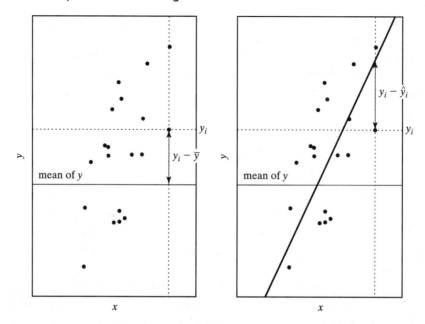

FIGURE 8.8: An illustration contrasting S_Y^2 and $S_{Y|x}^2$.

with Y. A detailed explanation of the reason that these particular values ($n-1$ and $n-2$) produce accurate estimates of the variance requires a sophisticated algebraic argument and is left to more theoretical texts.[23]

The estimated variance $S_{Y|x}^2$ measures variability about a straight line $\hat{y}_i$ with a nonzero slope (Figure 8.8). The sample variance S_Y^2 also measures variability but about a horizontal line $\bar{y}$ (Figure 8.8). Therefore, the fundamental difference between these two estimates is that $S_{Y|x}^2$ accounts for the role of the variable x in "explaining" the variability in Y and S_Y^2 does not.

The estimated variance of Y accurately measures the variability of the observations relative to the regression line as long as the sampled y-values randomly deviate from a straight line (requirement 5). In other words, it is assumed that all differences between y_i and $\hat{y}_i$ are due strictly to the randomness associated with the dependent variable Y and are not due to other factors such as nonlinearity of the xy-relationship or unequal variances among the populations sampled. If the relationship, for example, between x and Y is not linear, then $S_{Y|x}^2$ measures random variability plus the lack of linearity. The estimate of the variance then suffers from what might be called "*wrong model bias.*" Advanced regression analysis techniques exist to diagnose "wrong-model-bias" and, perhaps, suggest approaches to correct any deficiencies.[24]

A central quantity in a regression analysis is the residual sum of squares $\sum (y_i - \hat{y}_i)^2$, as mentioned. The direct calculation of the residual sum of squares becomes tedious when the number of estimates of $\hat{y}_i$ is large. A "shortcut" expression

$$\sum(y_i - \hat{y}_i)^2 = \sum(y_i - \overline{y})^2 - \hat{b}\sum(x_i - \overline{x})(y_i - \overline{y}) \qquad \text{see Box 8.5.}$$

is, therefore, sometimes helpful. Evaluating the residual sum of squares with this expression avoids calculating the estimated values $\hat{y}_i$ for each x_i, a total of n values. In addition, this relationship is useful in a theoretical context. For example, it demonstrates the expected property that $\sum(y_i - \hat{y}_i)^2 \leq \sum(y_i - \overline{y})^2$ since $\hat{b}\sum(x_i - \overline{x})(y_i - \overline{y}) = \hat{b}^2 S_X^2$ is always a positive number. Also, the "shortcut" expression shows that $\sum(y_i - \hat{y}_i)^2 = \sum(y_i - \overline{y})^2$ only when $\hat{b} = 0$.

Box 8.5. Computational Formula for $\sum(y_i - \hat{y}_i)^2$

$$\sum(y_i - \hat{y}_i)^2 = \sum(y_i - [\hat{a} + \hat{b}x_i])^2$$
$$= \sum(y_i - [\overline{y} + \hat{b}(x_i - \overline{x})])^2$$
$$= \sum[(y_i - \overline{y}) - \hat{b}(x_i - \overline{x})]^2$$
$$= \sum(y_i - \overline{y})^2 - 2\hat{b}\sum(x_i - \overline{x})(y_i - \overline{y}) + \hat{b}^2\sum(x_i - \overline{x})^2$$
$$= \sum(y_i - \overline{y})^2 - \hat{b}\sum(x_i - \overline{x})(y_i - \overline{y})$$

because $\hat{b}\sum(x_i - \overline{x})^2 = \sum(x_i - \overline{x})(y_i - \overline{y})$.

The assumption that the x-values are fixed (requirement 1) simplifies the linear regression model but is, in fact, unnecessary. More advanced regression analysis theory[17] reveals that the estimation of a straight line and the inferences drawn for its properties summarize the xy-relationship regardless of the nature of the independent variable. The x-values can be continuous, discrete, or even binary. For example, if the independent variable (x_i-value) is a binary zero/one variable, a simple linear regression analysis is the same as a two-sample t-test assessment of two mean values (Chapter 6). Regression methods, in general, allow the independent variable to be entirely unrestricted. This remarkable property is one of the reasons regression analysis is a widely used statistical tool and an effective approach to analyzing many kinds of data.

Assessing an estimated slope

The least squares estimated slope $\hat{b}$ viewed as a weighted sum of the observed y_i-values is

$$\hat{b} = \sum w_i y_i \quad \text{where the weights are} \quad w_i = \frac{x_i - \bar{x}}{\sum(x_i - \bar{x})^2} \quad \text{(Box 8.6)}.$$

Box 8.6. Another Weighted Sum Representation of the Slope $\hat{b}$

The estimate $\hat{b} = \dfrac{\sum(x_i - \bar{x})(y_i - \bar{y})}{\sum(x_i - \bar{x})^2} = \dfrac{\sum(x_i - \bar{x})y_i - \sum(x_i - \bar{x})\bar{y}}{\sum(x_i - \bar{x})^2}$

because $\bar{y}\sum(x_i - \bar{x}) = 0$ (Chapter 1), then

$$\hat{b} = \frac{\sum(x_i - \bar{x})y_i}{\sum(x_i - \bar{x})^2} = \sum\left[\frac{x_i - \bar{x}}{\sum(x_i - \bar{x})^2}\right]y_i$$

$$= \sum w_i y_i \quad \text{when} \quad w_i = \frac{x_i - \bar{x}}{\sum(x_i - \bar{x})^2}.$$

Weighted sums of normally distributed random variables are themselves normally distributed (Chapter 4). The slope $\hat{b}$ is a weighted sum of normally distributed y-values (requirement 3) and, therefore, the estimate $\hat{b}$ also has a normal distribution. The mean of the normal distribution that describes the variability of $\hat{b}$ is b. In symbols, $E(\hat{b}) = b$ (Box 8.7).

Box 8.7. $E(\hat{b}) = b$

To show that $E(\hat{b}) = b$; that is, the mean of the distribution of $\hat{b}$ is b

$$E(\hat{b}) = E\left[\sum w_i y_i\right] \quad \text{where} \quad w_i = \frac{x_i - \bar{x}}{\sum(x_i - \bar{x})^2} \quad \text{(Box 8.6)}$$

then

$$E\left(\hat{b}\right) = E(\sum w_i y_i) = \sum w_i E(Y_i \mid x_i) = \sum w_i (a + bx_i) \quad \text{(Chapter 4)}$$

$$= a\sum w_i + b\sum w_i x_i$$

$$= b$$

The sum of the weights $\sum w_i = 0$, because $\sum(x_i - \bar{x}) = 0$ and $\sum w_i x_i = 1$, because $\sum w_i x_i = \sum w_i(x_i - \bar{x}) = 1$.

The variance of the normal probability distribution that describes the variation of the estimate $\hat{b}$ is

$$\sigma_{\hat{b}}^2 = \frac{\sigma_{Y|x}^2}{\sum(x_i - \overline{x})^2} \qquad \text{(Box 8.8)}.$$

Box 8.8. Variance of the Slope $\hat{b}$

Note that $\sigma_{\hat{b}}^2 = \sigma_{\sum w_i y_i}^2 = \sum w_i^2 \sigma_{Y|x}^2 = \left(\sigma_{Y|x}^2\right) \sum w_i^2$

(Chapter 3 and requirement 4)

where again $\quad w_i = \dfrac{x_i - \overline{x}}{\sum(x_i - \overline{x})^2}$,

then

$$\sigma_{\hat{b}}^2 = \frac{\sigma_{Y|x}^2}{\sum(x_i - \overline{x})^2} \qquad \text{because} \qquad \sum w_i^2 = \sum \left[\frac{x_i - \overline{x}}{\sum(x_i - \overline{x})^2}\right]^2$$

$$= \frac{1}{\sum(x_i - \overline{x})^2}.$$

To summarize, the estimate $\hat{b}$ is an observation from a normal distribution with mean $= E(\hat{b}) = b$ and variance $= \sigma_{\hat{b}}^2$ when the collected data conform to the simple linear regression model (requirements 1–5).

Because the variance of the dependent variable $\sigma_{Y|x}^2$ is not known for most data sets, it is usually estimated using $S_{Y|x}^2$ giving an estimated variance of $\hat{b}$ as

$$S_{\hat{b}}^2 = \frac{S_{Y|x}^2}{\sum(x_i - \overline{x})^2}.$$

The estimated variance of an estimated mean value decreases as the sample size increases ($S_{\overline{x}}^2 = S_X^2/n$—Chapter 3). The variance of an estimated slope similarly decreases as the sample size increases. The denominator of the variance (sum of squares $\sum(x_i - \overline{x})^2$) increases with every additional value sampled and necessarily reduces the variance associated with $\hat{b}$. In addition, the variance of $\hat{b}$ is influenced by the spread of the independent variables (the range of the x-values). As noted, values close to the mean value $\bar{x}$ contribute more to the variability of the estimated slope than the more distant values. The spread of the distribution of the x-values is also directly reflected by the sum of squares $\sum(x_i - \bar{x})^2$. Thus, the sum of the squared deviations of the independent values from their mean value reflects both the number and spread of the x-values, which are both important components in determining the precision of an estimated slope.

Aside: When a sampled population is normally distributed and the variance is estimated, the statistical analysis frequently involves a Student's t-test. As before, the form of the t-test is

$$T = \frac{\hat{g} - g_0}{S_{\hat{g}}}$$

where $\hat{g}$ represents a normally distributed generic estimate of a summary value and g_0 represents a nonrandom expected value generated from a null hypothesis. The symbol $S_{\hat{g}}$ denotes the estimated standard deviation of the normal distribution describing the variability of the estimated value $\hat{g}$. The degrees of freedom associated with the test statistic T are a function of the sample size and are the denominator of the variance estimate $S_{\hat{g}}^2$.

Also, the bounds of a generic confidence interval based on the t-distribution are derived from the relationship

$$P(\hat{g} - t_{1-\alpha/2}S_{\hat{g}} < g < \hat{g} + t_{1-\alpha/2}S_{\hat{g}}) = 1 - \alpha$$

where $E(\hat{g}) = g$ is estimated by $\hat{g}$ and is again the mean of the normal distribution describing the variability of $\hat{g}$. The value of g is a fixed and unknown parameter. The value $t_{1-\alpha/2}$ is the $(1 - \alpha/2)^{\text{th}}$-percentile from a t-distribution.

These generic forms of a t-test and confidence interval are not new (Chapter 6) and, as before, are basic statistical tools used to assess the impact of sampling variation. The t-distribution, as might be expected, plays a central role in assessing the components of the simple linear regression model.

When the estimated slope $\hat{b}$ fulfills the requirements for the application of a t-test, then, parallel to the t-test associated with evaluating the sample mean $\bar{x}$, this estimate can be compared to a specified slope (denoted b_0) generated by a null hypothesis. The following table displays the elements of a t-test of the mean $\bar{x}$ (Chapter 6) and the parallel elements of a t-test of the slope $\hat{b}$, which differ in detail but not in principle:

	t-test: $\bar{x}$ versus μ_0	t-test: $\hat{b}$ versus b_0
expected values	$E(\overline{X}) = \mu$	$E(\hat{b}) = b$
population variances	σ_X^2	$\sigma_{Y\mid x}^2$
estimated variances	$S_X^2 = \dfrac{\sum (x_i - \bar{x})^2}{n-1}$	$S_{Y\mid x}^2 = \dfrac{\sum (y_i - \hat{y}_i)^2}{n-2}$
population variances	$\sigma_{\overline{X}}^2 = \dfrac{\sigma^2}{n}$	$\sigma_{\hat{b}}^2 = \dfrac{\sigma_{Y\mid x}^2}{\sum (x_i - \bar{x})^2}$
estimated variances	$S_{\bar{x}}^2 = \dfrac{S^2}{n}$	$S_{\hat{b}}^2 = \dfrac{S_{Y\mid x}^2}{\sum (x_i - \bar{x})^2}$
distributions	$\bar{x}$ is normally distributed	$\hat{b}$ is normally distributed
null hypotheses	$H_0: \mu = \mu_0$	$H_0: b = b_0$
test statistics	$T = \dfrac{\bar{x} - \mu_0}{S_{\overline{X}}}$	$T = \dfrac{\hat{b} - b_0}{S_{\hat{b}}}$
distributions of T	a t-distribution with $(n-1)$ degrees of freedom	a t-distribution with $(n-2)$ degrees of freedom

Succinctly, the estimate $\hat{b}$ is a special kind of mean value.

An important null hypothesis concerns a slope of $b_0 = 0$. A regression line with a slope equal to zero (horizontal line) occurs when x is not linearly related to Y or a change in x is not associated with a linear change in Y. Situations exist where the slope b is zero and x is related to Y but the relationship is not linear. Under the conditions of the simple linear regression model, the hypothesis $H_0: b = 0$ can be assessed using Student's t-distribution. An application of the generic t-test ($\hat{g} = \hat{b}$, $g_0 = b_0 = 0$ and $S_{\hat{g}} = S_{\hat{b}}$) gives

$$T = \frac{\hat{g} - g_0}{S_{\hat{g}}} = \frac{\hat{b} - 0}{S_{\hat{b}}},$$

which has a t-distribution with $n-2$ degrees of freedom when the null hypothesis is true ($b_0 = 0$).

A $(1 - \alpha)\%$ confidence interval for the slope b can be constructed from the estimates $\hat{b}$ and $S_{Y\mid x}^2$ also using the generic form (again, $\hat{g} = \hat{b}$ and $S_{\hat{g}} = S_{\hat{b}}$) and

$$P(\hat{b} - t_{1-\alpha/2} S_{\hat{b}} < b < \hat{b} + t_{1-\alpha/2} S_{\hat{b}}) = 1 - \alpha.$$

The interpretation of this confidence interval is same as the previous confidence interval for μ constructed from $\bar{x}$ and S_X^2 (Chapter 6).

Both the test of hypothesis and a confidence interval require the estimate $\hat{b}$ to have a normal distribution, which is the case when the sampled values are themselves normally distributed (requirement 3). Additionally, the estimated slope is a special kind of mean value (a weighted average of a sample of dependent values, as noted) and, therefore, typically has at least an approximate normal distribution regardless of the sampled distribution, particularly for large sample sizes (central limit theorem, Chapter 4).

EXAMPLE

The relationship between the amount of residual carbon monoxide (CO) measured in an individual's lungs and the time since that person last smoked a cigarette can be summarized using a linear regression approach. The following data (a small part of a large intervention trial called the Multi-risk Factor Intervention Trial—"MR. FIT")[25] recorded from 12 different smokers produce 12 pairs of observations (x_i, y_i):

$$x = \text{time since last smoked a cigarette (hours)}$$

$$Y = \text{amount of CO in parts per million (ppm)}$$

x	0.5	1.5	2.0	6.0	2.25	1.5	1.25	0.75	0.15	2.0	3.15	1.5
Y	53	22	38	17	28	32	35	40	61	22	28	31

The data represent $n = 12$ different (independent) individuals and the collected data are summarized by

$$x: \quad \sum x_i = 22.550 \quad \bar{x} = 1.879 \quad \sum(x_i - \bar{x})^2 = 25.757 \quad S_X^2 = 2.342$$

$$Y: \quad \sum y_i = 407 \quad \bar{y} = 33.917 \quad \sum(y_i - \bar{y})^2 = 1804.917 \quad S_Y^2 = 164.083$$

and $\sum(x_i - \bar{x})(y_i - \bar{y}) = -154.721$ giving $S_{XY} = -14.066$. The least squares estimated slope is then

$$\hat{b} = \frac{S_{XY}}{S_X^2} = \frac{-14.066}{2.342} = -6.007.$$

In words, the residual CO-levels in a person's lungs from smoking decrease an estimated rate of 6 ppm per hour. The estimated y-intercept is $\hat{a} = \bar{y} - \hat{b}\bar{x} = 33.917 - (-6.007)1.879 = 45.205$, making the estimated regression line (Figure 8.9)

$$\hat{y}_i = \hat{a} + \hat{b}x_i = 45.205 - 6.007x_i.$$

The residual sum of squares is $\sum(y_i - \hat{y}_i)^2 = 875.528$. The estimated variance of the normally distributed CO-measurements (Y) at each time since last smoked (x_i) is then $S^2_{Y|x} = 875.528/10 = 87.553$.

To test the null hypothesis that carbon monoxide levels are not linearly related to the time since last smoking a cigarette, the estimated slope $\hat{b} = -6.007$ is compared to $b_0 = 0$. In symbols,

$$H_0: b_0 = 0 \qquad \text{versus} \qquad H_1: b_0 < 0 \qquad \text{(one-tail alternative)}.$$

The estimated variance of $\hat{b}$ is $S^2_{\hat{b}} = 87.553/25.757 = 3.399$ making the standard deviation $S_{\hat{b}} = \sqrt{3.399} = 1.844$. For the selected level of significance $\alpha = 0.05$, the one-tail critical region is $T \leq -2.228$ based on a t-distribution with $n - 2 = 12 - 2 = 10$ degrees of freedom. The test statistic

$$T = \frac{\hat{b} - b_0}{S_{\hat{b}}} = \frac{-6.007}{1.844} = -3.258$$

falls in the critical region ($-3.258 < -2.228$), leading to the rejection of the null hypothesis. The p-value associated with the test statistic T is $P(T \leq -3.258 \,|\, b = 0) = 0.004$.

The following calculations are some of the details summarized in the regression analysis of the CO/smoking data:

	x	Y	$\hat{y}_i$	$y_i - \hat{y}_i$	$(y_i - \hat{y}_i)^2$
1	0.50	53	42.201	10.799	116.615
2	1.50	22	36.194	−14.194	201.477
3	2.00	38	33.191	4.809	23.128
4	6.00	17	9.163	7.837	61.413
5	2.25	28	31.689	−3.689	13.610
6	1.50	32	36.194	−4.194	17.592
7	1.25	35	37.696	−2.696	7.268
8	0.75	40	40.699	−0.699	0.489
9	0.15	61	44.304	16.696	278.771
10	2.00	22	33.191	−11.191	125.235
11	3.15	28	26.283	1.717	2.948
12	1.50	31	36.194	−5.194	26.980
Total	—	407	407	0	875.528

A 95% confidence interval for the slope b, based on its estimate $\hat{b}$, is

$$\hat{A} = upper\ bound = \hat{b} + t_{0.975}S_{\hat{b}} = -6.007 + 2.228(1.844) = -1.899$$

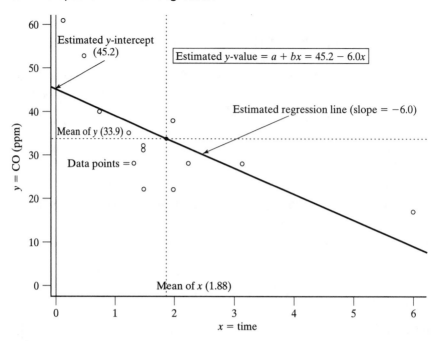

FIGURE 8.9: Plot of the carbon monoxide (Y) and time since smoking data (x) and the least squares estimated regression line ($\hat{y}$).

and

$$\hat{B} = lower\ bound = \hat{b} - t_{0.975}S_{\hat{b}} = -6.007 - 2.228(1.844) = -10.115.$$

Therefore, the population parameter b (estimated by $\hat{b} = -6.007$) is likely between -10.115 and -1.899 (confidence level $= 1 - \alpha = 0.95$). Both analytic approaches provide substantial evidence that the estimated slope $\hat{b} = -6.007$, despite the small sample size, is unlikely a result of random variation when no linear relationship exists ($b = 0$) between the time a cigarette was last smoked and the residual amount of CO measured in the smoker's lungs. ∎

Assessing an estimated regression line

An estimate of the dependent variable $E(Y \mid x)$ is sometimes desired for a specified value of the independent variable x. For a value denoted by x_0, the estimated $E(Y \mid x_0)$ is

$$\hat{y}_0 = \hat{a} + \hat{b}x_0.$$

In symbols, $\hat{y}_0$ estimates the expected value $E(Y \mid x_0)$ where, as before, $E(X \mid x)$ represents the mean of the distribution describing the variation of Y at the specified value of x. Like all estimates, the estimate $\hat{y}_0$ is subject to sampling variation.

When the assumptions of the simple linear regression model hold, the variation of $\hat{y}_0$ is described by a normal distribution ($\hat{a}$ and $\hat{b}$ are normally distributed and a sum of two random variables is also normally distributed, Chapter 4). The variance of this normal distribution is

$$\sigma_{\hat{y}_0}^2 = \sigma_{Y\,|\,x}^2 \left[\frac{1}{n} + \frac{(x_0 - \bar{x})^2}{\sum(x_i - \bar{x})^2} \right]$$

and, as before substituting $S_{Y\,|\,x}^2$ for $\sigma_{Y\,|\,x}^2$, is estimated by

$$S_{\hat{y}_0}^2 = S_{Y\,|\,x}^2 \left[\frac{1}{n} + \frac{(x_0 - \bar{x})^2}{\sum(x_i - \bar{x})^2} \right]. \qquad \text{See Box 8.9.}$$

Box 8.9. Variance of $\hat{y}_0$

Note that $\quad \hat{y}_0 = \hat{a} + \hat{b}x_0 = (\bar{y} - \hat{b}\bar{x}) + \hat{b}x_0 = \bar{y} + (x_0 - \bar{x})\hat{b}$

Then, the variance is

$$\sigma_{\hat{y}_0}^2 = \sigma_{\bar{y} + (x_0 - \bar{x})\hat{b}}^2 = \sigma_{\bar{y}}^2 + (x_0 - \bar{x})^2 \sigma_{\hat{b}}^2 \qquad \text{(Box 8.2)}$$

$$= \frac{\sigma_{Y\,|\,x}^2}{n} + (x_0 - \bar{x})^2 \frac{\sigma_{Y\,|\,x}^2}{\sum(x_i - \bar{x})^2} = \sigma_{Y\,|\,x}^2 \left[\frac{1}{n} + \frac{(x_0 - \bar{x})^2}{\sum(x_i - \bar{x})^2} \right].$$

This expression for the variance requires that the estimated mean $\bar{y}$ and slope $\hat{b}$ to be statistically independent, which is true but not shown.

Summarizing: the possible values of the estimate $\hat{y}_0$ are described by a normal distribution with mean $= E(Y\,|\,x_0) = a + bx_0$ and variance $\sigma_{\hat{y}_0}^2$.

The estimated intercept (value $\hat{a}$) is a special case of employing an estimated regression line to estimate a specific mean value. Namely, when $x_0 = 0$, $E(Y\,|\,x_0 = 0) = \hat{y}_0 = \hat{a}$ and the estimated variance measures the sampling variability associated with an estimated y-intercept ($S_{\hat{y}_0}^2 = S_{\hat{a}}^2$).

Just as in assessing the estimated slope $\hat{b}$, a t-test (using the generic form given earlier) provides an evaluation of the difference observed between an estimated point $\hat{y}_0$ and a null hypothesis generated expected value at x_0 [denoted $E(Y_0\,|\,x_0)$] or

$$T = \frac{\hat{y}_0 - E(Y_0\,|\,x_0)}{S_{\hat{y}_0}} \qquad \text{(specifically, } \hat{g} = \hat{y}_0,\ g_0 = E(Y_0\,|\,x_0),\ \text{and}\ S_{\hat{g}} = S_{\hat{y}_0}\text{).}$$

The test statistic T has a t-distribution with $n - 2$ degrees of freedom when the null hypothesis is true.

The bounds of a $(1 - \alpha)$-level confidence interval for the mean of the distribution of Y defined by a specific value x_0 are estimated from the relationship

$$P(\hat{y}_0 - t_{1-\alpha/2}S_{\hat{y}_0} < E(Y \mid x_0) < \hat{y}_0 + t_{1-\alpha/2}S_{\hat{y}_0}) = 1 - \alpha$$

and are, in principle, no different from the previously constructed confidence interval bounds. Such a confidence interval is called a *pointwise confidence interval*, because the confidence interval applies to a single estimated value x_0 and not the estimated line as a whole.

It is possible to construct a band about the estimated regression line $\hat{y}_i$ such that, with $(1 - \alpha)$-probability, the entire underlying regression line $E(Y \mid x)$ is likely contained between its boundaries, called a *confidence band*. It is not correct to connect the ends of the pointwise confidence intervals for a series of $E(Y \mid x)$-values to form a "confidence band." The correct confidence band is wider for all values of the independent variable x. An approximate 95% confidence band is $\hat{y}_x \pm f S_{\hat{y}_x}$ where $f = 2.44/(1 - 1.77/n)$ for a sample size of n observations ($n > 8$).

The variance of the estimated point $\hat{y}_0$ is minimum when $x_0 = \bar{x}$ and increases as x_0 moves further from $\bar{x}$. Therefore, the width of the pointwise confidence interval for $E(Y \mid x_0)$ and the width of a confidence band both increase as the difference between x and $\bar{x}$ increases. Figure 8.10 displays four 95% pointwise confidence intervals and a 95% confidence band for the CO/time regression analysis.

EXAMPLE

If the world was fair and just, then the 2000 presidential election dispute in Palm Beach County Florida would have been settled by a statistical analysis. The vote tabulations of the 67 Florida counties for presidential candidates George W. Bush and Pat Buchanan are

Bush	34062	5610	38637	5413	115185	177279	2873
Buchanan	262	73	248	65	570	789	90
Bush	10964	289456	4256	2697	152082	73029	12608
Buchanan	89	561	36	29	650	504	83
Bush	3546	2146	3764	4743	30646	20206	180713
Buchanan	71	23	30	22	242	127	845
Bush	1669	49963	106141	39053	6860	1316	3038
Buchanan	10	289	305	282	67	39	29
Bush	16404	52043	5058	134476	26212	68582	184884
Buchanan	90	267	43	446	145	570	1010
Bush	75293	39497	34705	12126	8014	4051	2332
Buchanan	194	229	124	114	108	27	29

Bush	35419	29744	41745	60426
Buchanan	182	270	186	122
Bush	2454	4750	3300	1840
Buchanan	33	39	29	9
Bush	4985	28635	9138	2478
Buchanan	76	105	102	29
Bush	57948	55141	33864	16059
Buchanan	272	563	108	47
Bush	90101	13439	36248	83100
Buchanan	538	147	311	305
Bush	82214	4511	12176	4983
Buchanan	396	46	120	88

Palm Beach County

| Bush | 152846 |
| Buchanan | 3407 |

Due to the exceptional form of the Palm Beach county ballot (so called "butterfly" ballot), voters claimed they mistakenly voted for Pat Buchanan when, in fact,

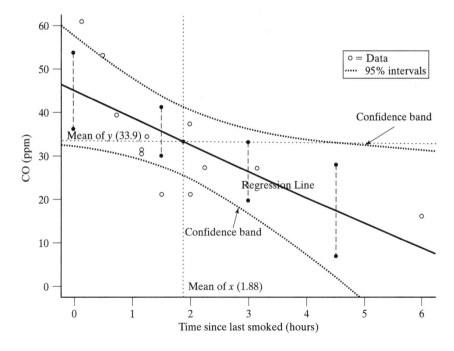

FIGURE 8.10: Pointwise 95% confidence intervals constructed from estimates $\hat{y}_0$ for four values of x_0 (hours = 0, 1.5, 3, and 4.5) and the estimated 95% confidence band.

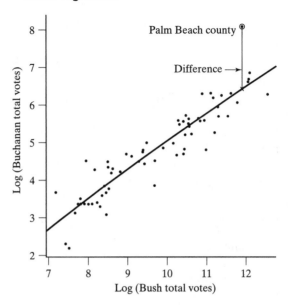

FIGURE 8.11: The 2000 presidential election: The log(Bush) votes plotted against log(Buchanan) votes for the 67 Florida counties.

they intended to vote for the Democratic candidate Al Gore. To explore this claim and estimate the number of votes that went to Buchanan that should have gone to Gore, a regression analysis is useful. The "correct" total of Buchanan votes in Palm Beach County can be estimated from the number of people who voted for Bush. The difference between this estimate and the actual votes estimates the number of mistaken votes recorded for Buchanan in Palm Beach County.

The logarithms of the Bush and Buchanan vote totals are plotted in the Figure 8.11 for each Florida county. The logarithms of the total vote counts are analyzed instead of the actual values because the relationship between the Bush log-vote (x-axis) and the Buchanan log-vote (y-axis) is more accurately summarized by a straight line (requirement 5). The correlation between the log-vote totals is 0.931 and the correlation between the vote totals is 0.624. A higher correlation (closer to one) indicates that the Buchanan log-vote total is more accurately predicted by straight line using the Bush log-vote total. (The interpretation of a correlation coefficient is taken up in detail in Chapter 9.) Using the logarithms of the Bush vote totals to estimate the logarithm of the total number of Buchanan votes rather than analyzing the directly reported counts presents no real problem. Once the logarithm of the number of votes is estimated, then exponentiating ("antilogarithm") this value gives an estimate of the total number votes (if $log(y) = x$, then $y = e^x$).

The least squares estimated line using the Bush log-vote totals (x) to predict the Buchanan log-vote totals (Y) excluding Palm Beach County has an estimated slope $\hat{b}$ of 0.730 and intercept $\hat{a}$ of -2.330 ($n = 66$). The regression line estimate of the log-number of Buchanan votes expected in each county is then $\hat{y}_i = -2.330 + 0.730x_i$ based on the log-number of votes (x_i) for Bush (solid line in Figure 8.11). From this regression line, it is possible to estimate the total Buchanan log-votes that would have occurred if Palm Beach county voters followed the same pattern as the rest of the state. Specifically, this estimate is

$$\hat{y}_0 = \hat{a} + \hat{b}x_0 = -2.330 + (0.730)[\log(152,846)] = 6.387$$

based on 152,846 Bush votes in Palm Beach County. The variance associated with this estimate is $S_{\hat{y}_0}^2 = 0.009$, which, as usual, is the key to assessing the precision of the estimate $\hat{y}_0 = 6.387$. The estimated number of total Buchanan "votes" is then $e^{\hat{y}_0} = e^{6.387} = 594.2$.

A 95% confidence interval based on the predicted log-estimate $\hat{y}_0$ is

$$\hat{A} = \textit{lower bound} = \hat{y}_0 - t_{0.975}S_{\hat{y}_0} = 6.3887 - 1.978(0.094) = 6.200$$

and

$$\hat{B} = \textit{upper bound} = \hat{y}_0 + t_{0.975}S_{\hat{y}_0} = 6.387 + 1.978(0.094) = 6.575$$

where $t_{0.975} = 1.998$ ($n - 2 = 66 - 2 = 64$ degrees of freedom). The estimated 95% confidence interval for the log-number of "Buchanan" votes is then (6.200, 6.575), which translates into a 95% confidence interval for the number of votes as $(e^{\hat{A}}, e^{\hat{B}}) = (e^{6.200}, e^{6.575}) = (492.7, 716.6)$. The estimation of the total "Buchanan" vote is $\hat{y}_0 = e^{6.387} = 594.2$. The confidence interval limits for this estimate are the same function of the lower and upper bounds calculated from the log-total. Clearly, the observed number of Buchanan votes (3407) lies outside the possibility of a random fluctuation from the estimated value. In other words, overwhelming evidence exists of a systematic difference between the observed (3407) and the estimated vote totals (594). The components of the estimated line and the estimated log-vote totals are displayed in Figure 8.11. The estimated difference (mistaken votes) is $3407 - 594 = 2813$. A historical note: G. W. Bush won the state of Florida by less than 600 votes. ∎

Assessing an estimated regression line with zero intercept

Occasionally, a situation arises where the y-intercept of a summary regression line must be zero ($a = 0$). For example, if the relationship is studied between inhabitable area and the size of the population living on a South Seas island, then necessarily an island with an area of zero has a population of zero. When it is known that the y-intercept value is zero, it frequently makes sense to incorporate this knowledge into the estimation of a line summarizing the relationship between an independent and a dependent variable. Such a summary regression line is

$$E(Y \mid x_i) = bx_i \qquad (a = 0).$$

When x_i is zero, the intercept $a = E(Y \mid x_i = 0)$ is zero.

Using the identical least squares logic (Appendix B.2), the slope of the line that minimizes the sum of the squared distances between a straight line with intercept zero and the observed values y_i is given by the expression

$$\hat{b} = \frac{\sum x_i y_i}{\sum x_i^2}.$$

That is, the estimate $\hat{b}$ minimizes the quantity $L = \sum (y_i - bx_i)^2$.

The estimated least squares line is then $\hat{y}_i = \hat{b}x_i$. When the simple regression model accurately represents the structure of the sampled population (requirements 1–5), the assessment of the slope and the values estimated from the regression line follow essentially the same pattern already discussed (a few minor details differ).

The estimated variance of Y is again a function of the differences between the observed values y_i and the values $\hat{y}_i$ estimated from the regression line at each value of x_i, namely

$$S_{Y|x}^2 = \frac{\sum (y_i - \hat{y}_i)^2}{n-1}.$$

The estimated variance of the estimate $\hat{b}$ is

$$S_{\hat{b}}^2 = \frac{S_{Y|x}^2}{\sum x_i^2},$$

which is similar to the previous case $(a \neq 0)$.

EXAMPLE

To define a relationship between price and size, a random sample of $n = 14$ pairs of observations was extracted from an extensive catalog advertising the sale of handmade prints from Japan. In the following table, the prices x in dollars and the sizes of the print Y in square inches are recorded for each observation in this sample:

x	50	100	100	100	150	150	150	200	200	200	250
Y	400	400	500	900	500	700	1200	900	1600	2000	625

x	250	250	250
Y	1200	1600	2000

To estimate a straight line summarizing the relationship between price and size, a least squares estimated line with intercept equal to zero has estimated slope

$$\hat{b} = \frac{2,816,250}{470,000} = 5.992$$

producing the estimated line $\hat{y}_i = 5.992 x_i$ (Figure 8.12). Each additional dollar buys an estimated additional six square inches. Implicit is the assumption that small prints have low prices and very small prints have very low prices; ultimately, a print of zero area has no cost (intercept = a = 0).

A confidence interval constructed to account for the impact of sampling variation on the estimated increase in area for each dollar spent ($\hat{b}$) requires an estimate of the variance associated with the distribution of the estimated slope. The estimated variance of $\hat{b}$ is

$$S_{\hat{b}}^2 = \frac{S_{Y|x}^2}{\sum x_i^2} = \frac{\sum (y_i - \hat{y}_i)^2/(n-1)}{\sum x_i^2} = \frac{2,445,595/13}{470,000} = 0.400$$

making the standard deviation $S_{\hat{b}} = \sqrt{0.400} = 0.633$. An estimated 95% confidence interval is then

$$\hat{A} = lower\ bound = \hat{b} - t_{0.975} S_{\hat{b}} = 5.992 - 2.160(0.633) = 4.625$$

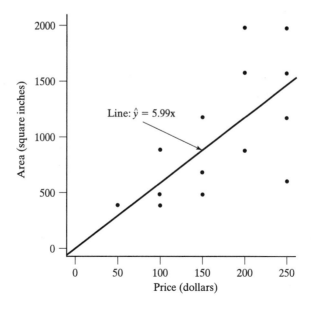

FIGURE 8.12: The relationship between area and price of a sample of Japanese prints (intercept = 0).

and

$$\hat{B} = upper\ bound = \hat{b} + t_{0.975}S_{\hat{b}} = 5.992 + 2.160(0.633) = 7.359$$

where $t_{0.975} = 2.160$ (degrees of freedom $= 13$). Therefore, it is unlikely (probability $= 0.05$) that the relationship between price and area for all the prints in the catalog is less than 4.63 dollars per square inch or higher than 7.36 dollars per square inch.   ∎

Assessing regression lines from two groups

Data are sometimes collected from two different populations to investigate differences in bivariate relationships between two variables but frequently the primary focus is on comparing adjusted mean values from the two sampled groups. The xy-relationship is summarized by estimating a regression line in each group. As might be expected, the t-test comparison of the estimated slopes from these two lines (denoted $\hat{b}_1$ and $\hat{b}_2$) parallels the t-test comparison of two sample mean values (Chapter 6), since an estimated slope, as noted earlier, is no more than a special kind of estimated mean value.

The quantities necessary to evaluate an observed difference between two estimated slopes are:

	Sample from population 1	Sample from population 2
sample sizes	n_1	n_2
dependent variables	y_{1j}	y_{2j}
independent variables	x_{1j}	x_{2j}
sums of squares (x)	$SS_1 = \sum(x_{1j} - \bar{x}_1)^2$	$SS_2 = \sum(x_{2j} - \bar{x}_2)^2$
estimated slopes	$\hat{b}_1$	$\hat{b}_2$
estimated y-values	$\hat{y}_{1j} = \hat{a}_1 + \hat{b}_1 x_{1j}$	$\hat{y}_{2j} = \hat{a}_2 + \hat{b}_2 x_{2j}$
estimated variances	$S^2_{Y_1\mid x} = \dfrac{\sum(y_{1j} - \hat{y}_{1j})^2}{n_1 - 2}$	$S^2_{Y_2\mid x} = \dfrac{\sum(y_{2j} - \hat{y}_{2j})^2}{n_2 - 2}$

The subscript "$1j$" denotes the jth-sampled observation from population 1 and similarly, "$2j$" denotes the jth-sampled observation from population 2. The estimated quantities are the same as those previously used to estimate a single regression line, simply repeated for each of two separate samples. A statistical comparison of the estimates $\hat{b}_1$ and $\hat{b}_2$ requires that both sampled populations conform to the simple linear regression model (requirements 1–5).

A test statistic to assess the null hypothesis that the slopes are equal ($b_1 = b_2 = b$ or $b_1 - b_2 = 0$) based on the estimated difference $\hat{b}_1 - \hat{b}_2$ is

$$T = \frac{(\hat{b}_1 - \hat{b}_2) - 0}{S_{\hat{b}_1 - \hat{b}_2}}.$$

Again, the test statistic T is a special case of the generic form of the t-statistic given earlier where $\hat{g} = (\hat{b}_1 - \hat{b}_2)$, $g_0 = (b_1 - b_2) = 0$ and the estimated standard deviation is $S_{\hat{g}} = S_{\hat{b}_1 - \hat{b}_2}$.

When populations are unrelated (independent), an estimated variance of the distribution of the estimated differences $(\hat{b}_1 - \hat{b}_2)$ is

$$S^2_{\hat{b}_1 - \hat{b}_2} = S^2_{\hat{b}_1} + S^2_{\hat{b}_2} = \frac{S^2_{Y_1 | x}}{\sum (x_{1j} - \bar{x}_1)^2} + \frac{S^2_{Y_2 | x}}{\sum (x_{2j} - \bar{x}_2)^2}.$$

Taking advantage of the assumption or knowledge that the variances of the two compared populations are equal and employing a combined (pooled) estimate of the variability of Y (denoted S^2_{pooled}) gives

$$S^2_{\hat{b}_1 - \hat{b}_2} = \frac{S^2_{pooled}}{\sum (x_{1j} - \bar{x}_1)^2} + \frac{S^2_{pooled}}{\sum (x_{2j} - \bar{x}_2)^2} = S^2_{pooled} \left[\frac{1}{SS_1} + \frac{1}{SS_2} \right].$$

The estimated variance S^2_{pooled} is again a weighted average (degrees of freedom = weights) of the estimated variances from each sample or

$$S^2_{pooled} = \frac{(n_1 - 2)S^2_{Y_1 | x} + (n_2 - 2)S^2_{Y_2 | x}}{(n_1 - 2) + (n_2 - 2)} = \frac{\sum (y_{1j} - \hat{y}_{1j})^2 + \sum (y_{2j} - \hat{y}_{2j})^2}{n_1 + n_2 - 4}.$$

Similar to comparing two sample mean values (Chapter 6), the quantity S^2_{pooled} is an estimate of the common population variance $\sigma^2_{Y | x}$ derived under the assumption that the variances are the same in both sampled populations. The degrees of freedom associated with the pooled variance are $(n_1 - 2) + (n_2 - 2) = n_1 + n_2 - 4$ and are the degrees of freedom associated with the t-test.

The test statistic becomes

$$T = \frac{(\hat{b}_1 - \hat{b}_2) - 0}{S_{pooled} \sqrt{\dfrac{1}{SS_1} + \dfrac{1}{SS_2}}}$$

and has a t-distribution with $n_1 + n_2 - 4$ degrees of freedom when no difference exists between slopes b_1 and b_2 (H_0: $b_1 = b_2 = b$ or $b_1 - b_2 = 0$ is true). As always, an extreme value of the test statistic T leads to the inference that random variation is not a plausible explanation of the observed difference (reject H_0).

In light of no evidence of a systematic difference between slopes b_1 and b_2, an estimate of the common value of the slope can be estimated by yet another weighted average or

$$\hat{b} = \frac{w_1 \hat{b}_1 + w_2 \hat{b}_2}{w_1 + w_2}$$

where the weights are sums of squares, $w_i = SS_i$. These weights reflect both the sample size and the spread of the x_i-values sampled from each population, directly accounting for the differences in the precision of each estimated value $\hat{b}_i$.

When a single slope plausibility describes both the xy-relationships, it is then possible to compare mean values from each of the two sampled populations free from any interfering (confounding) influence of the x-variable. Specifically, the regression line from population 1 produces an *adjusted mean value* given by

$$\bar{y}_1' = \hat{a}_1 + \hat{b}\bar{x} = \bar{y}_1 + \hat{b}(\bar{x} - \bar{x}_1).$$

The adjusted mean $\bar{y}_1'$ is an estimate of the mean value of the first population when the x-value is the overall mean ($\bar{x}$—the mean value of all $n_1 + n_2$ observed x-values). The second similarly adjusted mean value is

$$\bar{y}_2' = \hat{a}_2 + \hat{b}\bar{x} = \bar{y}_2 + \hat{b}(\bar{x} - \bar{x}_2),$$

and estimates the mean value of the second population, also at the overall mean $\bar{x}$. In symbols, the adjusted values estimate $E(Y_i \mid \bar{x})$.

These adjusted mean values are constructed so that $\bar{y}_2' - \bar{y}_1'$ measures the difference between the two sampled populations free of any influences from differences in the distributions of the x-values, because the two adjusted means are compared at exactly the same value, namely $\bar{x}$. Figure 8.13 displays the geometry of the comparison. The dots represent the sampled xy-pairs from population 1 and the circles represent the sampled xy-pairs from population 2. The locations of the two groups differ substantially causing $\bar{x}_1$ to differ from $\bar{x}_2$. A direct comparison of the unadjusted mean values ($\bar{y}_1$ directly compared to $\bar{y}_2$—the X's in Figure 8.13) is influenced by this difference in the distribution of the x-values. The sampled values from the first population are generally smaller than those from the second population, causing $\bar{y}_1$ to be smaller than $\bar{y}_2$ due, at least to some extent, to the differences in the distributions of the x-values. The observed mean difference $\bar{y}_2 - \bar{y}_1$ is a combination of the difference between the two groups and the difference between the two distributions of the independent variables. The important issue is typically the difference between groups.

The parallel lines based on the common slope $\hat{b}$ each summarize the relationship between x and Y within each group. Because these lines are parallel (same slope), the "distance" between the two populations is the same for any x-value. A common choice is to compare the two regression lines at the overall mean $\bar{x}$ (vertical dotted line). The difference between the adjusted mean values $\bar{y}_2' - \bar{y}_1'$, then, reflects differences between populations 1 and 2 unaffected by the differing distributions of the sampled x-values. Any influence of the x-values is said to be "removed".

If evidence exists that the lines summarizing each sample are not parallel ($H_0: b_1 = b_2$ is rejected), then the distance between estimated mean values

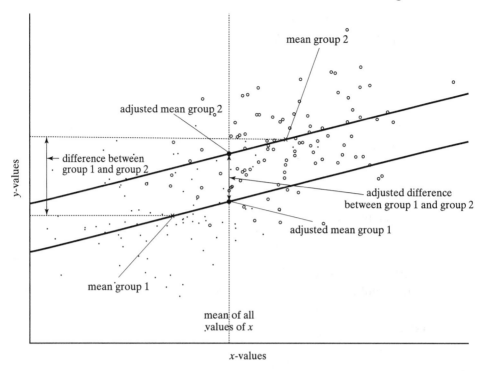

FIGURE 8.13: The comparison of two samples summarized by regression lines.

depends on the choice of the x-value and no single comparison summarizes the difference between populations, called an *interaction*. When an interaction is present (nonparallel regression lines), alternate approaches are necessary.

EXAMPLE

When data are collected to compare the birth weights of white infants to Asian infants, a problem arises. The prepregnancy weights of mothers of white infants are, by and large, greater than Asian mothers, making the birth weight of their infants also on average greater. If the purpose of a comparison is to understand how such things as environment, culture, and ethnic traditions influence birth weight, a direct comparison of mean birth weights is ineffective because it includes influences from the differences in maternal weight. Isolating other influences is not possible without further statistical analysis. A comparison of the adjusted mean values, however, estimates the difference between infant birth weights as if the two groups of sampled mothers do not, on average, differ with respect to maternal prepregnancy weight.

The birth weights of 21 (Figure 8.14) white infants ("o"-values) and 11 Asian infants ("+"-values), extracted from a large study of over 2000 women,[26] are plotted by their mother's prepregnancy weights. The maternal weights (denoted x, in kilograms) and the infant birth weights (denoted Y, in grams) for white and Asian samples are:

Whites:

	1	2	3	4	5	6	7
maternal weight (x)	63.4	58.5	79.7	60.4	62.8	51.6	70.7
birth weight (Y)	3330	3225	3475	3580	3380	3175	4085

	8	9	10	11	12	13	14
maternal weight (x)	56.9	67.3	70.8	50.4	87.6	56	93.3
birth weight (Y)	5015	2820	3996	2820	2745	2829	4169

	15	16	17	18	19	20	21
maternal weight (x)	51.7	69.7	71.9	64.2	73.3	81.2	60.6
birth weight (Y)	3430	3300	3515	3205	2880	3576	3860

Asians:

	1	2	3	4	5	6	7
maternal weight (x)	48.9	60.0	41.3	50.4	65.7	73.0	57.4
birth weight (Y)	3325	2206	3205	2318	3111	4140	2880

	8	9	10	11
maternal weight (x)	45.0	50.0	55.0	62.2
birth weight (Y)	4140	3040	3175	3070

Using these data, the following summary statistics allow the comparison of adjusted mean birth weights for white and Asian infants:

	Whites	Asians
number of observations	21	11
mean maternal weights (kilograms)—$\bar{x}$	66.8	55.4
mean birth weights (grams)—$\bar{y}$	3448.1	3146.4
sum of squares—$\sum(x_i - \bar{x})^2$	2742.0	890.8
sum of cross products—$\sum(x_i - \bar{x})(y_i - \bar{y})$	12907.7	4129.1
intercepts $(\hat{a})$	3133.8	2889.8
slopes $(\hat{b})$	4.707	4.635
standard deviations of Y $(S_{Y \mid x})$	563.9	637.0
standard deviations of the slopes $(S_{\hat{b}})$	10.769	21.342
adjusted mean birth weights $(\bar{y}')$	3429.7	3181.5

As expected, the white and Asian mean maternal prepregnancy weights differ considerably ($\bar{x}_1 = 66.8$ and $\bar{x}_2 = 55.4$ where white is coded as 1 and Asian is coded as 2). Also as expected, the white infants weigh more than the Asian infants ($\bar{y}_1 = 3448.1$ and $\bar{y}_2 = 3146.4$). This difference ($\bar{y}_1 - \bar{y}_2 = 3448.1 - 3146.4 = 301.7$ grams) is partly due to the differences in white and Asian maternal prepregnancy weight distributions (X's = mean values on Figure 8.14).

A regression line summarizing the relationship between maternal weight and infant birth weight from each of the two data sets produces estimated slopes of $\hat{b}_1 = 4.707$ (whites) and $\hat{b}_2 = 4.635$ (Asians). Since these two estimates hardly differ, a single estimate serves to summarize a linear relationship within both groups. Thus, a pooled slope $\hat{b} = 4.690$ produces two parallel summary regression lines (Figure 8.14) where

$$\text{white: } \hat{y}_i' = \hat{a}_1 + \hat{b}x_i = \bar{y}_1 - \hat{b}\bar{x}_1 + \hat{b}x_i$$

$$= 3448.1 - 4.690(66.762) + 4.690x_i = 3135.0 + 4.690x_i$$

and

$$\text{Asian: } \hat{y}_i' = \hat{a}_2 + \hat{b}x_i = \bar{y}_2 - \hat{b}\bar{x}_2 + \hat{b}x_i$$

$$= 3146.4 - 4.690(55.355) + 4.690x_i = 2886.8 + 4.690x_i.$$

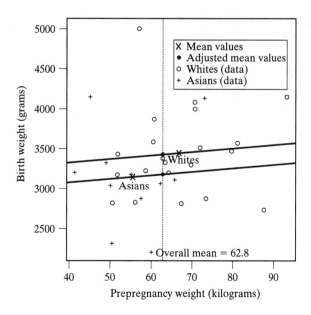

FIGURE 8.14: Birth weights of Asian and white infants plotted by maternal prepregnancy weights.

Adjusted means can be compared at any point on these parallel lines, that is, at any specific maternal prepregnancy weight x. The x-value chosen is $\bar{x} = 62.841$ (mean maternal weight of all 32 observations ignoring white/Asian status) giving adjusted mean values $\bar{y}_1' = 3135.0 + 4.690(62.841) = 3429.7$ for white infants and $\bar{y}_2' = 2886.8 + 4.690(62.841) = 3181.5$ for Asian infants. The comparison (vertical distance between the dots in Figure 8.14) $\bar{y}_1' - \bar{y}_2' = 3429.7 - 3181.5 = 248.2$ is not influenced by differences in maternal prepregnancy weight. The reduction in the mean difference in infant birth weight from 301.7 grams to 248.2 grams represents the "removal" of the influence from the difference in maternal prepregnancy weight distributions. The estimated white/Asian difference between groups of 248.2 is likely related to a variety of factors but it is not due to differences in maternal weights. The adjusted means are compared as if the mean maternal prepregnancy weight is the same for both white and Asian mothers. It is as if the mean values for both groups were $\bar{x} = 62.841$ kilograms.

The process of estimating a common slope for white and Asian mothers and using it to compare adjusted mean birth weights is an example of a general statistical technique called *analysis of covariance*.[27]   ∎

Assessing an estimated independent variable (linear calibration)

Sometimes a regression line is used "backwards." A line is established so that values of the independent variable X can be predicted from a specified value of the dependent variable y using the estimated line $\hat{y}_i = \hat{a} + \hat{b}x_i$. The procedure is called *linear calibration*. A predicted x-value (denoted $\hat{x}_0$) is estimated by rearranging the equation $y_0 = \hat{a} + \hat{b}x_0$ giving an estimated value $\hat{x}_0$ or

$$\hat{x}_0 = (y_0 - \hat{a})/\hat{b}.$$

The dependent variable y_0 is now the "input" value. The roles of x and y are reversed. A value of the independent variable x_0 is estimated (subject to sampling variation) from a specified value of the dependent variable y_0 (fixed—nonrandom). The variance associated with an estimate $\hat{x}_0$ is approximately

$$\sigma_{\hat{x}_0}^2 = \frac{\sigma_{Y|x}^2}{b^2}\left[1 + \frac{1}{n} + \frac{(\hat{x}_0 - \bar{x})^2}{\sum(x_i - \bar{x})^2}\right]$$

and the estimate of this variance becomes

$$S_{\hat{x}_0}^2 = \frac{S_{Y|x}^2}{\hat{b}^2}\left[1 + \frac{1}{n} + \frac{(\hat{x}_0 - \bar{x})^2}{\sum(x_i - \bar{x})^2}\right].$$

This approximation is most accurate when $(t_{1-\alpha/2}S_{\hat{b}}/\hat{b})^2$ is small.

Using the estimated standard deviation $S_{\hat{x}_0}$, an approximate $(1 - \alpha)\%$ confidence interval can be constructed from the usual consideration as

$$\hat{A} = lower\ bound = \hat{x}_0 + t_{1-\alpha/2}S_{\hat{x}_0}$$

and

$$\hat{B} = upper\ bound = \hat{x}_0 + t_{1-\alpha/2}S_{\hat{x}_0}$$

where

$$P(\hat{x}_0 - t_{1-\alpha/2}S_{\hat{x}_0} < x_0 < \hat{x}_0 + t_{1-\alpha/2}S_{\hat{x}_0}) = 1 - \alpha.$$

EXAMPLE

Linear calibration could apply to the previous carbon monoxide and smoking data. A line was established using CO-levels as the dependent variable and time since last smoking as the independent variable. Suppose, for a program to reduce smoking among teenagers, it is required to know when a participant last smoked. It is entirely possible that directly asking will not produce an accurate answer because some teenagers are likely to conceal the fact that they smoke. Therefore, using the previously estimated regression line allows an estimate of the time since last smoking a cigarette based not on the teenager's reply but based on the observed residual CO-level, which is a more objective measure.

Suppose a CO-level of $y_0 = 10$ parts per million is measured and it is desired to estimate the time since last smoking a cigarette, x_0 hours. The estimated time is

$$\hat{x}_0 = \frac{y_0 - \hat{a}}{\hat{b}} = \frac{10 - 45.205}{-6.007} = 5.861 \text{ hours}$$

and the estimated variance is

$$S_{\hat{x}_0}^2 = \frac{S_{Y|x}^2}{\hat{b}^2}\left[1 + \frac{1}{n} + \frac{(\hat{x}_0 - \overline{x})^2}{\sum(x_i - \overline{x})^2}\right]$$

$$= \frac{87.553}{(-6.007)^2}\left[1 + \frac{1}{12} + \frac{(5.861 - 1.879)^2}{25.757}\right] = 4.122$$

making the standard deviation $S_{\hat{x}_0} = \sqrt{4.122} = 2.030$. The approximate 95% confidence interval for the predicted time x_0, based on the estimated time $\hat{x}_0 = 5.861$, is $5.861 \pm 2.228(2.030)$ or $(\hat{A}, \hat{B}) = (1.337, 10.384)$ where $t_{0.975} = 2.228$ (degrees of freedom $= n - 2 = 12 - 2 = 10$). ∎

A last example: In the early part of the 20th century considerable scientific effort was focused on measuring genetic inheritance as part of a new field, called *biometrics*. To study genetic variation in human populations, a large data set (over 1000 pairs) of fathers' heights and their sons' heights was collected.[28] A small ($n = 30$) sample of these data is given in Table 8.1.

TABLE 8.1: Father's height and son's height.

	1	2	3	4	5	6	7	8	9	10
father (x)	5.6	5.8	5.7	5.8	5.9	5.8	5.8	6.0	5.4	5.6
son (y)	5.5	5.9	5.4	5.6	6.0	5.9	6.1	5.9	5.6	5.4

	11	12	13	14	15	16	17	18	19	20
father (x)	5.3	5.6	5.4	5.4	5.8	5.6	5.6	5.5	5.5	6.0
son (y)	5.4	5.3	5.4	5.4	5.7	5.6	6.2	5.4	5.4	5.9

	21	22	23	24	25	26	27	28	29	30
father (x)	6.0	5.8	5.3	6.0	5.7	5.5	5.7	5.7	5.7	5.6
son (y)	5.8	5.9	5.4	5.7	5.5	5.7	5.8	5.8	5.6	5.8

These 30 father/son observations are from different families and are, therefore, essentially independent pairs. Of primary interest is the change in height from one generation to the next. If differences are only due to chance, then a straight line with slope of one ($b = 1$) describes the relationship between the heights of fathers and sons. For example, fathers who are six feet tall will, on average, have sons who are also six feet tall.

For the $n = 30$ pairs of observations where x = father's height (feet) and Y = son's height (feet), the summary values

$$\bar{x} = 5.670 \qquad\qquad \bar{y} = 5.667$$
$$\sum(x_i - \bar{x})^2 = 1.203 \qquad \sum(x_i - \bar{x})(y_i - \bar{y}) = 0.880$$
$$\hat{b} = 0.732 \qquad\qquad \hat{a} = 1.519$$

produce the least square estimated line

$$\hat{y}_i = \hat{a} + \hat{b}x_i = 1.519 + 0.732x_i.$$

The sum of the squared deviations of each observation from its estimate (residual sum of squares) is

$$\sum(y_i - \hat{y}_i)^2 = 1.063$$

producing an estimated variance of Y equal to 0.038 ($S_{Y|x}^2 = 1.063/28 = 0.038$).

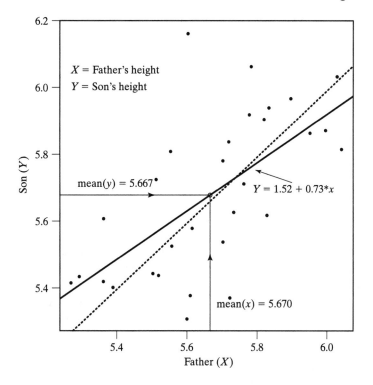

FIGURE 8.15: Fathers' heights and sons' heights for $n = 30$ individuals.

Figure 8.15 displays the 30 pairs of observations (dots) and the estimated line (solid line). For comparison, a dotted line is included with intercept $= 0$ and slope $= 1$.

Test of the slope

To test the consistency of these data with the conjecture that the slope b is 1.0, the null hypothesis becomes H_0: $b_0 = 1$ versus H_1: $b_0 < 1$. Selecting $\alpha = 0.05$ gives $t_{0.05} = -1.701$ (degrees of freedom $= 28$) making the critical region $T < -1.701$. Using $S_{Y|x}^2 = 0.038$, the estimated variance associated with at least the approximate normal distribution describing the variation of the estimate $\hat{b}$ becomes

$$S_{\hat{b}}^2 = \frac{0.038}{1.203} = 0.032 \quad \text{with standard deviation } S_{\hat{b}} = \sqrt{0.032} = 0.178.$$

The T-statistic to evaluate the hypothesis that only random changes in heights occurred between generations ($b_0 = 1$) is

$$T = \frac{0.732 - 1.0}{0.178} = -1.511.$$

Therefore, the null hypothesis is not rejected since the test statistic T is not in the critical region $(-1.701 < -1.511)$, but the p-value is $P(T \le -1.511 \,|\, b_0 = 1) = 0.07$.

A 95% confidence interval for the slope

Since $t_{0.975} = 2.048$ (degrees of freedom $= 28$), a 95% confidence interval is

$$\text{lower bound} = \hat{A} = \hat{b} - t_{0.975}(S_{\hat{b}}) = 0.732 - 2.048(0.178) = 0.429$$

and

$$\text{upper bound} = \hat{B} = \hat{b} + t_{0.975}(S_{\hat{b}}) = 0.732 + 2.048(0.178) = 1.034.$$

The estimated interval $(\hat{A}, \hat{B}) = (0.429, 1.034)$ indicates the likely range of the parameter b and shows that a slope of $b = 1.0$ is near the upper limit.

In fact, a slope of less than 1.0 is expected. A slope of considerably less than 1.0 was observed in the original data indicating that in general the sons' heights were, on average, closer to the overall mean value than their fathers' heights, then called "regression of mediocrity." This observation leads to the dilemma that each successive generation should be, on average, smaller, which was obviously not the case. Today, a slope of less than 1.0 is recognized as a statistical phenomenon called *regression to the mean*.

Regression to the mean arises because extreme values do not tend to be repeated. An extremely tall father is not likely to have an even taller son because an even more extreme height is unlikely. It is simply more likely that very tall fathers will have somewhat shorter sons, on average. Similarly, sons of extremely short fathers will tend to be taller, on average, than their fathers, because again it is unlikely that an extremely short father will have an even shorter son. The tendency of a second measurement to be more like the overall mean than a first extreme measurement produces a regression line with a slope of less than one. Consecutive and correlated measurements such as fathers' and sons' heights are called *repeated measurements* and accounting for the impact of regression to the mean from repeated measurements is an advanced statistical topic.[29]

Review

Chapters 6 (assessment of an estimated mean) and 8 (assessment of an estimated slope) differ considerably in detail and focus but underlying the statistical details is a general pattern. Suppose a sample of n independent observations is collected from a population. Then, from this sample a summary value is calculated, denoted in a generic form as $\hat{g}$. The estimated quantity $\hat{g}$ has three properties that lead to a statistical test or a $(1 - \alpha)$-level confidence interval. They are:

Distribution: When the summary value $\hat{g}$ is a mean value (in a broad sense—a weighted average or a weight sum of observed values) estimated from a moderately

TABLE 8.2: The basic expressions for statistical inference (tests) and construction of confidence intervals.

Statistic	Estimate	Expected Value	Variance
mean	$\bar{x}$	μ	σ_X^2/n
proportion	$\hat{p}$	p	$\dfrac{p(1-p)}{n}$
difference in means	$\bar{x}_1 - \bar{x}_2$	$\mu_1 - \mu_2$	$\sigma_X^2\left[\dfrac{1}{n_1} + \dfrac{1}{n_2}\right]$
difference in proportions	$\hat{p}_1 - \hat{p}_2$	$p_1 - p_2$	$p(1-p)\left[\dfrac{1}{n_1} + \dfrac{1}{n_2}\right]$
slope	$\hat{b}$	b	$\dfrac{\sigma_{Y\,|\,x}^2}{\sum (x_i - \bar{x})^2}$
estimated y-value	$\hat{y}_0$	$E(Y\,|\,x_0)$	$\sigma_{Y\,|\,x}^2\left[\dfrac{1}{n} + \dfrac{(x_0 - \bar{x})^2}{\sum (x_i - \bar{x})^2}\right]$
estimated y-intercept	$\hat{a}$	a	$\sigma_{Y\,|\,x}^2\left[\dfrac{1}{n} + \dfrac{\bar{x}^2}{\sum (x_i - \bar{x})^2}\right]$
difference in slopes	$\hat{b}_1 - \hat{b}_2$	$b_1 - b_2$	$\sigma_{Y\,|\,x}^2\left[\dfrac{1}{SS_1} + \dfrac{1}{SS_2}\right]$
generic	$\hat{g}$	g or $E(\hat{g})$	$\sigma_{\hat{g}}^2$

large sample data, the value $\hat{g}$ typically has an approximate normal distribution (central limit theorem). When the data are sampled from a normal distribution, the estimated value $\hat{g}$ has an exact normal distribution for any sample size.

Mean value: The normal distribution describing the variability of the estimate $\hat{g}$ has a mean value denoted g or $E(\hat{g})$. This value is frequently generated from theoretical considerations such as a null hypothesis (denoted g_0).

Variance: The estimate $\hat{g}$ is subject to sampling variation. To evaluate the impact of this sampling variation, an estimate of the variance of the normal distribution that describes the likelihood of possible values of the estimate $\hat{g}$ is derived.

In short, the summary estimate $\hat{g}$ typically has at least an approximate normal distribution with mean value g and estimated variance $S_{\hat{g}}^2$.

Table 8.2 lists eight previously encountered statistical summaries. All eight summaries have associated variances that depend on the population variability [for example, σ^2, $p(1 - p)$ or $\sigma^2_{Y|x}$] and the number of sampled observations. Clearly, details differ in the application but the pattern of the analysis is the same. A test statistic

$$T \text{ or } Z = \frac{\hat{g} - g_0}{S_{\hat{g}}}$$

is used to assess a null hypothesis (g_0) and a $(1 - \alpha)$-level confidence interval

$$\hat{g} \pm t_{1-\alpha/2} S_{\hat{g}} \qquad \text{or} \qquad \hat{g} \pm z_{1-\alpha/2} S_{\hat{g}}$$

is constructed without reference to a null hypothesis. Both approaches account for the impact of random variation on the estimated summary value, providing a basis for statistical inferences about the sampled population. This pattern appears frequently as part of many kinds of both simple and complex statistical analyses.

Having given the number of instances respectively in which things are both thus and so, in which they are thus but not so, in which they are so but not thus, and in which they are neither thus nor so, it is required to eliminate the general quantitative relativity inherent in the mere thingness of the things, and to determine the special quantitative relativity subsisting between the thusness and the soness of the things.

M. H. Doolittle

PROBLEM SET 8

For problems 1 and 2, assume the requirements for the simple linear regression model (requirements 1–5 in Chapter 8) are fulfilled, then

(a) Plot the data.
(b) Estimate the least squares line summarizing the relationship between Y and x.
(c) Draw the estimated regression line.
(d) For the selected value of x (denoted x_0) estimate the corresponding value of $\hat{y}$ (denoted $\hat{y}_0$) from the line on the graph and from the estimated equation.
(e) Compute the standard deviation $S_{Y|x}$.
(f) Does the intercept $\hat{a}$ have a useful interpretation? Why or why not?

	White		African American	
bwt (Y)	gestation (x)	bwt (Y)	gestation (x)
3.84	282	2.66	244
2.89	266	2.89	272
3.13	259	3.05	284
3.77	252	3.21	272
2.66	248	2.55	221
4.02	290	3.66	292
4.55	286	3.63	280
3.78	248	2.77	222
2.56	227	3.11	268
3.33	269	2.34	216

1. For whites, the variable x is the days of gestation and Y is an infant's birth weight (measured in kilograms). Find $\hat{y}_0$ at $x_0 = 290$.

2. For African Americans, again the variable x is the days of gestation and Y is an infant's birth weight (measured in kilograms). Find $\hat{y}_0$ at $x_0 = 290$.

A study* was conducted to identify the relationship of risk factors in the development of gallstones. Gallstones are less common among males than females. Part of the study focused on the relationship of age and sex to bile acid synthesis. Partial results are given below for a group of 17 healthy non-obese adults.

		Males	Females
sample sizes	n	10	7
AGE			
means	$\bar{x}$	38.0	38.0
variances	S_X^2	188.9	200.0
BILE ACID SYNTHESIS			
means	$\bar{y}$	600.0	400.0
variances	S_Y^2	30411.1	11000.0
AGE/BILE			
covariances	S_{XY}	−1700.0	−1000.0

*Adapted from an article: *New England Journal of Medicine*.

(a) For male subjects:

3. Estimate a line summarizing the relationship between age and rate of bile acid synthesis.
4. Plot this estimated regression line.

(a) For the female patients:

5. Estimate a line summarizing the relationship between age and rate of bile acid synthesis.
6. Add this estimated regression line to the previous plot.
7. Construct a 95% confidence interval for the intercept (denoted a) for male subjects.
8. Is the rate of synthesis related to age in male subjects? Find the p-value.
9. Construct 95% confidence intervals for $E(Y \mid x_0)$ at $x_0 = 25$ and $x_0 = 65$ years for males.
10. Test the hypothesis that the intercept $a = 0$ for the females.
11. Find the 95% confidence interval for the slope b in the females.

The following data are two samples of San Francisco Bay Area commuters, smokers, and nonsmokers. The variable x represents the carbon monoxide concentration in expired air as measured by a laboratory test and Y represents the CO concentration in expired air as measured by a breath analyzer (similar to the method used to detect alcohol levels).

Smokers		Nonsmokers	
x	Y	x	Y
22	25	6	10
23	22	7	7
24	24	8	10
24	26	9	6
25	24	9	9
25	28	11	8
26	26	11	11
27	22	12	10
27	25	13	11
27	28	14	8

12. Estimate the regression line for smokers.
13. Estimate the regression line for nonsmokers.
14. Plot the points for both sets of data on the same axes and draw each estimated regression line.
15. Estimate the regression line for the combined (total) sample of 20 observations. Add this third estimated regression line to the previous plot.
16. Why are the results in (d) entirely different from (a) and (b)? When is it a good idea to combine the samples?

CHAPTER 9

Correlation

Informally, it is has long been known that "birds of a feather flock together." Formally, however, the statistical analysis of similarity began with Karl Pearson's creation of the correlation coefficient around the turn of the 20th century.

Linear regression analysis treats the independent variable as a nonrandom quantity that "explains" the dependent variable. For example, the volume of a fish tank x "explains" the size of the fish Y. There is a natural direction from x to Y. A correlation approach summarizes the relationship between two variables in a symmetric fashion where both have equal roles and both are random variables. For example, the relationship between the IQ of the first born child X and the IQ of the second born child Y has no natural direction from X to Y or from Y to X. A correlation coefficient, therefore, would be used to indicate the agreement between the two IQ scores. A number of similarities exist, as might be suspected, between simple linear regression (Chapter 8) and correlation analyses because both techniques are different kinds of assessments of the linear association between two variables.

Product-moment correlation

The estimated *correlation coefficient* (denoted r) measuring the degree of linear relationship between two random variables X and Y is estimated by

$$estimated\ correlation\ coefficient = r = \frac{\sum (x_i - \bar{x})(y_i - \bar{y})}{\sqrt{\sum (x_i - \bar{x})^2}\sqrt{\sum (y_i - \bar{y})^2}}$$

$$= \frac{S_{XY}}{S_X S_Y}$$

where again S_{XY} represents the estimated covariance between X and Y, S_X represents the estimated standard deviation associated with the distribution of X, and S_Y represents the estimated standard deviation associated with the distribution of Y. The estimate r is called the product-moment correlation coefficient or sometimes the Pearson correlation coefficient. The correlation coefficient, as with the slope of a line, is a standardized covariance producing a single statistical summary with a useful and sometimes elegant interpretation of the relationship between X and Y.

The value r is a sample estimate of the population correlation coefficient (denoted ρ) where

$$population\ correlation\ coefficient = \rho = \frac{\sigma_{XY}}{\sigma_X \sigma_Y}.$$

The product-moment correlation coefficient r is the estimate of ρ created by replacing the population standard deviations σ_X, σ_Y and covariance σ_{XY} in the definition of the population correlation coefficient with the corresponding sample estimates.

The standardization of the covariance (dividing by the standard deviations of X and Y) guarantees that r (or ρ) is always greater than or equal to -1 and less than or equal to $+1$ or

$$-1 \le r \le +1 \qquad \text{and} \qquad -1 \le \rho \le +1. \qquad \text{See Box 9.1.}$$

Box 9.1. Bounds on a Correlation Coefficient r

$$0 \le \sum \left[\frac{(x_i - \bar{x})}{S_X} + \frac{(y_i - \bar{y})}{S_Y} \right]^2$$

$$= \frac{1}{S_X^2} \sum (x_i - \bar{x})^2 + \frac{1}{S_Y^2} \sum (y_i - \bar{y})^2 + \frac{2}{S_X S_Y} \sum (x_i - \bar{x})(y_i - \bar{y})$$

$$= \frac{1}{S_X^2}(n-1)S_X^2 + \frac{1}{S_Y^2}(n-1)S_Y^2 + 2(n-1)r$$

$$= 2(n-1)(1+r) \qquad (n \text{ is the number of observations} \ge 1).$$

Therefore, $0 \le 2(n-1)(1+r)$ implies that $0 \le 1+r$ and $r \ge -1$. Similarly,

$$0 \le \sum \left[\frac{(x_i - \bar{x})}{S_X} - \frac{(y_i - \bar{y})}{S_Y} \right]^2 \qquad \text{yields } r \le 1.$$

Therefore, $-1 \le r \le 1$. A parallel argument applies to ρ, yielding $-1 \le \rho \le 1$.

An estimated correlation coefficient of $r = 1$ or $r = -1$ occurs when all sampled pairs of observations X and Y fall exactly on a straight line. A correlation of $r = 0$ indicates that a straight line is useless as a summary of the relationship between two variables. Other values of r measure the degree to which a straight line summarizes the relationship between X and Y. For example, a correlation coefficient of ± 0.9 indicates that the data generally have a linear pattern while a correlation coefficient of ± 0.1 indicates that the pattern of the data is not accurately summarized by a straight line.

Three "benchmark" values of the correlation coefficient (r close to 1, 0, and -1) are

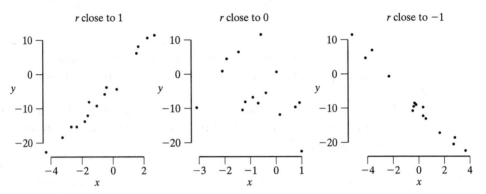

Two sets of points with the same sample correlation coefficient ($r = 0.5$).

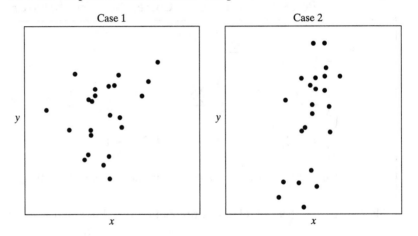

The interpretation of r, like any single summary of sampled observations, must be done cautiously. For example, the variables X and Y can have a large covariance as well as relatively large variances yielding a small value of r. On the other hand, a small covariance between variables X and Y with limited variability also can yield a small value of r. Since similar values of a correlation coefficient do not necessarily indicate similar underlying situations, it must be kept in mind that a correlation coefficient measures the degree of linear association between X and Y, but other influences are frequently relevant to its interpretation. Like all summary statistics, the correlation coefficient also does not tell the "whole story" but provides a summary description that frequently reflects essential features of the collected data.

The product-moment correlation coefficient does not depend on the units used to measure the variables X or Y. This valuable property expressed in symbols is

if $U = aX + b$ and $V = cY + d$, then $|r_{UV}| = |r_{XY}|$.   See Box 9.2.

Box 9.2. Invariance of Estimated Correlation Coefficient r

Let $U = aX + b$ and $V = cY + d$ where a, b, c, and d are constant values, then

$$r_{UV} = \frac{\sum (u_i - \bar{u})(v_i - \bar{v})}{\sqrt{\sum (u_i - \bar{u})^2}\sqrt{\sum (v_i - \bar{v})^2}}$$

$$= \frac{\sum [(ax_i + b) - (a\bar{x} + b)][(cy_i + d) - (c\bar{y} + d)]}{\sqrt{\sum [(ax_i + b) - (a\bar{x} + b)]^2}\sqrt{\sum [(cy_i + d) - (c\bar{y} + d)]^2}}$$

$$= \frac{ac \sum (x_i - \bar{x})(y_i - \bar{y})}{\sqrt{a^2 \sum (x_i - \bar{x})^2}\sqrt{c^2 \sum (y_i - \bar{y})^2}}$$

$$= \frac{ac \sum (x_i - \bar{x})(y_i - \bar{y})}{ac\sqrt{\sum (x_i - \bar{x})^2}\sqrt{\sum (y_i - \bar{y})^2}} = \frac{ac}{ac} r_{XY} = r_{XY}.$$

Thus, r_{UV} and r_{XY} are either equal or differ only in sign.

If X is measured in pounds and Y in inches, the correlation between X and Y is identical to the correlation between U measured in kilograms ($U = 2.205X$) and V measured in centimeters ($V = 0.394Y$). The correlation coefficient is a unitless value regardless of the units of the variables summarized.

A slope $\hat{b}$ measures the linear response in Y for a one-unit change in x while r measures the degree of the linear association between X and Y as a number between -1 and $+1$. The estimated correlation coefficient, nevertheless, is directly related to the estimated slope of a regression line. In symbols,

$$r = \hat{b}\frac{S_X}{S_Y}.$$ See Box 9.3.

Box 9.3. Relationship between r and $\hat{b}$

$$r = \frac{S_{XY}}{S_X S_Y} = \frac{S_{XY}}{S_X S_Y} \cdot \frac{S_X}{S_X} = \frac{S_{XY}}{S_X^2} \cdot \frac{S_X}{S_Y} = \hat{b} \cdot \frac{S_X}{S_Y}$$

The relationship between the correlation coefficient r and the estimated slope $\hat{b}$ shows why two correlation coefficients with similar values may reflect different underlying situations. The correlation r combines three quantities $(\hat{b}, S_X, S_Y)$ into a single summary value. For example, if $\hat{b} = 0.2$, $S_X = 1.0$, and $S_Y = 2.0$, then $r = 0.1$; however, if $\hat{b} = 4$, $S_X = 1.0$, and $S_Y = 40$, then the correlation coefficient remains the same $(r = 0.1)$. On the other hand, if $r = 0$, then necessarily $\hat{b} = 0$ and vice versa.

The similarities and differences between the estimated correlation coefficient r and the estimated slope $\hat{b}$ are contrasted for four rather extreme cases in Figure 9.1: (1) large $\hat{b}$ and large r, (2) large $\hat{b}$ and small r, (3) small $\hat{b}$ and large r, and (4) small $\hat{b}$ and small r.

Testing a correlation coefficient

Similar to the previous statistical tests, a null hypothesis generates the question: What is the likelihood that a particular value of the estimated correlation

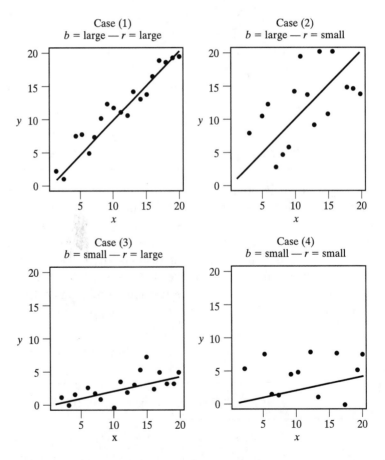

FIGURE 9.1: Four cases illustrating different possibilities for r and $\hat{b}$.

coefficient r occurs by chance alone when X and Y are not linearly related ($\sigma_{XY} = 0$ or $\rho = 0$ or $b = 0$)? A t-test is one way to assess the likelihood that an observed value of r reflects no more than random variation when the underlying value is zero.

Formally, the null and alternative hypotheses are

$$H_0\text{: } \rho = 0 \text{ or } X \text{ and } Y \text{ are not linearly related}$$

versus

$$H_1\text{: } \rho \neq 0 \text{ or } X \text{ and } Y \text{ are linearly related.}$$

For a t-test, like the previous t-tests, two basic requirements are necessary. The pairs of observations are required to be independently sampled. The independence of the sampled pairs (x_i, y_i) should not be confused with the issue of independence within each pair. It is exactly the within-pair relationship that a correlation coefficient is designed to measure. Also, the random variables X and Y must be sampled from a bivariate normal distribution. When these two requirements are met, a t-test applies (the generic form is given in Chapter 8).

An estimate of the variance of the distribution of the estimated correlation coefficient is needed to evaluate an estimate r with a t-test. Such an estimate of the variance is given by the expression

$$S_r^2 = \frac{1 - r^2}{n - 2}.$$

This estimated variance is derived under the assumption that the null hypothesis is true ($\rho = 0$). When $\rho \neq 0$, the variance of r is not estimated by S_r^2. A considerably more complex general expression exists (not given) but is not necessary because the t-test, as always, is conducted and interpreted as if the null hypothesis is true. The variance used as part of the test of a sample proportion is another example of a variance that is useful only when the null hypothesis is true (Chapter 6).

The test statistic T, under the null hypothesis of no linear association (H_0: $\rho = 0$), becomes

$$T = \frac{r - 0}{S_r} = \frac{r - 0}{\sqrt{(1 - r^2)/(n - 2)}}.$$

The components of the generic t-test expression (Chapter 8) are: $\hat{g} = r$, $g_0 = \rho = 0$, and $S_{\hat{g}} = S_r$. The possible values of the test statistic T are described by Student's t-distribution with $n - 2$ degrees of freedom when no linear association exists between variables labeled X and Y ($\rho = 0$).

This version of a *t*-test is identical to the *t*-test used to assess the null hypothesis that the slope of a regression line is zero (H_0: $b = 0$—Chapter 8). In symbols,

$$T = \frac{r - 0}{S_r} = \frac{\hat{b} - 0}{S_{\hat{b}}}.$$ See Box 9.4.

The two identical *t*-tests address the identical question: Does a straight line with a nonzero slope ($\rho \neq 0$ or $b \neq 0$) reflect a linear relationship between variables X and Y, at least to some extent?

Box 9.4. T-test of r and $\hat{b}$

$$T = \frac{\hat{b} - 0}{S_{\hat{b}}} = \frac{\hat{b}}{\sqrt{\dfrac{S^2_{Y\,|\,x}}{\sum(x_i - \bar{x})^2}}} = \frac{\hat{b}\sqrt{\sum(x_i - \bar{x})^2}}{\sqrt{\dfrac{\sum(y_i - \hat{y})^2}{n - 2}}}$$

$$= \frac{\hat{b}\sqrt{\sum(x_i - \bar{x})^2} \Big/ \sqrt{\sum(y_i - \bar{y})^2}}{\sqrt{\dfrac{\sum(y_i - \hat{y})^2}{n - 2}} \Big/ \sqrt{\sum(y_i - \bar{y})^2}}$$

$$= \frac{\hat{b}\dfrac{S_X}{S_Y}}{\sqrt{\dfrac{\sum(y_i - \bar{y})^2 - \hat{b}\sum(x_i - \bar{x})(y_i - \bar{y})}{\sum(y_i - \bar{y})^2}} \Big/ (n - 2)}$$

$$= \frac{r}{\sqrt{\left[1 - \dfrac{\left[\sum(x_i - \bar{x})(y_i - \bar{y})\right]^2}{\sum(x_i - \bar{x})^2 \sum(y_i - \bar{y})^2}\right] \Big/ (n - 2)}}$$

$$= \frac{r}{\sqrt{(1 - r^2)/(n - 2)}} = \frac{r - 0}{S_r}$$

Inferences about a correlation coefficient ρ (estimated by r) are, therefore, the same as inferences about a slope b (estimated by $\hat{b}$) with regard to the impact of random variation. Or, when the observed value of the estimated correlation coefficient r is unlikely to have occurred by chance (small p-value), the slope $\hat{b}$ estimated from the same data is equally unlikely to have occurred by chance (same small p-value).

EXAMPLE

A correlation coefficient provides a summary of the linear relationship between height and weight for a sample of $n = 10$ five-year-old children (from a large child development study[2]—Chapter 1) where

Height (in inches)—X	40.9	44.0	44.1	44.6	42.5	46.3	43.3	46.2	43.9	43.0

$\bar{X} = 43.9$

Weight (in pounds)—Y	35.2	40.7	46.5	39.2	44.0	50.2	45.0	48.0	42.2	37.0

$\bar{Y} = 42.8$

The three components necessary to estimate the correlation coefficient are

$$\sum (x_i - \bar{x})^2 = 23.716 \qquad (S_X^2 = 2.635),$$

$\frac{\sum (x_i - \bar{x})^2}{n-1}$

$$\sum (y_i - \bar{y})^2 = 210.900 \qquad (S_Y^2 = 23.433)$$

$\frac{\sum (y_i - \bar{y})^2}{n-1}$

and

$$\sum (x_i - \bar{x})(y_i - \bar{y}) = 52.750 \qquad (S_{XY} = 5.861).$$

$1.87 \quad 14.52$ $\frac{}{n-1} \longrightarrow$

The estimated correlation coefficient becomes

$$r = \frac{S_{XY}}{S_x S_Y} = \frac{52.750}{\sqrt{23.716}\sqrt{210.900}} = \frac{5.861}{\sqrt{2.635}\sqrt{23.433}} = 0.746.$$

No reason exists for assigning height as X and weight as Y; the reverse yields the same estimate and analysis. Parenthetically, the correlation also equals 0.746 when height is measured in centimeters and weight in kilograms.

Although the estimate $r = 0.746$ is large (close to 1), the impact of sampling variation is potentially a factor because the sample size is small ($n = 10$). To assess the possibility that a more extreme estimated correlation coefficient ($|r| \geq 0.746$) would occur by chance alone, when in fact height and weight are not linearly related, a t-test of the hypothesis $\rho = 0$ is helpful. The null hypothesis and an alternative hypothesis are

$$H_0: \rho = 0 \qquad \text{versus} \qquad H_1: \rho \neq 0.$$

Select $\alpha = 0.05$, then $t_{0.975} = 2.306$ (from a t-distribution with degrees of freedom $= n - 2 = 8$) yields the two-tail critical region of $T \leq -2.306$ and

$T \geq 2.306$. The test statistic is

$$T = \frac{0.746 - 0}{\sqrt{[1 - (0.746)^2]/8}} = 3.167.$$

The null hypothesis is rejected because $T = 3.167$ falls within the critical region ($2.306 < 3.167$), implying that the estimate $r = 0.746$ is unlikely a result of random variation alone. To further evaluate the null hypothesis, since $P(T \geq 3.167 \,|\, \rho = 0)$ is 0.007, the two tail p-value $= P(|T| \geq 3.138 \,|\, \rho = 0) = 0.007 + 0.007 = 0.01$. Based on a small sample of five-year-old children, both the α-level test and the p-value indicate that a straight line ($b \neq 0$) is likely an effective summary of the relationship between height and weight. ∎

A short cut

The expression for the t-test of $\rho = 0$ can be solved for the smallest value of r necessary to reject the null hypothesis of no linear relationship. Continuing the height/weight example, when the sample size is $n = 10$, a value (denoted r_c) can be calculated such that all estimated values of r more extreme than r_c (c for critical point) give a t-value greater than $t_{0.975} = 2.306$ or less than $t_{0.025} = -2.306$ and, therefore, all such values of r lead to rejecting H_0. More concisely, if $|r|$ exceeds $r_c = 0.632$, then $|T|$ exceeds 2.306 (Box 9.5).

Box 9.5. The Relationship between $t_{1-\alpha/2}$ and r_c

If

$$|T| = \frac{|r|}{\sqrt{(1 - r^2)/(n - 2)}} \geq t_{1-\alpha/2},$$

the null hypothesis is rejected (T is found in one of the two tails of an α-level critical region). Therefore, H_0 is rejected when

$$r^2(n - 2) \geq (1 - r^2)t^2_{1-\alpha/2} \quad \text{or} \quad r^2(t^2_{1-\alpha/2} + n - 2) \geq t^2_{1-\alpha/2}$$

or, when

$$|r| \geq \frac{t_{1-\alpha/2}}{\sqrt{t^2_{1-\alpha/2} + n - 2}} = r_c.$$

That is, when $|r| > r_c$, then $|T| > t_{1-\alpha/2}$ and, conversely.

Specifically, for an estimated correlation coefficient based on a sample of 10 observations (degrees of freedom $= 8$)

$$r_c = \frac{t_{0.975}}{\sqrt{t_{0.975}^2 + n - 2}} = \frac{2.306}{\sqrt{(2.306)^2 + 8}} = 0.632$$

and the estimate $|r|$ has a probability (p-value) of less than 0.05 of exceeding 0.632 by chance alone when no linear association exists. In symbols, for $n = 10$, then $P(|r| \geq 0.632 \mid \rho = 0) = P(|T| \geq 2.306 \mid \rho = 0)$. Because the estimated correlation coefficient $r = 0.746$ exceeds $r_c = 0.632$ ($r \geq r_c$), it is likely that a straight line is not a misleading description of the weight and height relationship for these five-year-old children, as noted before.

Values of r_c for testing $\rho = 0$ are given in Table A.4 (two-tail tests) listed by degrees of freedom, not sample sizes. Instead of calculating a value of T, the observed value r is simply compared to the table value of r_c to test H_0: $\rho = 0$ at a selected significance level. The table values are no more than redefining a t-test into a more convenient form to evaluate the values of r.

EXAMPLE

For a sample of $n = 20$ observations, any estimated correlation coefficient $|r|$ that exceeds $r_c = 0.444$ is declared significantly different from zero (5% level). Or, any value of $|r|$ less than 0.444 lacks sufficient evidence to declare the measured association substantially different from zero (again at the 5% level). The value $r_c = 0.444$ comes from Table A.4 but, in fact, is calculated entirely from a sample size ($n = 20$) and a t-value ($t_{0.975} = 2.101$ with 18 degrees of freedom) producing $r_c = 2.101/\sqrt{(2.101)^2 + 18} = 0.444$. ∎

Confidence interval for a correlation coefficient

Previously $(1 - \alpha)$-level confidence intervals were constructed from estimates that had at least approximate normal distributions. Such estimates as $\bar{x}$, $\hat{p}$, $\hat{b}$, and $\hat{y}_0$ (all weighted averages) usually have at least approximate normal distributions leading directly to the calculation of approximate $(1 - \alpha)$-level confidence intervals. Because the estimated correlation coefficient r is bounded between -1 and $+1$ and is not a weighted average, it typically does not have even an approximate normal distribution, making it necessary to modify the usual approach to constructing a confidence interval. The influence of this lack of normality is minimal when the correlation is close to zero but is more of an issue as ρ differs from zero, becoming particularly acute for values of ρ approaching $+1$ or -1. Figure 9.2 illustrates, showing the asymmetric probability distribution describing the possible values of the estimated correlation coefficient r when $\rho = 0.5$ and

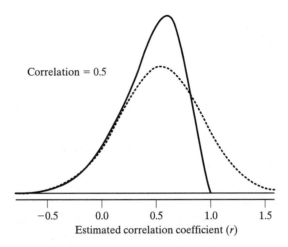

Correlation = 0.5

−0.5	0.0	0.5	1.0	1.5

Estimated correlation coefficient (r)

FIGURE 9.2: The probability distribution describing the estimated correlation coefficient r (solid line) and the approximate normal distribution of the transformed value s (dotted line) when $\rho = 0.5$ and $n = 20$.

$n = 20$. In addition, an easily calculated estimate of the variance of r is only readily available when ρ is zero.

To construct a confidence interval based on the estimate r, for the underlying correlation coefficient ρ, a transformation is used. When r is transformed to s where

$$s = \tfrac{1}{2} \log \left(\frac{1+r}{1-r} \right),$$

the value s has an approximate normal probability distribution with mean $= E(S) = \tfrac{1}{2} \log[(1 + \rho)/(1 - \rho)]$ and variance $= \sigma_S^2 = 1/(n - 3)$. For example, for $\rho = 0.5$ and $n = 20$ observations, the possible values of variable s are described by an approximate normal distribution with an expected value of $E(S) = \tfrac{1}{2} \log(1.5/0.5) = 0.549$ and variance of $1/17 = 0.059$ (dotted line—Figure 9.2).

The transformation of the sample correlation coefficient from r to the value s enables the determination of probabilities associated with an observed value of s directly and accurately using a normal distribution and, therefore, the probabilities associated with r itself. This transformation is used primarily to construct confidence intervals for ρ. It can also be used to test various hypotheses about ρ (H_0: $\rho = \rho_0$). A null hypothesis that generates a value of ρ other than zero, however, is only rarely encountered in practice.

The demonstration that this rather complex transformation has surprisingly simple statistical properties is beyond the scope of this text and is found elsewhere.[30] Nevertheless, the properties are familiar. The transformed value s has (1) an approximate normal distribution, with (2) a mean value of $E(S) = \tfrac{1}{2} \log[(1 + \rho)/(1 - \rho)]$, which can be determined by postulating values of ρ, and

(3) a standard deviation of $\sigma_S = 1/\sqrt{n-3}$ entirely determined by the sample size n. These three properties make the construction of a confidence interval based on the estimate s straightforward. An approximate $(1-\alpha)$-level confidence interval is, as usual, $s \pm z_{1-\alpha/2}\sigma_S$ (Chapter 5).

EXAMPLE

Suppose a sample of $n = 20$ pairs of observations yields an estimated correlation coefficient of $r = 0.7$, then $s = \frac{1}{2}\log[(1+0.7)/(1-0.7)] = 0.867$. The value of s is then a single observation from an approximate normal distribution with standard deviation $= \sigma_S = 1/\sqrt{n-3} = 1/\sqrt{17} = 0.243$ (Figure 9.2). Constructed from the observed value of $s = 0.867$, an approximate 95% confidence interval for $E(S)$ is $0.867 \pm 1.960(0.243)$ or $(0.392, 1.343)$. ∎

The confidence interval for $E(S)$ is not of much interest but it is the first step in constructing a confidence interval for ρ. An approximate $(1-\alpha)\%$ confidence interval for ρ based on r follows the previous pattern (Chapters 5 and 6) but requires a bit of algebraic manipulation. As always, from a standard normal distribution,

$$P(z_{\alpha/2} \leq Z \leq z_{1-\alpha/2}) = 1 - \alpha$$

and the fact that the random variable S has an approximate normal distribution means that

$$P(-z_{1-\alpha/2} \leq \frac{s - E(S)}{\sigma_S} \leq z_{1-\alpha/2}) = 1 - \alpha$$

or, as before (Chapter 5),

$$P(s - z_{1-\alpha/2}\sigma_S \leq E(S) \leq s + z_{1-\alpha/2}\sigma_S) = 1 - \alpha.$$

Now, the estimated confidence bounds are

$$\hat{A} = lower\ bound = s - z_{1-\alpha/2}\sigma_S = \frac{1}{2}\log\left(\frac{1+r}{1-r}\right) - z_{1-\alpha/2}\frac{1}{\sqrt{n-3}}$$

and

$$\hat{B} = upper\ bound = s + z_{1-\alpha/2}\sigma_S = \frac{1}{2}\log\left(\frac{1+r}{1-r}\right) + z_{1-\alpha/2}\frac{1}{\sqrt{n-3}},$$

where $\hat{A}$ and $\hat{B}$ form the bounds of an approximate $(1-\alpha)$-level confidence interval for the mean of the normal distribution $E(S)$ based on the observed value s and a sample size n. In symbols,

$$P(\hat{A} \le E(S) \le \hat{B}) = P\left[\hat{A} \le \tfrac{1}{2}\log\left(\frac{1+\rho}{1-\rho}\right) \le \hat{B}\right] = 1 - \alpha$$

where $\hat{A}$ and $\hat{B}$ are estimated entirely from the sampled observations.

Algebraically manipulating the confidence interval limits for $E(S)$ so that ρ is bounded by upper and lower limits yields an approximate $(1-\alpha)\%$ confidence interval for ρ based on the sample generated limits $\hat{A}$ and $\hat{B}$. The result is

$$P\left[\frac{e^{2\hat{A}} - 1}{e^{2\hat{A}} + 1} \le \rho \le \frac{e^{2\hat{B}} - 1}{e^{2\hat{B}} + 1}\right] = 1 - \alpha.$$

Therefore, the estimated confidence interval bounds are

$$lower\ bound = \frac{e^{2\hat{A}} - 1}{e^{2\hat{A}} + 1}$$

and

$$upper\ bound = \frac{e^{2\hat{B}} - 1}{e^{2\hat{B}} + 1}$$

and these bounds form an approximate $(1-\alpha)\%$ confidence interval for ρ, based on the estimate r.

The estimated endpoints for this approximate confidence interval for ρ are a bit tedious to calculate. Charts are created to avoid this calculation and also show the relationship between the estimate r and the confidence interval bounds for selected sample sizes n. Such a chart is found in Appendix (Chart A.6). As anticipated, the confidence interval becomes narrower as the sample size n increases (values of $n = 4, 5, 6, 10 \cdots 400$—A.6). Perhaps less anticipated, the length of the confidence interval is widest when $\rho = 0$ and becomes smaller as values of ρ approach -1 or $+1$ for all sample sizes.

EXAMPLE

For the previous height and weight data, the estimate $r = 0.746$ for $n = 10$ five-year-old children, the approximate 95% confidence interval is

lower bound $= \hat{A} = 0.22$ from the chart A.6 in the appendix

upper bound $= \hat{B} = 0.94$ from the chart A.6 in the appendix.

More exactly, using $r = 0.746$ gives $s = 0.964$, producing a symmetric confidence interval for $E(S)$ based on the normal distribution of $(\hat{A}, \hat{B}) =$

(0.223, 1.704). From these bounds, the estimated endpoints for an approximate 95% confidence interval for ρ become (0.219, 0.936). The 95% confidence interval clearly shows the considerable impact of sampling variation on the estimate r based on only 10 observations. ∎

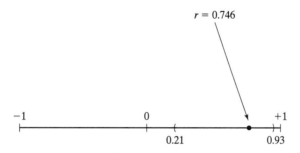

The confidence interval for ρ, unlike the previously encountered intervals, is not symmetric around the estimated value r. The interpretation, nevertheless, is the same. There exists an approximate $1 - \alpha$ probability that the underlying population correlation coefficient ρ, estimated by the sample correlation coefficient r, is between the estimated interval bounds (between 0.219 and 0.936, for example). As always, the estimated confidence interval varies from sample to sample, not the parameter ρ.

The role of a correlation coefficient in linear regression

The Pearson correlation coefficient takes on a rich meaning in the context of simple linear regression analysis. The key role of the estimated correlation coefficient r in a regression analysis context arises from the comparison of two sums of squared values, namely $\sum(y_i - \hat{y}_i)^2$ and $\sum(y_i - \overline{y})^2$, called, as before, the *residual sum of squares* and the *total sum of squares*, respectively. The difference between these two sums of squares is a simple function of the estimated correlation coefficient. Specifically, the total sum of squares multiplied by $1 - r^2$ equals the residual sum of squares or

$$\sum(y_i - \overline{y})^2(1 - r^2) = \sum(y_i - \hat{y}_i)^2 \qquad \text{see Box 9.6.}$$

From another point of view, the same expression shows that r^2 is a proportional decrease in the comparison of these two sum of squares, or

$$r^2 = \frac{\sum(y_i - \overline{y})^2 - \sum(y_i - \hat{y}_i)^2}{\sum(y_i - \overline{y})^2}.$$

Box 9.6. Relationship between a Correlation Coefficient and Regression Residual Sum of Squares

$$\sum (y_i - \hat{y}_i)^2 = \sum (y_i - [\hat{a} + \hat{b}x_i])^2$$

$$= \sum ([y_i - \bar{y}] - \hat{b}[x_i - \bar{x}])^2$$

$$= \sum (y_i - \bar{y})^2 - 2\hat{b} \sum (y_i - \bar{y})(x_i - \bar{x}) + \hat{b}^2 \sum (x_i - \bar{x})^2$$

$$= \sum (y_i - \bar{y})^2 - 2r^2 \sum (y_i - \bar{y})^2 + r^2 \sum (y_i - \bar{y})^2$$

$$= \sum (y_i - \bar{y})^2 (1 - r^2)$$

since $\hat{b} \sum (x_i - \bar{x})(y_i - \bar{y}) = \hat{b}^2 \sum (x_i - \bar{x})^2 = r^2 \sum (y_i - \bar{y})^2$.

The two sums of squared deviations differ because of the way the mean values $\hat{y}_i$ and $\bar{y}$ are estimated. For the residual sum of squares $\sum (y_i - \hat{y}_i)^2$, the values $\hat{y}_i$ are estimated from the least square estimated line $\hat{y}_i = \hat{a} + \hat{b}x_i$ based entirely on the values of x_i. That is, the sample mean $\hat{y}_i$ estimates the population mean $E(Y \mid x_i) = a + bx_i$. For the total sum of squares $\sum (y_i - \bar{y})^2$, the mean value $\bar{y}$ is estimated entirely without regard to the values of x. That is, the sample mean $\bar{y}$ estimates the population mean $E(Y)$. The difference between these two sums of squares directly reflects the influence of the variable x on the dependent variable Y. That is, the comparison of these two sums of squares measures the effectiveness of the independent variable x to "explain" the dependent variable Y using a linear regression equation. The word "explain" is in quotes because the correlation coefficient only applies to a linear relationship as an "explanation" and other nonlinear "explanations" could also accurately describe the relationship between X and Y.

When a straight line based on x is absolutely useless in predicting the values of Y ($b = 0$), then $\sum (y_i - \hat{y}_i)^2$ equals $\sum (y_i - \bar{y})^2$ (Chapter 8). When a straight line based on x perfectly predicts the value of Y, then $y_i = \hat{y}_i$ and $\sum (y_i - \hat{y}_i)^2$ equals zero. In terms of a correlation coefficient, when a straight line is absolutely useless, $r^2 = 0$ (r equals 0) and when a straight line perfectly predicts Y, $r^2 = 1$ (r equals $+1$ or -1). Between these two extremes, the quantity r^2 measures the proportional reduction in the total sum of squares $\sum (y_i - \bar{y})^2$ associated with accounting for the linear influence of the variable x. For example, if $r = 0.7$, then the reduction in variability associated with Y, achieved by using a straight line that incorporates values of x to estimate the values Y ($\hat{y}_i$), is $r^2 = (0.7)^2 = 0.49$ or about 50%.

The squared correlation coefficient r^2 indicates the proportion of the variability of the dependent variable Y "explained" by the independent variable x

and, conversely, $1 - r^2$ indicates the proportion not "explained" by using a straight line to summarize the relationship between x and Y. The squared Pearson correlation coefficient, therefore, answers the question: *How important is the variable* x *in "explaining" the variation in the variable* Y *using the least squares estimated line* $\hat{y}_i = \hat{a} + \hat{b} x_i$?

Maybe the simplest interpretation of the correlation coefficient r in the context of a linear regression analysis comes from a specific application of the fact that the *correlation* $(ax + b, cy + d) = correlation(x, y) = r$ (Box 9.2). An estimated regression line is the linear function $\hat{y} = \hat{a} + \hat{b} x$ of x; therefore,

$$correlation(\hat{y}, y) = correlation(\hat{a} + \hat{b} x, y) = correlation(x, y) = r.$$

In words, an estimated correlation coefficient summarizes the degree of linear relationship between the estimated values $\hat{y}$ (based strictly on the independent variables x) and the observed values y. The value r indicates how well a value y can be predicted from a value x. Once again the estimate r summarizes the effectiveness of using a straight line based on x to describe the dependent variable Y.

There is one last note on the interpretation of a Pearson correlation coefficient. A small or zero value of r does not imply that two variables are unrelated. A correlation coefficient in the neighborhood of zero means that two values are not linearly related, but the possibility remains that X and Y are related in a nonlinear fashion. The following extreme case illustrates:

X	0	2	4	6	8
Y	16	4	0	4	16

giving $r = 0$, but $Y = (X - 4)^2$, certainly showing that X and Y are related.

Rank correlation coefficient

Pearson's product-moment correlation coefficient is frequently calculated from pairs of specific kinds of variables and treated as a "new" correlation coefficient. One such example occurs when the observed values are replaced by their ranks. The Pearson correlation coefficient applied to ranks is called the *Spearman rank correlation coefficient*.

EXAMPLE

The previous data on height and weight of five-year-old children can be ranked and a Pearson correlation coefficient calculated using these ranks in place of the original observed values. The observation 40.9 inches is the smallest sampled height and is ranked 1; 42.5 inches is the next largest and is ranked 2; $\cdots$ and 46.3 inches is the largest value and is ranked 10. The observed weights are similarly ranked. All 10 pairs of observations and their ranks are

Height
(in inches)—X   40.9 44.0 44.1 44.6 42.5 46.3 43.3 46.2 43.9 43.0
rank x_i 1   6   7   8   2   10   4   9   5   3

Weight
(in pounds)—Y   35.2 40.7 46.5 39.2 44.0 50.2 45.0 48.0 42.2 37.0
rank y_i 1   4   8   3   6   10   7   9   5   2

The value of Spearman's correlation coefficient is found by calculating r in the usual way but using the ranks instead of the actual data values (denoted r_S—S for Spearman). Applying this process to the height/weight ranks gives

$$\sum(x_i - \bar{x})^2 = 82.5 \qquad \sum(y_i - \bar{y})^2 = 82.5 \quad \text{and}$$

$$\sum(x_i - \bar{x})(y_i - \bar{y}) = 54.5 \text{ making}$$

$$r_S = \frac{\sum(x_i - \bar{x})(y_i - \bar{y})}{\sqrt{\sum(x_i - \bar{x})^2}\sqrt{\sum(y_i - \bar{y})^2}} = \frac{54.5}{\sqrt{82.5}\sqrt{82.5}} = 0.661.$$

The product moment correlation coefficient is $r = 0.746$. ∎

Four reasons for using a Spearman rank correlation r_S instead of the product-moment correlation r are:

1. The data may not consist of numeric measurements. It is possible to rank observations that cannot be measured on a numeric scale. Two experts, for example, can rank bottles of wine by quality of the taste (a nonnumeric but ordinal scale) and the degree of agreement summarized by a rank correlation coefficient.

2. A rank correlation is not highly affected by large nonstatistical errors (outliers). For example, if the observed weight 48 lbs was accidentally recorded as 84 lbs, the rank correlation decreases from 0.661 to 0.648 (a 2% decrease), where the product-moment correlation decreases from 0.746 to 0.669 (a 10% decrease). As with the median value, a rank correlation coefficient minimizes the impact of extreme observations.

3. A rank correlation can be calculated with a simple computational formula. The rank correlation (r_S) is easily found using the expression

$$r_S = 1 - \frac{6\sum d_i^2}{n(n^2 - 1)} \qquad \text{see Box 9.7.}$$

where $d_i = rank\ y_i - rank\ x_i$ and n equals the number of pairs of observations (x_i, y_i).

To illustrate, consider again the height/weight data. The differences d_i between ranks are:

Pair	1	2	3	4	5	6	7	8	9	10	Total
d_i	0	−2	1	−5	4	0	3	0	0	−1	0
d_i^2	0	4	1	25	16	0	9	0	0	1	56

Since $n = 10$, then $r_S = 1 - 6(56)/[10(10^2 - 1)] = 0.661$, as before.

4. The estimated variance and the t-test associated with testing $\rho = 0$ using Pearson's correlation coefficient r depends on the assumption that X and Y come from a bivariate normal distribution. Once the sampled values are replaced with their ranks, the original distribution of the observed values is no longer relevant to any subsequent calculations. The properties of sampled population do not influence the estimation or assessment of a rank correlation coefficient. For example, whatever the mean and the variance of the sampled population, the mean and variance of n ranks are always $(n + 1)/2$ and $(n^2 - 1)/12$ (Chapter 4). Exact tests of a rank correlation coefficient, nevertheless, exist and require only that the pairs of observations are sampled independently.

The first three reasons for using a rank correlation coefficient are not as important as the last. The fact that an exact statistical test exists regardless of the properties of the parent distribution sampled is the primary reason a rank correlation is valuable. A Spearman rank correlation coefficient is, therefore, frequently called a *nonparametric* or *distribution-free* measure of association. A cost, however, is incurred. There is a slight loss of statistical efficiency when the data are replaced by their ranks. Of more importance, when the data are sampled from a bivariate normal distribution, the Pearson correlation coefficient is statistically optimum and is related to linear regression, providing an efficient summary with a sophisticated interpretation of the xy-relationship. The rank correlation coefficient r_S has no such interpretation. It is simply a single summary value bounded between -1 and $+1$ reflecting the degree of agreement between two sets of ranks.

To test the hypothesis that random variables X and Y are not associated, values of r_S (calculated from the ranked data) are compared to tabled values. If the absolute value of the rank correlation r_S exceeds the tabled value (denoted r_C—C for critical point), then the null hypothesis is rejected (H_0: no association exists between ranked values of X and Y) in favor of the alternative hypothesis (H_1: an association exists). Selected values of r_C are given in Table A.5 for two-tail tests for sample sizes 5 to 30. The values r_C for each sample size are not calculated but are found from a computer-generated list of all possible rank

---

Box 9.7. Computational form of r_S

1. $\sum x_i = \sum i = n(n+1)/2$ and $\bar{x} = (n+1)/2$

2. $\sum y_i = \sum i = n(n+1)/2$ and $\bar{y} = (n+1)/2$

3. $\sum x_i^2 = \sum y_i^2 = \dfrac{n(n+1)(2n+1)}{6}$ (a result from algebra)

4. $\sum(x_i - \bar{x})^2 = \sum x_i^2 - \left(\sum x_i\right)^2 / n = \dfrac{n(n+1)(2n+1)}{6}$

$$- \dfrac{(n(n+1)/2)^2}{n} = \dfrac{n(n^2-1)}{12} \quad \text{(Chapter 3)}$$

Also, $\sum(y_i - \bar{y})^2 = n(n^2 - 1)/12$ because the y-ranks are the same as the x-ranks.
Additionally,

5. $\sum d_i^2 = \sum(x_i - y_i)^2 = \sum x_i^2 - 2\sum x_i y_i + \sum y_i^2$

then $\sum x_i y_i = \dfrac{1}{2}\left[\sum x_i^2 + \sum y_i^2 - \sum d_i^2\right]$.

Therefore,

$$r_S = \frac{\sum x_i y_i - \sum x_i \sum y_i / n}{\sqrt{\sum x_i^2 - \left(\sum x_i\right)^2 / n}\sqrt{\sum y_i^2 - \left(\sum y_i\right)^2 / n}}$$

$$= \frac{\left[\dfrac{n(n+1)(2n+1)}{6} - \dfrac{\sum d_i^2}{2}\right] - ([n(n+1)/2]^2)/n}{\sqrt{\dfrac{n(n^2-1)}{12}}\sqrt{\dfrac{n(n^2-1)}{12}}}$$

$$= \frac{\dfrac{n(n^2-1)}{12} - \dfrac{\sum d_i^2}{2}}{\dfrac{n(n^2-1)}{12}} = 1 - \frac{6\sum d_i^2}{n(n^2-1)}.$$

correlations coefficients. A more complete explanation of how tables such as A.5 are constructed is a topic for a more extensive discussion of nonparametric statistics.[31] For a sample size n greater than 30, the table for testing the Pearson correlation coefficient (Table A.4) can be used since only small differences exist between the tabled values for the tests of r ($df = n - 2$) and r_S for moderately large sample sizes ($r_c \approx r_C$). For example, when $n = 20$, $r_c = 0.378$ (95%—Table A.4), and $r_C = 0.377$ (95%—Table A.5). In general, as the sample size increases ($n > 30$), the distinctions between a rank correlation (r_S) and a Pearson correlation coefficient (r) become less and less.

EXAMPLE

Continuing the height/weight example, a rank correlation of $|r_S|$ greater $r_C = 0.636$ (Table A.5; $\alpha = 0.05$ for a two-tail alternative) is necessary to reject the null hypothesis of no association based on $n = 10$ pairs of ranked observations. Because $|r_S| = 0.661 > 0.636$, the null hypothesis is rejected. It is inferred that chance is not a plausible explanation for a Spearman rank correlation as large as 0.661 when no association exists between height and weight (H_0) and likely indicates an underlying systematic association between height and weight reflected in the sample of five-year-old children. ∎

Correlation in a 2 by 2 table

The ϕ-correlation (read "phi-correlation") measures the degree of the association between two variables when both variables take on only two alternatives (coded as 0 and 1). The association between two binary variables was explored previously by applying a chi-square test to counts contained in a 2 by 2 table (Chapter 7). A chi-square statistic, however, is not a summary measure of an association.

EXAMPLE

Suppose two binary variables X and Y record the presence and absence of two specific species of insects where

$$x_i = \begin{cases} 0 & \textit{absence of species A} \\ 1 & \textit{presence of species A} \end{cases}$$

and

$$y_i = \begin{cases} 0 & \textit{absence of species B} \\ 1 & \textit{presence of species B} \end{cases}$$

describe the ith-observation (pair). The question to be investigated is whether species A associates with species B (perhaps, it is suspected that A is a predator of B). Eighteen observations from different locations are

Locations	1	2	3	4	5	6	7	8	9	10	11	12	13	14
species A (X)	0	1	0	1	1	0	1	0	1	0	1	1	1	0
species B (Y)	0	1	0	0	1	0	0	0	1	1	1	0	0	1

Locations	15	16	17	18
species A (X)	0	1	1	1
species B (Y)	0	1	0	1

The same $n = 18$ pairs of binary observations classified into a 2 by 2 table give

	Presence of B $(Y = 1)$	Absence of B $(Y = 0)$	Total
presence of A $(X = 1)$	6	5	11
absence of A $(X = 0)$	2	5	7
Total	8	10	18

The following summary statistics are calculated directly from either the pairs of observations or the counts in the 2 by 2 table:

$$\sum x_i = 11 \quad \sum x_i^2 = 11 \quad \sum y_i = 8 \quad \sum y_i^2 = 8 \quad \sum x_i y_i = 6$$

$$\sum (x_i - \bar{x})^2 = \sum x_i^2 - \left(\sum x_i\right)^2 / n$$

$$= 11 - (11)^2/18 = \frac{11}{18}(18 - 11) = \frac{(11)(7)}{18}$$

$$\sum (y_i - \bar{y})^2 = \sum y_i^2 - \left(\sum y_i\right)^2 / n$$

$$= 8 - (8)^2/18 = \frac{8}{18}(18 - 8) = \frac{(8)(10)}{18}$$

$$\sum (x_i - \bar{x})(y_i - \bar{y}) = \sum x_i y_i - \sum x_i \sum y_i / n = 6 - (11)(8)/18$$

$$= \frac{(18)(6) - 8(11)}{18}$$

since x_i is either a one or zero and y_i is also either a one or zero. Again, using the product-moment expression produces a specialized correlation coefficient summarizing the relationship between two binary variables (denoted r_ϕ). Applying the expression for the Pearson correlation coefficient gives

$$r_\phi = \frac{\sum (x_i - \bar{x})(y_i - \bar{y})}{\sqrt{\sum (x_i - \bar{x})^2}\sqrt{\sum (y_i - \bar{y})^2}} = \frac{[(18)(6) - 8(11)]/18}{\sqrt{(11)(7)/18}\sqrt{(8)(10)/18}} = 0.255. \quad \blacksquare$$

In general, for n pairs of binary variables classified into a 2 by 2 table,

	$Y = 1$	$Y = 0$	Total
$X = 1$	f_{11}	f_{12}	n_1
$X = 0$	f_{21}	f_{22}	n_2
Total	m_1	m_2	n

the ϕ-correlation coefficient is

$$r_\phi = \frac{\sum (x_i - \bar{x})(y_i - \bar{y})}{\sqrt{\sum (x_i - \bar{x})^2}\sqrt{\sum (y_i - \bar{y})^2}} = \frac{f_{11} f_{22} - f_{12} f_{21}}{\sqrt{n_1 n_2}\sqrt{m_1 m_2}}. \qquad \text{See Box 9.8.}$$

As all Pearson correlation coefficients, the value of r_ϕ is bounded between -1 and $+1$, or $-1 \le r_\phi \le 1$. The expression for r_ϕ is again no more than Pearson's product-moment correlation coefficient expression applied to a specific kind of data.

Continuing the insect example, the ϕ-correlation expression yields a summary measure of the association between species A and B and, as required,

$$r_\phi = \frac{(6)(5) - (2)(5)}{\sqrt{(11)(7)}\sqrt{(8)(10)}} = 0.255.$$

The chi-square test of the association between the binary variables X and Y classified into a 2 by 2 table (Chapter 7) is directly related to the calculated value r_ϕ. Specifically, the transformation

$$nr_\phi^2 = \frac{n(f_{11} f_{22} - f_{12} f_{21})^2}{m_1 m_2 n_1 n_2} = X^2$$

has a chi-square distribution with one degree of freedom when no association exists (Chapter 7). For the example data, $r_\phi = 0.255$, then $nr_\phi^2 = 18(0.255)^2 = 1.169$, which has a chi-square distribution with one degree of freedom when the presence and absence of species A and B are unrelated. The corresponding p-value is $P(X^2 \ge 1.169 \mid no\ association) = 0.28$, which is directly calculated from nr_ϕ^2 and, therefore, is also exactly the probability that applies to the correlation coefficient r_ϕ. Thus, $P(|r_\phi| \ge 0.255 \mid no\ association) = 0.28$.

Box 9.8. Computational form of r_ϕ

1. $\sum x_i = \sum x_i^2 = n_1$ $\sum y_i = \sum y_i^2 = m_1$ $\sum x_i y_i = f_{11}$

2. $\sum (x_i - \bar{x})^2 = \sum x_i^2 - \left(\sum x_i\right)^2/n = n_1 - n_1^2/n = \dfrac{n_1}{n}(n - n_1) = \dfrac{n_1 n_2}{n}$

3. $\sum (y_i - \bar{y})^2 = \sum y_i^2 - \left(\sum y_i\right)^2/n = m_1 - m_1^2/n = \dfrac{m_1}{n}(n - m_1) = \dfrac{m_1 m_2}{n}$

4. $\sum (x_i - \bar{x})(y_i - \bar{y}) = \sum x_i y_i - \sum x_i \sum y_i/n = f_{11} - n_1 m_1/n$

$$= \frac{1}{n}(n f_{11} - n_1 m_1) = \frac{1}{n}(f_{11} f_{22} - f_{12} f_{21})$$

Applying the results 1–4, then

$$r_\phi = \frac{\sum (x_i - \bar{x})(y_i - \bar{y})}{\sqrt{\sum (x_i - \bar{x})^2}\sqrt{\sum (y_i - \bar{y})^2}} = \frac{f_{11} f_{22} - f_{12} f_{21}}{\sqrt{n_1 n_2}\sqrt{m_1 m_2}}.$$

The ϕ-correlation, like most statistical summaries, plays a dual role in describing the properties of a data set. A ϕ-correlation provides a summary value between -1 and $+1$ reflecting the degree of association within a 2 by 2 table. Additionally, it can be transformed into a test statistic to produce a significance probability (p-value), which reflects the plausibility of the conjecture that no association exists between the two binary variables. As with the rank correlation, this measure of association is not related to linear regression.

Point biserial correlation coefficient

Another special application of the Pearson product-moment correlation coefficient to a specific kind of data is called a *point biserial correlation coefficient*. This application involves one variable that is binary and another that is continuous. For example, a group might be divided into two categories (for example, male or female, or $X = 0$ or $X = 1$) and within each group a variable Y is measured (for example, $Y =$ the final score in a statistics class—Chapter 6).

The notation is

	X	Observations (Y)	Total numbers	Mean values
group 1	$X = 0$	$y_{11}, y_{12}, \cdots, y_{1n_1}$	n_1	$\bar{y}_1$
group 2	$X = 1$	$y_{21}, y_{22}, \cdots, y_{2n_2}$	n_2	$\bar{y}_2$

For the measurement denoted y_{ij}, the first subscript indicates one of the two categories (for group 1, $i = 1$ and for group 2, $i = 2$). The second subscript identifies different individual observations within each category. The data displayed as pairs of observations would look like

Group $= 1$ $X = 0$	Group $= 2$ $X = 1$
$(0, y_{11})$	$(1, y_{21})$
$(0, y_{12})$	$(1, y_{22})$
.	.
.	.
.	.
$(0, y_{1n_1})$	$(1, y_{2n_2})$

There are a total of $n_1 + n_2 = n$ pairs and the overall mean of the y-observations is a weighted average of the two group mean values or $\bar{y} = \sum\sum y_{ij}/n = (n_1\bar{y}_1 + n_2\bar{y}_2)/n$.

The point biserial correlation coefficient (denoted r_{pb}) is

$$r_{pb} = \frac{\sum\sum(x_{ij} - \bar{x})(y_{ij} - \bar{y})}{\sqrt{\sum\sum(x_{ij} - \bar{x})^2}\sqrt{\sum\sum(y_{ij} - \bar{y})^2}}$$

$$= \frac{\bar{y}_2 - \bar{y}_1}{\sqrt{\sum\sum(y_{ij} - \bar{y})^2}}\sqrt{\frac{n_1 n_2}{n}}. \qquad \text{See Box 9.9.}$$

Because this correlation coefficient is again a special case of the Pearson product-moment correlation coefficient, the estimated value r_{pb} is bounded between -1 and $+1$.

Box 9.9. Point Biserial Correlation Coefficient r_{pb}

1. $\sum x_i = \sum x_i^2 = n_2$ ($x_i = 0$ or 1) and $\sum\sum(x_{ij} - \bar{x})^2 = n_2 n_1/n$

2. $\sum\sum x_i y_{ij} = 0 \cdot y_{11} + \cdots + 0 \cdot y_{1n_1} + 1 \cdot y_{21} + \cdots + 1 \cdot y_{2n_2}$

$$= \sum y_{2j} = n_2 \bar{y}_2$$

3. $\sum\sum y_{ij}/n = \bar{y}$

4. $\sum\sum(x_{ij} - \bar{x})(y_i - \bar{y}) = n_2\bar{y}_2 - n_2\bar{y} = n_2\bar{y}_2 - n_2(n_1\bar{y}_1 + n_2\bar{y}_2)/n$

$$= n_1 n_2 (\bar{y}_2 - \bar{y}_1)/n$$

Applying results 1–4, then

$$r_{pb} = \frac{\sum\sum(x_{ij} - \bar{x})(y_i - \bar{y})}{\sqrt{\sum\sum(x_{ij}-\bar{x})^2}\sqrt{\sum\sum(y_{ij}-\bar{y})^2}} = \frac{n_1 n_2(\bar{y}_2 - \bar{y}_1)}{n\sqrt{n_1 n_2/n}\sqrt{\sum\sum(y_{ij}-\bar{y})^2}}$$

$$= \frac{n_1 n_2(\bar{y}_2 - \bar{y}_1)}{\sqrt{n(n_1 n_2)}\sqrt{\sum\sum(y_{ij}-\bar{y})^2}} = \frac{\bar{y}_2 - \bar{y}_1}{\sqrt{\sum\sum(y_{ij}-\bar{y})^2}}\sqrt{\frac{n_2 n_1}{n}}$$

EXAMPLE

For the male/female statistics class data (Chapter 6), again

male scores: $\bar{y}_1 = 85.738$ from the $n_1 = 37$ male student scores,

female scores: $\bar{y}_2 = 89.400$ from $n_2 = 30$ female student scores,

and $\sum\sum(y_{ij} - \bar{y})^2 = 8172.076$ from $n = n_1 + n_2 = 67$ observations. The point biserial correlation coefficient is then

$$r_{pb} = \frac{(89.400 - 85.738)}{\sqrt{8172.076}}\sqrt{\frac{(37)(30)}{67}} = 0.165. \qquad \blacksquare$$

Like the rank correlation and ϕ-correlation coefficients, the identical point biserial correlation could have been calculated directly from the 67 pairs of observations using the Pearson expression directly.

As with the ϕ-correlation, the point biserial correlation coefficient r_{pb} is a specific function of a test statistic. The t-test of the difference between two mean values (Chapter 6) is related to the point biserial correlation coefficient. This relationship is

$$T = \frac{\bar{y}_2 - \bar{y}_1}{\sqrt{S_{pooled}^2 \left(\dfrac{1}{n_1} + \dfrac{1}{n_2} \right)}}$$

$$= \frac{r_{pb}}{\sqrt{(1 - r_{pb}^2)/(n - 2)}}$$ (Box 9.4 contains a parallel argument).

For example, when $r_{pb} = 0.165$, then

$$T = \frac{r_{pb}}{\sqrt{(1 - r_{pb}^2)/(n - 2)}} = \frac{0.165}{\sqrt{[1 - (0.165)^2]/65}} = 1.348$$

and the test statistic T has a t-distribution with $n - 2 = 67 - 2 = 65$ degrees of freedom when no association exists between the sex and exam score. The identical T-value can be calculated directly from the two-sample t-test approach (Chapter 6).

A point biserial correlation t-test has the same form as the product-moment correlation coefficient t-test. Therefore, Table A.4 equally provides the critical points for estimates r_{pb}. For example, for the male and female exam scores the degrees of freedom are $n_1 + n_2 - 2 = 65$, making the critical point $r_c = 0.240$ (that is, $r_c = 1.997/\sqrt{(1.977)^2 + 65} = 0.240$ where $t_{0.975} = 1.977$). For samples with less than 30 observations, critical points can be read directly from Table A.4. Since the observed correlation $|r_{pb}| = 0.165$ is less than 0.240, the null hypothesis not rejected. The values represented by X (sex) and Y (scores) that produce the correlation $r_{pb} = 0.165$ show no strong evidence of a linear association. To repeat, this process of comparing the estimated value r_{pb} to r_c is exactly the same as performing a two-tail t-test comparing two mean values calculated from normally distributed data sampled from two independent populations.

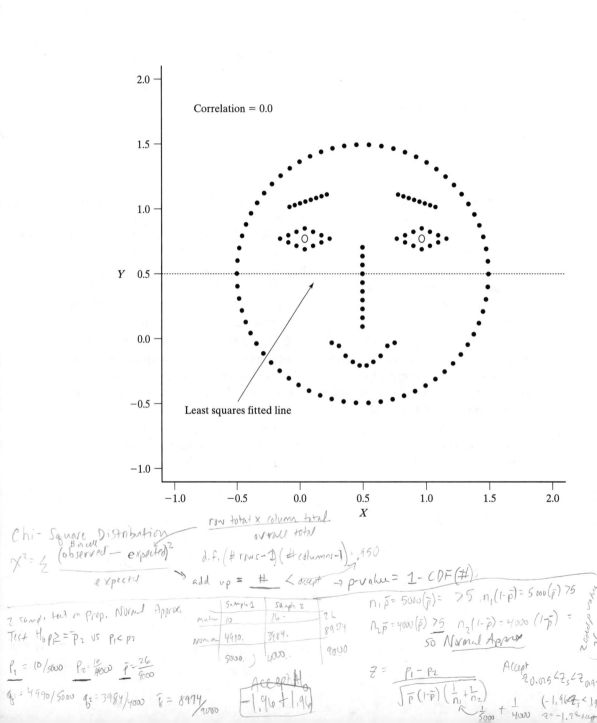

Correlation = 0.0

Y   0.5

Least squares fitted line

X

Chi- Square Distribution

$\chi^2 = \sum \dfrac{(\text{observed} - \text{expected})^2}{\text{expected}}$ # in cell

$\dfrac{\text{row total} \times \text{column total}}{\text{overall total}}$

d.f. $(\text{\# rows} - 1)(\text{\# columns} - 1) = .950$

add up = __#__ < accept → p-value = $1 - CDF(\text{\#})$

2 sample test on Prop. Normal Approx

Test $H_0 \, p_1 \geq = \bar{p}_2$ vs $p_1 < p_2$

	Sample 1	Sample 2	
mutur	10	16	26
Normal	4990.	3984.	8974
	5000.)	4000.	9000

$n_1 \bar{p} = 5000(\bar{p}) = \; > 5 \;, \; n_1(1-\bar{p}) = 5000(\bar{p}) \; 75$

$n_2 \bar{p} = 4000(\bar{p}) \; 75 \quad n_2(1-\bar{p}) = 4000 (1-\bar{p}) =$

so Normal Approx

$P_1 = 10/5000 \quad P_2 = \dfrac{10}{4000} \quad \bar{p} = \dfrac{26}{9000}$

$q_1 = 4990/5000 \quad q_2 = 3984/4000 \quad \hat{q} = 8974/9000$

Accept H_0

$\boxed{-1.96 \; +1.96}$

$Z = \dfrac{P_1 - P_2}{\sqrt{\bar{p}(1-\bar{p})\left(\dfrac{1}{n_1} + \dfrac{1}{n_2}\right)}}$

Accept $-z_{0.025} < z_s < z_{0.975}$

$(-1.96 < z_s < 1.96)$

$z = -1.78$ accept

PROBLEM SET 9

$z = \frac{x - \mu}{\sigma}$

A sample of $n = 12$ birth weights (grams) of fraternal (dizygotic) unlike sex twins are:

males: 2850, 2530, 2590, 2130, 3180, 2730, 3040, 2270, 2360, 2440, 2820, 3130

$\rho = \frac{y_1 + y_2}{n_1 + n_2} = \#$

females: 2140, 2531, 2580, 2370, 3220, 2970, 3080, 2820, 2690, 2470, 2280, 3000.

1. Calculate the Pearson correlation coefficient (r).
2. Test the hypothesis that $\rho = 0$.

$\# \times n > 5$
use N.A.

3. Construct a 95% confidence interval based on the estimated value of r.
4. Ten applications for graduate school were ranked by two faculty members:

Normal App
need $\bar{x}$, $\frac{\sigma}{n}$

1 sample t-test

Application	Rank given by Dr. S	Rank given by Dr. J
A	6	7
B	10	8
C	5	5
D	1	4
E	7	6
F	2	3
G	8	9
H	9	10
I	3	1
J	4	2

① Look up $t_{.975} @ n-1$
② $-t < \frac{\bar{x} - \mu_0}{s \sqrt{n}} < t$
③ multiply $-t$ and t by $s.e.$
④ Subtract $\bar{x}$ from both $t + -t$
⑤ multiply by -1 $-\mu$
    $t - \mu < t \rightarrow = \mu_0$ $\angle$ be twen those

find

$t = \dfrac{\bar{x} - \mu_0}{\left(\frac{s}{\sqrt{n}}\right) \cdot s.e.}$

P-value → $2 CDF \left(\frac{entire}{answer}\right) =$

Calculate the rank correlation coefficient and test the conjecture of no association at $\alpha = 0.05$.

5. The following samples are weights of five-year-olds from a study* of growth in children. Assess the evidence of an association between weight and sex at $\alpha = 0.05$ using both a point biserial correlation coefficient and a two-sample t-test ($x = 0$ for males and $x = 1$ for females).

Goodness Poisson ratio χ^2 / $Y_i \{\ln(y_i) - \ln(\hat{y})\}$

1 sample test on proportions

① Point estimate of $\pi = p = \frac{\mathscr{L}_{well}}{n}$ happen in a given total

Subject	Sex	Weight (in kilograms)
1	1	36.1
2	0	29.5
3	1	30.1
4	0	33.2
5	1	49.5
6	1	44.9
7	0	30.9
8	0	40.7
9	0	35.5
10	1	33.1

N eggs N nm2

0	5
1	3
2	1
3	1
4	0

$1\{\ln(1) - \ln(\hat{y})\} = \#$ $\times 3$
$2\{\ln(2) - \ln(\hat{y})\} = \#$ $\times 1$
3

compute mean $= \bar{y}$

② 95% C.L. for π
   If $N\hat{\pi} > 5 \cdot N(1-\hat{\pi}) > 5$ use N.A.

$z_s = \dfrac{p - \pi_o}{\sqrt{\dfrac{\pi_o(1-\pi_o)}{n}}}$ ← .5 → true proportion
   solve

③ $\hat{\pi} \pm z_{.975} \sqrt{\dfrac{\pi(1-\pi)}{n}}$

$\dfrac{\pi_o(1-\pi_o)}{n}$

$z = \dfrac{x - .5^n}{\sqrt{n \cdot .5(1-.5)}}$ 2 given #'s $= \bar{x} \pm \#$

④ Plug in $\dfrac{n - .5^n}{\sqrt{.5(1-.5)} \cdot n} = \#$

$\rightarrow$ p-value $= 2 CDF \# = $ if pvalue is less than reject
if pvalue > 0.05 accept H_0

$2\left(\frac{\#}{}\right) = \underline{\quad}$

p-value $= 1 - CDF$ chi-square $(.05, \underline{\quad})$

*Adapted from: R. Tuddenham and M. Snyder: *Physical Growth of California Boys and Girls from Birth to Eighteen Years.*

Binomial Test

$\pi\% = \#\left(\frac{1}{2}\right) = <$ if use bino

p-value $= 2 CDF$ (1)
$2(Pr(0) + Pr(1)) = 2C$

$F = \dfrac{S_1^2}{S_2^2} = $ testing equality of variances

$\dfrac{1}{2} \dfrac{S_1^2}{S_2^2}$ p-value $2[1 - CDF_{F\#, \#}(\#)]$
accept $ST.D.$
if $> .05$ Reject equal variance

6. The following data on the occurrence of hip fractures in women were collected during a study in Kensington, N.Y.

Age group	No hip fracture	Hip fracture	Total
45–65	4276	41	4317
over 65	2549	36	2585
Total	6825	77	6902

Calculate the phi-correlation coefficient to measure the association between age group and hip fractures in older women. Test the hypothesis that no association exists between age and hip fracture status (find the p-value).

Home health care is an alternative to institutional care for elderly patients who can look after themselves. The data below give the length of stay in the home health program for 10 patients and the mean cost-per-day per patient to the program.

Patient	Length of stay (days)	Average cost per day (dollars)
1	10	64.50
2	150	15.25
3	143	10.21
4	25	32.75
5	132	16.92
6	65	37.50
7	118	10.75
8	129	33.50
9	70	25.35
10	92	20.52

7. Plot these data. Do you expect a correlation coefficient greater or less than zero? Why?
8. What correlation coefficient is most appropriate? Why? Calculate it.
9. Test for evidence of an association; select $\alpha = 0.05$.

A P P E N D I X   A

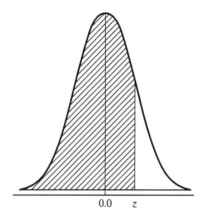

TABLE A.1: Normal Distribution

z	Area	z	Area	z	Area	z	Area	Area	z
−2.500	0.006	−1.250	0.106	0.000	0.500	1.250	0.894	0.0001	−3.719
−2.475	0.007	−1.225	0.110	0.025	0.510	1.275	0.899	0.0010	−3.090
−2.450	0.007	−1.200	0.115	0.050	0.520	1.300	0.903	0.0050	−2.576
−2.425	0.008	−1.175	0.120	0.075	0.530	1.325	0.907	0.0100	−2.326
−2.400	0.008	−1.150	0.125	0.100	0.540	1.350	0.911	0.0150	−2.170
−2.375	0.009	−1.125	0.130	0.125	0.550	1.375	0.915	0.0200	−2.054
−2.350	0.009	−1.100	0.136	0.150	0.560	1.400	0.919	0.0250	−1.960
−2.325	0.010	−1.075	0.141	0.175	0.569	1.425	0.923	0.0500	−1.645
−2.300	0.011	−1.050	0.147	0.200	0.579	1.450	0.926	0.0750	−1.440
−2.275	0.011	−1.025	0.153	0.225	0.589	1.475	0.930	0.1000	−1.282
−2.250	0.012	−1.000	0.159	0.250	0.599	1.500	0.933	0.1250	−1.150
−2.225	0.013	−0.975	0.165	0.275	0.608	1.525	0.936	0.1500	−1.036
−2.200	0.014	−0.950	0.171	0.300	0.618	1.550	0.939	0.1750	−0.935
−2.175	0.015	−0.925	0.177	0.325	0.627	1.575	0.942	0.2000	−0.842

TABLE A.1: (*continued*)

z	Area	z	Area	z	Area	z	Area	Area	z
−2.150	0.016	−0.900	0.184	0.350	0.637	1.600	0.945	0.2250	−0.755
−2.125	0.017	−0.875	0.191	0.375	0.646	1.625	0.948	0.2500	−0.674
−2.100	0.018	−0.850	0.198	0.400	0.655	1.650	0.951	0.2750	−0.598
−2.075	0.019	−0.825	0.205	0.425	0.665	1.675	0.953	0.3000	−0.524
−2.050	0.020	−0.800	0.212	0.450	0.674	1.700	0.955	0.3250	−0.454
−2.025	0.021	−0.775	0.219	0.475	0.683	1.725	0.958	0.3500	−0.385
−2.000	0.023	−0.750	0.227	0.500	0.691	1.750	0.960	0.3750	−0.319
−1.975	0.024	−0.725	0.234	0.525	0.700	1.775	0.962	0.4000	−0.253
−1.950	0.026	−0.700	0.242	0.550	0.709	1.800	0.964	0.4250	−0.189
−1.925	0.027	−0.675	0.250	0.575	0.717	1.825	0.966	0.4500	−0.126
−1.900	0.029	−0.650	0.258	0.600	0.726	1.850	0.968	0.4750	−0.063
−1.875	0.030	−0.625	0.266	0.625	0.734	1.875	0.970	0.5000	0.000
−1.850	0.032	−0.600	0.274	0.650	0.742	1.900	0.971	0.5250	0.063
−1.825	0.034	−0.575	0.283	0.675	0.750	1.925	0.973	0.5500	0.126
−1.800	0.036	−0.550	0.291	0.700	0.758	1.950	0.974	0.5750	0.189
−1.775	0.038	−0.525	0.300	0.725	0.766	1.975	0.976	0.6000	0.253
−1.750	0.040	−0.500	0.309	0.750	0.773	2.000	0.977	0.6250	0.319
−1.725	0.042	−0.475	0.317	0.775	0.781	2.025	0.979	0.6500	0.385
−1.700	0.045	−0.450	0.326	0.800	0.788	2.050	0.980	0.6750	0.454
−1.675	0.047	−0.425	0.335	0.825	0.795	2.075	0.981	0.7000	0.524
−1.650	0.049	−0.400	0.345	0.850	0.802	2.100	0.982	0.7250	0.598
−1.625	0.052	−0.375	0.354	0.875	0.809	2.125	0.983	0.7500	0.674
−1.600	0.055	−0.350	0.363	0.900	0.816	2.150	0.984	0.7750	0.755
−1.575	0.058	−0.325	0.373	0.925	0.823	2.175	0.985	0.8000	0.842
−1.550	0.061	−0.300	0.382	0.950	0.829	2.200	0.986	0.8250	0.935
−1.525	0.064	−0.275	0.392	0.975	0.835	2.225	0.987	0.8500	1.036
−1.500	0.067	−0.250	0.401	1.000	0.841	2.250	0.988	0.8750	1.150
−1.475	0.070	−0.225	0.411	1.025	0.847	2.275	0.989	0.9000	1.282
−1.450	0.074	−0.200	0.421	1.050	0.853	2.300	0.989	0.9250	1.440
−1.425	0.077	−0.175	0.431	1.075	0.859	2.325	0.990	0.9500	1.645
−1.400	0.081	−0.150	0.440	1.100	0.864	2.350	0.991	0.9750	1.960
−1.375	0.085	−0.125	0.450	1.125	0.870	2.375	0.991	0.9800	2.054
−1.350	0.089	−0.100	0.460	1.150	0.875	2.400	0.992	0.9850	2.170
−1.325	0.093	−0.075	0.470	1.175	0.880	2.425	0.992	0.9900	2.326
−1.300	0.097	−0.050	0.480	1.200	0.885	2.450	0.993	0.9950	2.576
−1.275	0.101	−0.025	0.490	1.225	0.890	2.475	0.993	0.9990	3.090
−1.250	0.106	0.000	0.500	1.250	0.894	2.500	0.994	0.9999	3.719

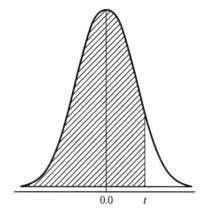

0.0 t

TABLE A.2: t-distribution

$df/area$	0.750	0.900	0.950	0.975	0.990	0.995	0.999
1	1.000	3.078	6.314	12.706	31.821	63.657	318.309
2	0.816	1.886	2.920	4.303	6.965	9.925	22.327
3	0.765	1.638	2.353	3.182	4.541	5.841	10.215
4	0.741	1.533	2.132	2.776	3.747	4.604	7.173
5	0.727	1.476	2.015	2.571	3.365	4.032	5.893
6	0.718	1.440	1.943	2.447	3.143	3.707	5.208
7	0.711	1.415	1.895	2.365	2.998	3.499	4.785
8	0.706	1.397	1.860	2.306	2.896	3.355	4.501
9	0.703	1.383	1.833	2.262	2.821	3.250	4.297
10	0.700	1.372	1.812	2.228	2.764	3.169	4.144
11	0.697	1.363	1.796	2.201	2.718	3.106	4.025
12	0.695	1.356	1.782	2.179	2.681	3.055	3.930
13	0.694	1.350	1.771	2.160	2.650	3.012	3.852
14	0.692	1.345	1.761	2.145	2.624	2.977	3.787
15	0.691	1.341	1.753	2.131	2.602	2.947	3.733
16	0.690	1.337	1.746	2.120	2.583	2.921	3.686
17	0.689	1.333	1.740	2.110	2.567	2.898	3.646
18	0.688	1.330	1.734	2.101	2.552	2.878	3.610
19	0.688	1.328	1.729	2.093	2.539	2.861	3.579
20	0.687	1.325	1.725	2.086	2.528	2.845	3.552
21	0.686	1.323	1.721	2.080	2.518	2.831	3.527
22	0.686	1.321	1.717	2.074	2.508	2.819	3.505
23	0.685	1.319	1.714	2.069	2.500	2.807	3.485
24	0.685	1.318	1.711	2.064	2.492	2.797	3.467
25	0.684	1.316	1.708	2.060	2.485	2.787	3.450
26	0.684	1.315	1.706	2.056	2.479	2.779	3.435
27	0.684	1.314	1.703	2.052	2.473	2.771	3.421

TABLE A.2: (*continued*)

$df/area$	0.750	0.900	0.950	0.975	0.990	0.995	0.999
28	0.683	1.313	1.701	2.048	2.467	2.763	3.408
29	0.683	1.311	1.699	2.045	2.462	2.756	3.396
30	0.683	1.310	1.697	2.042	2.457	2.750	3.385
31	0.682	1.309	1.696	2.040	2.453	2.744	3.375
32	0.682	1.309	1.694	2.037	2.449	2.738	3.365
33	0.682	1.308	1.692	2.035	2.445	2.733	3.356
34	0.682	1.307	1.691	2.032	2.441	2.728	3.348
35	0.682	1.306	1.690	2.030	2.438	2.724	3.340
36	0.681	1.306	1.688	2.028	2.434	2.719	3.333
37	0.681	1.305	1.687	2.026	2.431	2.715	3.326
38	0.681	1.304	1.686	2.024	2.429	2.712	3.319
39	0.681	1.304	1.685	2.023	2.426	2.708	3.313
40	0.681	1.303	1.684	2.021	2.423	2.704	3.307
50	0.679	1.299	1.676	2.009	2.403	2.678	3.261
60	0.679	1.296	1.671	2.000	2.390	2.660	3.232
70	0.678	1.294	1.667	1.994	2.381	2.648	3.211
80	0.678	1.292	1.664	1.990	2.374	2.639	3.195
90	0.677	1.291	1.662	1.987	2.368	2.632	3.183
100	0.677	1.290	1.660	1.984	2.364	2.626	3.174
200	0.676	1.286	1.653	1.972	2.345	2.601	3.131
500	0.675	1.283	1.648	1.965	2.334	2.586	3.107
1000	0.675	1.282	1.646	1.962	2.330	2.581	3.098
10000	0.675	1.282	1.645	1.960	2.327	2.576	3.091

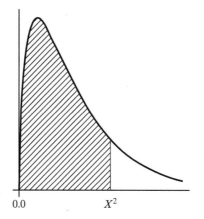

0.0 X^2

$0.05 < p\text{-value} < 0.1$

yes

less than accept

TABLE A.3: Chi-square Distribution

df/area	0.025	0.050	0.500	0.800	0.900	0.950	0.975	0.990
1	0.001	0.004	0.455	1.642	2.706	3.841	5.024	6.635
2	0.051	0.103	1.386	3.219	4.605	5.991	7.378	9.210
3	0.216	0.352	2.366	4.642	6.251	7.815	9.348	11.345
4	0.484	0.711	3.357	5.989	7.779	9.488	11.143	13.277
5	0.831	1.145	4.351	7.289	9.236	11.070	12.833	15.086
6	1.237	1.635	5.348	8.558	10.645	12.592	14.449	16.812
7	1.690	2.167	6.346	9.803	12.017	14.067	16.013	18.475
8	2.180	2.733	7.344	11.030	13.362	15.507	17.535	20.090
9	2.700	3.325	8.343	12.242	14.684	16.919	19.023	21.666
10	3.247	3.940	9.342	13.442	15.987	18.307	20.483	23.209
11	3.816	4.575	10.341	14.631	17.275	19.675	21.920	24.725
12	4.404	5.226	11.340	15.812	18.549	21.026	23.337	26.217
13	5.009	5.892	12.340	16.985	19.812	22.362	24.736	27.688
14	5.629	6.571	13.339	18.151	21.064	23.685	26.119	29.141
15	6.262	7.261	14.339	19.311	22.307	24.996	27.488	30.578
16	6.908	7.962	15.338	20.465	23.542	26.296	28.845	32.000
17	7.564	8.672	16.338	21.615	24.769	27.587	30.191	33.409
18	8.231	9.390	17.338	22.760	25.989	28.869	31.526	34.805
19	8.907	10.117	18.338	23.900	27.204	30.144	32.852	36.191
20	9.591	10.851	19.337	25.037	28.412	31.410	34.170	37.566
21	10.283	11.591	20.337	26.171	29.615	32.671	35.479	38.932
22	10.982	12.338	21.337	27.301	30.813	33.924	36.781	40.289
23	11.689	13.091	22.337	28.429	32.007	35.172	38.076	41.638
24	12.401	13.848	23.337	29.553	33.196	36.415	39.364	42.980
25	13.120	14.611	24.337	30.675	34.382	37.652	40.646	44.314
26	13.844	15.379	25.336	31.795	35.563	38.885	41.923	45.642

(#rows −1)(#columns −1)

TABLE A.3: (*continued*)

df/area	0.025	0.050	0.500	0.800	0.900	0.950	0.975	0.990
27	14.573	16.151	26.336	32.912	36.741	40.113	43.195	46.963
28	15.308	16.928	27.336	34.027	37.916	41.337	44.461	48.278
29	16.047	17.708	28.336	35.139	39.087	42.557	45.722	49.588
30	16.791	18.493	29.336	36.250	40.256	43.773	46.979	50.892
31	17.539	19.281	30.336	37.359	41.422	44.985	48.232	52.191
32	18.291	20.072	31.336	38.466	42.585	46.194	49.480	53.486
33	19.047	20.867	32.336	39.572	43.745	47.400	50.725	54.776
34	19.806	21.664	33.336	40.676	44.903	48.602	51.966	56.061
35	20.569	22.465	34.336	41.778	46.059	49.802	53.203	57.342
36	21.336	23.269	35.336	42.879	47.212	50.998	54.437	58.619
37	22.106	24.075	36.336	43.978	48.363	52.192	55.668	59.892
38	22.878	24.884	37.335	45.076	49.513	53.384	56.896	61.162
39	23.654	25.695	38.335	46.173	50.660	54.572	58.120	62.428
40	24.433	26.509	39.335	47.269	51.805	55.758	59.342	63.691
41	25.215	27.326	40.335	48.363	52.949	56.942	60.561	64.950
42	25.999	28.144	41.335	49.456	54.090	58.124	61.777	66.206
43	26.785	28.965	42.335	50.548	55.230	59.304	62.990	67.459
44	27.575	29.787	43.335	51.639	56.369	60.481	64.201	68.710
45	28.366	30.612	44.335	52.729	57.505	61.656	65.410	69.957
46	29.160	31.439	45.335	53.818	58.641	62.830	66.617	71.201
47	29.956	32.268	46.335	54.906	59.774	64.001	67.821	72.443
48	30.755	33.098	47.335	55.993	60.907	65.171	69.023	73.683
49	31.555	33.930	48.335	57.079	62.038	66.339	70.222	74.919
50	32.357	34.764	49.335	58.164	63.167	67.505	71.420	76.154
60	40.482	43.188	59.335	68.972	74.397	79.082	83.298	88.379
70	48.758	51.739	69.334	79.715	85.527	90.531	95.023	100.425
80	57.153	60.391	79.334	90.405	96.578	101.879	106.629	112.329

TABLE A.4: Values for Testing Correlations (conversion of t-values)

$df/area$	0.900	0.950	0.975	0.990
2	0.800	0.900	0.950	0.980
3	0.687	0.805	0.878	0.934
4	0.608	0.729	0.811	0.882
5	0.551	0.669	0.754	0.833
6	0.507	0.621	0.707	0.789
7	0.472	0.582	0.666	0.750
8	0.443	0.549	0.632	0.715
9	0.419	0.521	0.602	0.685
10	0.398	0.497	0.576	0.658
11	0.380	0.476	0.553	0.634
12	0.365	0.458	0.532	0.612
13	0.351	0.441	0.514	0.592
14	0.338	0.426	0.497	0.574
15	0.327	0.412	0.482	0.558
16	0.317	0.400	0.468	0.543
17	0.308	0.389	0.456	0.529
18	0.299	0.378	0.444	0.516
19	0.291	0.369	0.433	0.503
20	0.284	0.360	0.423	0.492
21	0.277	0.352	0.413	0.482
22	0.271	0.344	0.404	0.472
23	0.265	0.337	0.396	0.462
24	0.260	0.330	0.388	0.453
25	0.255	0.323	0.381	0.445
26	0.250	0.317	0.374	0.437
27	0.245	0.311	0.367	0.430
28	0.241	0.306	0.361	0.423
29	0.237	0.301	0.355	0.416
30	0.233	0.296	0.349	0.409
31	0.229	0.291	0.344	0.403
32	0.225	0.287	0.339	0.397
33	0.222	0.283	0.334	0.392
34	0.219	0.279	0.329	0.386
35	0.216	0.275	0.325	0.381
36	0.213	0.271	0.320	0.376
37	0.210	0.267	0.316	0.371
38	0.207	0.264	0.312	0.367
39	0.204	0.260	0.308	0.362
40	0.202	0.257	0.304	0.358

TABLE A.4: (*continued*)

df/area	0.900	0.950	0.975	0.990
50	0.181	0.231	0.273	0.322
60	0.165	0.211	0.250	0.295
70	0.153	0.195	0.232	0.274
80	0.143	0.183	0.217	0.257
90	0.135	0.173	0.205	0.242
100	0.128	0.164	0.195	0.230
200	0.091	0.116	0.138	0.164
500	0.057	0.073	0.088	0.104
1000	0.041	0.052	0.062	0.073
10000	0.013	0.016	0.020	0.023

TABLE A.5: Values for Testing Rank Correlations

n/area	0.950	0.990
5	0.900	—
6	0.829	0.943
7	0.714	0.893
8	0.643	0.833
9	0.600	0.783
10	0.564	0.745
11	0.523	0.736
12	0.497	0.703
13	0.475	0.745
14	0.457	0.716
15	0.441	0.623
16	0.425	0.601
17	0.412	0.582
18	0.399	0.564
19	0.388	0.549
20	0.377	0.534
21	0.368	0.521
22	0.359	0.508
23	0.351	0.496
24	0.343	0.485
25	0.336	0.475
26	0.329	0.465
27	0.323	0.456
28	0.317	0.448
29	0.311	0.440
30	0.305	0.432

Chart A.6: 95% Confidence intervals for a correlation coefficient

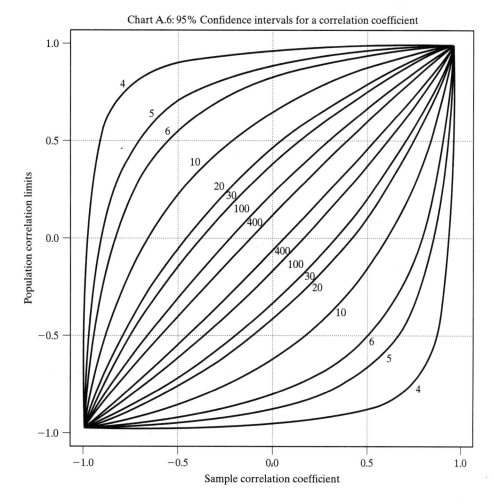

A P P E N D I X   B

B.1 SUMMATION NOTATION

A sum of a series of values can be tedious to represent especially when more than a few values are involved, making a notation that symbolizes the entire process useful. The Greek letter capital *sigma* denotes the process of summation or

$$\sum_{i=1}^{n}$$

where i indicates the starting point and n indicates the last term of the sum. The symbol following the sigma ($\sum$) represents the variable summed. For example,

$$\sum_{i=1}^{5} x_i = x_1 + x_2 + x_3 + x_4 + x_5$$

or

$$\sum_{i=1}^{3} c_i = c_1 + c_2 + c_3.$$

Rules for summation notation:

(i) $\displaystyle\sum_{i=1}^{n} ax_i = a \sum_{i=1}^{n} x_i$ *distributive law*

Example: $\displaystyle\sum_{i=1}^{4} ax_i = ax_1 + ax_2 + ax_3 + ax_4 = a(x_1 + x_2 + x_3 + x_4) = a \sum_{i=1}^{4} x_i$

(ii) $\displaystyle\sum_{i=1}^{n}(x_i + y_i) = \sum_{i=1}^{n} x_i + \sum_{i=1}^{n} y_i$ *associative law*

Example: $\displaystyle\sum_{i=1}^{3}(x_i + y_i) = (x_1 + y_1) + (x_2 + y_2) + (x_3 + y_3)$

$$= (x_1 + x_2 + x_3) + (y_1 + y_2 + y_3)$$

$$= \sum_{i=1}^{3} x_i + \sum_{i=1}^{3} y_i$$

(iii) $\displaystyle\sum_{i=1}^{n} c = nc$

Example: $\displaystyle\sum_{i=1}^{5} c = c + c + c + c + c = 5c$

The sigma-notation is flexible enough to denote a wide variety of kinds of sums. Seven examples are:

1. $\displaystyle\sum_{i=5}^{10} y_i = y_5 + y_6 + y_7 + y_8 + y_9 + y_{10}$

2. $\displaystyle\sum_{i=0}^{4} z_i^2 = z_0^2 + z_1^2 + z_2^2 + z_3^2 + z_4^2$

3. $\displaystyle\sum_{i=1}^{3} x_i y_i = x_1 y_1 + x_2 y_2 + x_3 y_3$

4. $\displaystyle\sum_{i=1}^{4}(x_i - c) = (x_1 - c) + (x_2 - c) + (x_3 - c) + (x_4 - c) = \sum_{i=1}^{4} x_i - 4c$

5. $\displaystyle\sum_{i=1}^{3}(y_i - m)^2 = (y_1 - m)^2 + (y_2 - m)^2 + (y_3 - m)^2$

6. $\displaystyle\sum_{i=1}^{5} i = 1 + 2 + 3 + 4 + 5 = 15$

7. $\displaystyle\sum_{i=1}^{5} p^i = p^1 + p^2 + p^3 + p^4 + p^5$

The subscript i is simply an index and can be any letter:

$$\sum_{i=1}^{n} x_i = \sum_{j=1}^{n} x_j = \sum_{l=1}^{n} x_l = x_1 + x_2 + x_3 + \cdots + x_n.$$

Double summation

It is occasionally necessary to sum values that depend on two subscripts. For example,

$$\sum_{i=1}^{2}\sum_{j=1}^{3} x_{ij} = \sum_{i=1}^{2}(x_{i1} + x_{i2} + x_{i3}) = (x_{11} + x_{12} + x_{13}) + (x_{21} + x_{22} + x_{23})$$

$$= \sum_{j=1}^{3}(x_{1j} + x_{2j}) = (x_{11} + x_{21}) + (x_{12} + x_{22}) + (x_{13} + x_{23})$$

$$= x_{11} + x_{12} + x_{13} + x_{21} + x_{22} + x_{23}.$$

Rules similar to the single summation apply to double summation.

(i) $\displaystyle\sum_{i=1}^{n}\sum_{j=1}^{m} ax_{ij} = a\sum_{i=1}^{n}\sum_{j=1}^{m} x_{ij}$

and

$$\sum_{i=1}^{n}\sum_{j=1}^{m} a_i x_{ij} = \sum_{i=1}^{n} a_i \sum_{j=1}^{m} x_{ij}$$

(ii) $\displaystyle\sum_{i=1}^{n}\sum_{j=1}^{m}(x_{ij} + y_{ij}) = \sum_{i=1}^{n}\sum_{j=1}^{m} x_{ij} + \sum_{i=1}^{n}\sum_{j=1}^{m} y_{ij}$

(iii) $\displaystyle\sum_{i=1}^{n}\sum_{j=1}^{m} x_{ij} = \sum_{j=1}^{m}\sum_{i=1}^{n} x_{ij}$

(iv) $\displaystyle\sum_{i=1}^{n}\sum_{j=1}^{m} c = \sum_{i=1}^{n} mc = \sum_{i=1}^{m} nc = nmc$

Five examples:

1. $\displaystyle\sum_{j=1}^{2}\sum_{i=1}^{3} p_{ij} = p_{11} + p_{21} + p_{31} + p_{12} + p_{22} + p_{32}$

2. $\displaystyle\sum_{i=1}^{3} p_{ij} = p_{1j} + p_{2j} + p_{3j}$

3. $\displaystyle\sum_{i=5}^{6}\sum_{j=1}^{3} x_{ij} = x_{51} + x_{52} + x_{53} + x_{61} + x_{62} + x_{63}$

4. $\displaystyle\sum_{i=1}^{2}\sum_{j=1}^{2}(z_{ij} - c)^2 = (z_{11} - c)^2 + (z_{12} - c)^2 + (z_{21} - c)^2 + (z_{22} - c)^2$

5. $\displaystyle\sum_{i=1}^{2}\sum_{j=1}^{3}(y_{ij} - a)(w_{ij} - b) = (y_{11} - a)(w_{11} - b) + (y_{12} - a)(w_{12} - b)$
$$+ (y_{13} - a)(w_{13} - b) + (y_{21} - a)(w_{21} - b)$$
$$+ (y_{22} - a)(w_{22} - b) + (y_{23} - a)(w_{23} - b)$$

B.2   DERIVATION OF THE NORMAL EQUATIONS FOR SIMPLE LINEAR REGRESSION

The following describes the least squares estimation of the parameters a and b for the simple linear regression model. The question addressed is: What values of a and b produce the minimum value of L where L is defined as

$$L = \sum (y_i - [a + bx_i])^2?$$

Using calculus

To answer this question, the partial derivatives of L with respect to a and b are set equal to zero and the resulting equations solved:

1. $\displaystyle\frac{\partial L}{\partial a} = -2\sum (y_i - [a + bx_i])$

then

$$\sum(y_i - [\hat{a} + \hat{b}x_i]) = 0$$

or

$$\sum y_i = n\hat{a} + \hat{b}\sum x_i \qquad \textit{(first normal equation)}$$

giving

$$\overline{y} = \hat{a} + \hat{b}\overline{x} \qquad \text{and} \qquad \hat{a} = \overline{y} - \hat{b}\overline{x}.$$

2. $\dfrac{\partial L}{\partial b} = -2\sum(y_i - [a + bx_i])x_i$

$$\sum(y_i - [\hat{a} + \hat{b}x_i])x_i = 0$$

or

$$\sum x_i y_i - \hat{a}\sum x_i - \hat{b}\sum x_i^2 = 0$$

giving

$$\sum x_i y_i = \hat{a}\sum x_i + \hat{b}\sum x_i^2 \qquad \textit{(second normal equation)}.$$

Substituting $\hat{a} = \overline{y} - \hat{b}\overline{x}$ from the first normal equation into the second normal equation gives

$$\sum x_i y_i = (\overline{y} - \hat{b}\overline{x})\sum x_i + \hat{b}\sum x_i^2$$

$$\sum x_i y_i = \overline{y}\sum x_i + \hat{b}\left(\sum x_i^2 - \overline{x}\sum x_i\right)$$

therefore,

$$\hat{b} = \left(\sum x_i y_i - \overline{y}\sum x_i\right) \Big/ \left(\sum x_i^2 - \overline{x}\sum x_i\right)$$

$$= \sum(x_i - \overline{x})(y_i - \overline{y}) \Big/ \sum(x_i - \overline{x})^2$$

$$= \frac{S_{XY}}{S_X^2}.$$

The estimates $\hat{a}$ and $\hat{b}$ are the least squares estimates of the parameters a and b and only these values minimize the quantity $L = \sum(y_i - [a + bx_i])^2$ (Chapter 8).

Using algebra

In general, for any quadratic equation $F = Ax^2 + Bx + C = \left(x + \frac{B}{2A}\right)^2 A - \frac{B^2}{4A} + C$. Therefore, the minimum value of F occurs at $x = -\frac{B}{2A}$ when $A > 0$.

Now, $L = \sum(y_i - [a + bx_i])^2$ can be written in two ways where each expression is a quadratic equation.

1. $L = \sum(y_i - [a + bx_i])^2 = (n)a^2 + (2b\sum x_i - 2\sum y_i)a + \sum(y - bx_i)^2$

then

$$\hat{a} = -\frac{B}{2A} = \frac{-(2\hat{b}\sum x_i - 2\sum y_i)}{2n}$$

or

$$n\hat{a} = \sum y_i - \hat{b}\sum x_i$$

or

$$\sum y_i = n\hat{a} + \hat{b}\sum x_i \qquad \textit{(first normal equation)}$$

2. $L = \sum(y_i - [a + bx_i])^2 = \left(\sum x_i^2\right)b^2$

$$+ \left(2a\sum x_i - 2\sum x_i y_i\right)b + \sum(y_i - a)^2$$

or

$$\hat{b} = -\frac{B}{2A} = \frac{-(2\hat{a}\sum x_i - 2\sum x_i y_i)}{2\sum x_i^2}$$

or

$$\hat{b}\sum x_i^2 = \sum x_i y_i - \hat{a}\sum x_i$$

or

$$\sum x_i y_i = \hat{a}\sum x_i + \hat{b}\sum x_i^2 \qquad \textit{(second normal equation).}$$

Again, solving these two normal equations for the estimates $\hat{a}$ and $\hat{b}$ give the least squares estimates of the parameters a and b and only these values minimize the quantity $L = \sum(y_i - [a + bx_i])^2$ (Chapter 8).

B.3 POISSON PROBABILITY DISTRIBUTION

A Poisson probability distribution (named after the French mathematician Simeon Denis Poisson) is related to the binomial distribution and can be justified from the following.

Starting with a binomial probability,

$$P(X = k) = \binom{n}{k}p^k(1 - p)^{n-k} = \frac{n(n-1)(n-2)\cdots(n-k+1)}{k!}$$

$$\times p^k \left(1 - \frac{np}{n}\right)^{n-k}$$

and

$$P(X = k) = \frac{1\left(1 - \frac{1}{n}\right)\left(1 - \frac{2}{n}\right) \cdots \left(1 - \frac{k-1}{n}\right)}{k!} (np)^k \left(1 - \frac{np}{n}\right)^{n-k}.$$

If n is large and p is small, then $(1 - \frac{np}{n})^{n-k} \approx e^{-np}$, which is a special case of the definition of the mathematical constant $e = 2.7182818$. Then, as n becomes large, the Poisson probability distribution becomes

$$P(X = k) = \frac{(np)^k e^{-np}}{k!} = \frac{\lambda^k e^{-\lambda}}{k!}$$

and is completely defined by a single parameter λ. The Greek letter $\lambda = np$ is traditional notation associated with a Poisson distribution. This expression shows the Poisson probabilities viewed as a limiting case of the binomial distribution. That is, the binomial distribution becomes indistinguishable from the Poisson distribution when n (the number of binary X_i-values) is large and $P(X_i = 1) = p$ is small. The Poisson distribution can also be derived from a number of other considerations.[9] Like the binomial distribution, the Poisson distribution plays an important role in analyzing count data (Chapters 3 and 7).

References

[1] J. W. Tukey, *Exploring Data Analysis*. Addison-Wesley Publishing Co., Reading, MA, 1977.

[2] "Child Health and Development Study." Division of Biostatistics, School of Public Health, University of California, Berkeley. J. Yersushalmy, Director.

[3] D. Huff and I. Geis, *How to Take a Chance*. Norton & Company, New York, NY, 1959.

[4] E. Robert, J. A. Harris, O. Robert, and S. Selvin, "Case-control study on maternal residential proximity to high-voltage power lines and congenital anomalies in France." *Paediatric and Perinatal Epidemiology*, 10:32–38 (1996).

[5] University of California Wellness Letter. Volume 18, Issue 4, Jan. 2002.

[6] L. H. Tribe, "Trial by mathematics: precision and ritual in the legal process." *Harvard Law Review*, 84(6):1329–1393 (1971).

[7] S. Selvin, Letter to the Editor—"Monty Hall" problem. *American Statistician*, 29(3):74 (1976).

[8] L. Gonick and W. Smith, *The Cartoon Guide to Statistics*. HarperCollins, New York, NY, 1993.

[9] C. C. Chiang, *Introduction to Stochastic Process in Biostatistics*. John Wiley & Sons, New York, NY, 1968.

[10] W. Feller, *An Introduction to Probability Theory and Its Applications* (Volume 1). John Wiley & Sons, New York, NY, 1966.

[11] R. M. Coates, *The Law in The World of Mathematics* (editor: J. R. Newman). Simon and Schuster, New York, NY, 1956.

[12] W. G. Cochran, *Sampling Techniques*. John Wiley & Sons, New York, NY, 1965.

[13] M. G. Kendall and A. Stuart, *The Advanced Theory of Statistics*. Charles Griffin & Co., London, UK, 1969.

[14] R. A. Fisher, *The Design of Experiments*. Oliver & Boyd, Edinburgh, UK, 1935.

[15] D. Salsberg, *The Lady Tasting Tea: How Statistics Revolutionized Science in the Twentieth Century*. W. H. Freeman, New York, NY, 2001.

[16] R. C. Spear, S. Selvin, J. Schulman, and M. Francis, "Benzene exposure in the petroleum industry." *Applied Industrial Hygiene*, 2:155–163 (1987).

[17] J. Neer, W. Wasserman, and M. H. Kutner, *Applied Linear Statistical Models*. Irwin, Boston, MA, 1990.

[18] R. G. Miller, *Beyond ANOVA, Basics of Applied Statistics*. John Wiley & Sons, New York, NY, 1986.

[19] S. M. Brown, S. Selvin, and W. Winkelstein Jr. "The association of economic status with the occurrence of lung cancer." *Cancer*, 36:1903–1911 (1975).

[20] D. H. Freeman, *Applied Categorical Data*. Marcel Dekker, Inc., New York, NY, 1987.

[21] W. G. Cochran, "Some methods for strengthening the common chi-square test." *Biometrics*, 10:417–451 (1954).

[22] E. Gunderson, B. Abrams, and S. Selvin, "The relative importance of gestation Al gain and maternal characteristics associated with becoming overweight after pregnancy." *International Journal of Obesity*, 20:134–139 (2000).

[23] R. V. Hogg and A. T. Craig, *Introduction to Mathematical Statistics* (5th edition). Prentice Hall, Upper Saddle River, NJ, 1994.

[24] D. A. Belsley, E. K. Kuh, and R. E. Welsch, *Regression Diagnostics*. John Wiley & Sons, New York, NY, 1980.

[25] T. Vogt, S. B. Hulley, S. Selvin, and G. Widdowson, "Expired air carbon monoxide and serum thiocyanate as objective measures of cigarette exposure." *American Journal of Public Health*, 67:545–549 (1977).

[26] B. Abrams and S. Selvin, "Maternal weight gain pattern and birth weight." *Obstetrics and Gynecology*, 86(2):163–169 (1995).

[27] O. J. Dunn and V. A. Clark, *Applied Statistics: Analysis of Variance and Regression*. John Wiley & Sons, New York, NY, 1974.

[28] C. C. Li, *Human Genetics, Principles and Methods*. McGraw-Hill Book Company, New York, NY, 1961.

[29] D. J. Hand and C. C. Taylor, *Multivariate Analysis of Variance and Repeated Measures*. Chapman & Hill, New York, NY, 1987.

[30] O. Kempthorne, *Design and Analysis of Experiments*. John Wiley & Sons, New York, NY, 1952.

[31] E. L. Lehmann, *Nonparametrics: Statistical Methods Based on Ranks*. McGraw-Hill International Book Company, New York, NY, 1975.

Partial Solutions to Most Problems

Problem Set 1

(1) $\bar{x}_A = 17.0$ min. $M_A = 16.5$ min. $S_A = 11.8$ min.
$\bar{x}_B = 17.0$ min. $M_B = 16.5$ min. $S_B = 6.8$ min.

(5) $\bar{x} = 35.2$ yrs. $M_d = 34.19$ yrs. $S = 6.31$ yrs.
$\bar{x} = 34.8$ yrs. $M_d = 34.0$ yrs. $S = 6.24$ yrs.

(7) 31, 34, 39   **(10)** 38.2, 37.2, 6.31

13–20 sometimes, sometimes, always, sometimes, never, sometimes, sometimes, and sometimes

Problem Set 2

(15) 5/36, 4/36   **(16)** 1/6   **(17)** 10/36   **(18)** 1/36   **(19)** 10/36   **(20)** 0

(21) $P[yy \mid Yellow] = 1/3$

(22) $P(HH) = 1/4$

(23) $P[B \mid \overline{A}] = 40/75 = 0.533$

(24) **(a)** 0.0821   **(b)** 0.684

(25) **(a)** 1/9   **(b)** 4/9   **(c)** 4/5

(26) 0.5, 0.0, 0.5; 0.25, 0.50, 0.25; 0.325, 0.350, 0.325, and 0.25, 0.50, 0.25

(27) 1/5

(28) 2/3

(29) d, f, a, h, g, e, c, and b

(30) 0.03125   **(31)** 0.03125   **(32)** 0.96875   **(33)** 0.5   **(34)** 0.5

(35) $(3/52)^8$ **(36)** $4(3/52)^8$ **(37)** 0.070

(38) 0.123, 0.294, 0.309, 0.185, 0.070, 0.017, 0.003, 0.0002, 0.00001

(39) **(a)** 17,576,000   **(d)** 1/26   **(g)** 1/26
(b) 11,232,000   **(e)** 1/10   **(h)** 1/10
(c)   1,872,000   **(f)** 1/260

(40) 0.01196   **(45)** 0.2618

(41) 0.00226   **(46)** 0.3576

(42) 0.01422   **(47)** 0.8391

(43) 0.01562   **(48)** 0.2197

(44) 0.98445   **(49)** 0.7803

(50) $P(X = 0) = 0.814506$
$P(X = 1) = 0.171475$
$P(X = 2) = 0.013538$
$P(X = 3) = 0.000475$
$P(X = 4) = 0.000006$

(51) $P(X = 0) = 0.95^{20} = 0.3585$
$P(X \geq 1) = 1 - 0.3585 = 0.6415$

(52)   **(a)** 0.633   **(b)** 0.474   **(c)** 0.625

(53) $(1 - p_0) + p_0(1 - p_1) + p_0 p_1(1 - p_2)$
$= 1 - p_0 p_1 p_2$

(54–61) never, always, sometimes, sometimes, sometimes, always, always, and sometimes

Problem Set 3

1.   0, 1, 2, and 3

2.   0.512, 0.384, 0.96, and 0.008

3. $E(X) = 0.6$

4. $\text{Var}(X) = 0.48$

5.   0.692

6.   9 weeks

7. $1/49$ (weeks)^2

8. $1/7$ weeks

9. $E(T) = 2$ $\text{Var}(T) = 1$

10. $E(W) = 4$ $\text{Var}(W) = 4$

11. $E(D) = 28$ $\text{Var}(D) = 196$

13. $\sigma_T = 1$ treatment $\sigma_W = 2$ weeks $\sigma_D = 14$ days

14. $E(D + 7) = 35$ $\text{Var}(D + 7) = 196$

15. $E(T_1 + T_2) = 4$ $\text{Var}(T_1 + T_2) = 2$

16. $E(T_1 + T_2 + \cdots + T_{10}) = 20$ $\text{Var}(T_1 + T_2 + \cdots + T_{10}) = 10$

PART I: **(19)** 3 and 3 **(20)** 1.5

PART II: **(22)** 0.05 and 0.05 **(23)** 0.5 **(24)** 0.25

PART III: **(26)** 3.0 **(27)** 1.5

Problem Set 4

(1) $\hat{p} = 0.34$

(2)

X	Expected
0	71.9
1	111.1
2	57.2
3	9.8
Total	250.00

(4–6) $\hat{p} = 0.2325$

X	$p_0 = 0.25$	$\hat{p}$
0	45.2	49.6
1	60.3	60.1
2	30.2	27.3
3	6.7	5.5
4	0.6	0.4

(8–9) $\hat{\lambda} = 0.5$

Number of typhoons (X)	0	1	2	3	4	5	≥ 6
Observed freq.	149	24	15	5	4	3	0
Expected freq.	121.3	60.7	15.2	2.5	0.3	0.0	0.0

(11) 0.3413 **(12)** 0.95 **(13)** 0.05

(14) 0 **(15)** 1.645 **(16)** 1.645

(17) 0.50 **(18)** 0.9544 **(19)** 43.6, 47.4, 50, 53.4, 58.2

(20) 0.0228 **(21)** 0.1359 **(22)** 67 **(23)** 74.653

(24) 0.0005 **(25)** 0.0062

(27) 0.9876 **(28)** 0.6826 **(29)** 0.9544

Problem Set 5

(1) $c = 103.29$ $1 - \beta = 0.968$
(2) $c = 104.652$ $1 - \beta = 0.880$
(3) $c = 102.056$ $1 - \beta = 0.999$
(4) $n = 18$

(5)

Type I Error	$\alpha = 0.05$	$\alpha = 0.10$	$\alpha = 0.05$	$\alpha = 0.05$	$\alpha = 0.05$
Type II Error	$\beta = 0.10$	$\beta = 0.10$	$\beta = 0.05$	0.3613	0.0093
Critical Point	655.2	649.7	649.3	682.3	641.1
Sample Size	$n = 20$	$n = 15$	$n = 25$	$n = 9$	$n = 36$

(7–10) decrease, increase, increase and decrease

(11) $Z = -4.04$

(12) $Z = -2.667$

(13) 0.4514   **(14)** 0.9281   **(15)** 2.178   **(16)** 1.827

(17) 8.54, 7.68

Problem Set 6

(1) $T = 1.799$

(2) $T = -0.63$

(3) (4.377, 4.623),   **(4)** (4.294, 4.706)

(7) $Z = -15.0$ **(8)** (0.290, 0.335)

(9) $Z = -2.50$

(10) $Z = -1.60$

Calculated values of test statistic only:

(11) $T = -2.555$

(12) $T = 5.375$

(13) $T = -9.549$

(14) $T = 7.434$

(15) $Z = 2.76$

(16) $Z = -2.28$

(17) $Z = 5.82$

(19) $P(C \mid S) = 0.0001634$ $P(C \mid \bar{S}) = 0.0000607$

(20) Relative Risk $= 2.69$

Problem Set 7

(1) $X^2 = 7.64$ **(2)** $X^2 = 5.21$ **(3)** $X^2 = 33.84$

(4) $X^2 = 64.92$

(5) $X^2 = 12.37$ without pooling and df $= 12$

(9) $X^2 = 56.47$

(10) runners: $S^2 = 166.0$, 95%CI: $(78.5, 553.3)$
controls: $S^2 = 134.2$, 95%CI: $(63.5, 447.3)$

(13) $X^2 = 62.5$

(14) $X^2 = 40.5$

(15) $X^2 = 0.724$

(16) $\hat{\lambda} = 2$

(17) $X^2 = 3.4$ with 4 df if pooled the last 4 categories so that $E_i > 5$

(18) $X^2 = 186.0$, p-value $= 0.74$

Problem Set 8

(1) $\hat{b} = 0.023$. $\hat{y}_0 = 4.087$

(2) $\hat{b} = 0.013$. $\hat{y}_0 = 3.418$

(3) Males: $S_{xy} = -1700$ **(4)** $\hat{y}_M = 942 - 9x$

(5) Females: $S_{xy} = -1000$ **(6)** $\hat{y}_F = 590 - 5x$

(7) 95%CI: $(649.0, 1235.0)$

(8) $T = -2.85$

(9) 95% CI: $(582.7, 851.3)$ 95% CI: $(138.4, 575.7)$

(10) $T = 5.99$

(11) 95% CI: $(-11.3, 1.3)$

(12) Smokers: $\hat{y} = 18.75 + 0.25x$

(13) Nonsmokers: $\hat{y} = 7.71 + 0.13x$

(15) Total: $\hat{y} = -0.5 - x$

Problem Set 9

(1) $r = 0.479$

(2) 1.724

(3) 95%CI: $(-0.131, 0.826)$

(4) $r_s = 0.842$

(5) $r_{pb} = 0.377$

(6) $r_\phi = 0.020$

(8) $r = -0.798$

Index